D1086040

TRANSPLANTATION NURSING SECRETS

TRANSPLANTATION NURSING SECRETS

Sandra A. Cupples, DNSc, RN
Heart Transplant Coordinator
Washington Hospital Center
Washington, DC

Linda Ohler, MSN, RN, CCTC, FAAN
Editor, Progress in Transplantation
Arlington, Virginia

Nursing Secrets Series Editor ————

Linda J. Scheetz, EdD, RN, CS, CEN
Assistant Professor, College of Nursing
Rutgers, The State University of New Jersey
Newark, New Jersey

HANLEY & BELFUS
An Affiliate of Elsevier

BP45

HANLEY & BELFUS, INC.
An *Affiliate of* Elsevier

The Curtis Center
Independence Square West
Philadelphia, Pennsylvania 19106

Note to the reader: Although the techniques, ideas, and information in this book have been carefully reviewed for correctness, the authors, editors, and publisher cannot accept any legal responsibility for any errors or omissions that may be made. Neither the publisher nor the editors make any guarantee, expressed or implied, with respect to the material contained herein.

This book is designed to provide information about the background and modalities used frequently in transplantation nursing and how they are applied by practitioners in the field. It is not intended to be exhaustive, nor should patients use it as a substitute for the advice of their physician. It is strongly recommended that you talk with your own physician about any treatments you use personally, and research the area further for safety as it applies to the person you are treating. Before trying/recommending any treatment, the reader should review dosages, accepted indications, and other information pertinent to the safe and effective use of the therapies described.

Library of Congress Control Number: 2002112992

TRANSPLANTATION NURSING SECRETS
ISBN 1-56053-519-9

Printed in the United States of America

Last digit is the print number: 9 8 7 6 5 4

2/8/07

CONTENTS

CONTRIBUTORS

Sharon M. Augustine, RN, CRNP
Clinical Manager, Thoracic Transplant Program, Cardiovascular Surgery, University of Maryland, Baltimore, Maryland

Jamie D. Blazek, RN, MPH, CCTC, FNP-C
Transplant Nurse Practitioner, Abdominal Transplant, Ochsner Multi-organ Transplant Center, Ochsner Clinic Foundation, New Orleans, Louisiana

Robert A. Bray, PhD, Diplomate (ABHI)
Professor of Pathology, Department of Pathology and Laboratory Medicine, Emory University, Atlanta Georgia

Franki Chabalewski, RN, MS
Professional Services Coordinator, Department of Professional Services, United Network for Organ Sharing, Richmond, Virginia

Lori Coleman, RN, CPTC
Heart Transplant and Ventricular Assist Device Coordinator, Division of Cardiothoracic Surgery, University Hospitals of Cleveland, Cleveland, Ohio

Jacqueline M. Corsini, MS, ANP, CCRN
Clinical Nurse Specialist, National Institutes of Health Solid Organ Transplant Program, Bethesda, Maryland; Nursing Department, National Institutes of Health Clinical Center, Bethesda, Maryland

Sandra A. Cupples, DNSc, RN
Heart Transplant Coordinator, Washington Hospital Center, Washington, DC

Terri Allison Donaldson, RN, MN, ACNP
Lecturer, School of Nursing, Vanderbilt University, Nashville, Tennessee

Debi H. Dumas-Hicks, RN, BS, CCTC
Head, Post-Heart Transplant Division, Ochsner Cardiomyopathy and Heart Transplant Center, Ochsner Clinic Foundation, New Orleans, Louisiana

Maureen P. Flattery, RN, MSN, C-ANP
Medical College of Virginia, Virginia Commonwealth University Health System, Richmond, Virginia

Bridget M. Flynn, BSN, RN, CCTC
Clinical Transplant Coordinator, Thomas E. Starzl Transplantation Institute, Pittsburgh, Pennsylvania

Elizabeth Ann Sparks Ford, BSN, RN
National Institute of Diabetes and Digestive and Kidney Diseases, Transplant Autoimmunity Branch, National Institutes of Health, Bethesda, Maryland

Jeanie Haines, BScN, RN
Nurse Coordinator, Medical Psychiatry Nursing, University Health Network, Toronto, Ontario, Canada

Jane D. Harrison, LCSW, C-ASWCM
Social Work Supervisor, Case Management Department, Inova Fairfax Hospital, Falls Church, Virginia

Mary Jo Holechek, MS, CRNP, CNN
Adult Abdominal Organ Transplant Nurse Practitioner, Department of Surgery, Johns Hopkins Hospital, Johns Hopkins University, Baltimore Maryland

Ann Lee, RN, CRNP, MSN, CCTC
Cardiothoracic Transplant Coordinator, Department of Cardiothoracic Surgery, University of Pittsburgh Medical Center, Pittsburgh, Pennsylvania

Mary E. Leshko, RN, BSN, CCRN, CNN
Clinical Research Nurse, National Institutes of Health, Bethesda, Maryland

Jan D. Manzetti, RN, PhD, CCTC
Adjunct Assistant Professor, Department of Nursing, University of Pittsburgh, Pittsburgh, Pennsylvania; Coordinator of Cardiothoracic Transplantation, University of Pittsburgh Medical Center, Pittsburgh, Pennsylvania

Brenda McQuarrie, BScN, RN(EC)
Primary Care Nurse Practitioner, Multiorgan Transplant Program, University Health Network, Toronto, Ontario, Canada

Janet B. Mize, RN, BSN, CCTC, CCM
Clinical Transplant Coordinator, Multi-Organ Transplant Center, Methodist Hospital, Houston, Texas

Linda Ohler, MSN, RN, CCTC, FAAN
Editor, Progress in Transplantation, Arlington, Virginia

Marian O'Rourke, RN, CCTC
Senior Clinical Coordinator, Recanati/Miller Transplantation Institute, Mount Sinai Medical Center, New York, New York

Melinda Paredes, RN, MS
Transplant Clinical Nurse Specialist, Johns Hopkins Hospital, Baltimore, Maryland

Beverly Kosmach Park, MSN, CRNP
Clinical Nurse Specialist, Department of Transplant Surgery, Starzl Transplantation Institute, Children's Hospital of Pittsburgh, Pittsburgh, Pennsylvania

Lisa S. Pearlman, RN, MN, ACNP
Clinical Nurse Specialist/Nurse Practitioner, Pediatric Academic Multi-organ Transplant Program, Hospital for Sick Children, Toronto, Ontario, Canada

Jade K. Perdue, MPA
Public Health Analyst, Department of Health and Human Services, Division of Transplantation, Rockville, Maryland

Lori A. Purdie, MS, RN
Nurse Manager, Solid and Tissue Transplant Program, National Institutes of Health, Bethesda, Maryland

Debbie Seem, RN, CPTC
Professional Services Coordinator, Department of Professional Services, United Network for Organ Sharing, Richmond, Virginia

Leslie C. Sweet, RN, BSN
Ventricular Assist Device Coordinator, Washington Hospital Center, Washington, DC

Connie White-Williams, RN, MSN, FNP
Cardiothoracic Transplant Coordinator, Cardiology Services, University of Alabama at Birmingham Medical Center, Birmingham, Alabama

Linda Wright, MHSc, MSW
Bioethicist, University Health Network, Toronto, Ontario, Canada

PREFACE

Although there are many books on solid organ transplantation, few are exclusively written for nurses. *Transplantation Nursing Secrets* fills this gap in the literature. Written by a variety of experienced transplant professionals (nurses, nurse practitioners, and social workers), this book focuses on the complex issues that transplant nurses face on a daily basis. Our book features the classic question-and-answer format of the Nursing Secrets Series® and places sensible tips and pearls of wisdom at the reader's fingertips.

The chapters span a broad range of transplant-related topics. All types of solid organ transplant procedures are addressed, along with practical information about the nursing care of transplant recipients and living donors. In addition, two chapters are devoted to the unique psychosocial issues faced by living donors and transplant candidates. We are confident that the collective wisdom shared in this book will enhance transplant-nursing practice.

We gratefully acknowledge the contributions of our authors, who so willingly shared their knowledge and expertise, and our reviewers, who were instrumental in fine-tuning our chapters. Both our contributors and reviewers are busy transplant professionals, and we genuinely appreciate the time and effort that they devoted to this endeavor!

We would like to thank Stan Ward at Hanley & Belfus for his patience and good humor. His wise advice kept us calm during the final production days.

Above all, we extend our gratitude to Linda Scheetz, our Editor-in-Chief, and Linda Belfus, our publisher, for providing us with this opportunity—and for their encouragement, guidance, and support.

Sandra A. Cupples, DNSc, RN
Linda Ohler, MSN, RN, CCTC, FAAN

DEDICATION

We dedicate this book to our husbands, Howard P. Cupples, MD and Richard Knight, JD, for their patience, support and dedication to our goals

and

to our parents (Elizabeth and Alexander Aino, Elizabeth and Dominic Russo) for their inspiration, guidance, and encouragement in helping us to achieve our dreams to be nurses, authors, and editors.

1. THE U.S. NATIONAL TRANSPLANTATION SYSTEM

Franki Chabalewski, RN, MS, *and Debbie Seem*, RN, CPTC

1. How many people with end-stage organ disease need an organ for transplantation?

As of May 3, 2002, 85,134 people were waiting for an organ transplant. In 2001, there were 12,580 organ donors (6081 cadaveric and 6499 living donors), and 24,075 transplantations were performed. The number of patients waiting for an donor organs continues to rise annually, whereas the number of organs available for transplantation remains relatively static. Unfortunately, during that same year, 6096 deaths were reported of patients on the waiting list because of this shortfall. Many lives could have been saved if an organ had been available for transplantation.[4]

2. Who can be considered an organ and tissue donor?

Anyone who dies should be considered a potential organ and tissue donor. However, patients who have extracerebral malignancies, are human immunodeficiency virus (HIV)-positive, or have unresolved transmissible infections may not be acceptable as organ donors. With every patient death, one should always contact the local organ procurement organization (OPO) or tissue recovery agency so that a procurement coordinator may perform a thorough evaluation and determine whether the patient is an appropriate candidate.

3. Which organs and tissues can be donated for transplantation?

One individual's donation can benefit more than 75 others by saving or dramatically improving their quality of life. The following organs and tissues can be donated for transplantation:
- Organs—kidneys, heart, pancreas, liver, lungs, and small intestine.
- Tissues—corneas, skin, heart valves, bone, bone marrow, veins, tendons, cartilage, ligaments, fascia, and dura.

4. What organs can be transplanted from living donors?

Living donation is the donation of an organ (e.g., kidney) or part of an organ (e.g., liver, lung, intestine, pancreas) from a healthy individual. The individual may be a family member, friend, or someone unknown to the person who needs the organ. Living donor transplants are a viable alternative for patients in need of new organs. In 2001, 6499 living donations occurred (5958 kidneys, 37 lung segments, 2 pancreas segments, 1 kidney with pancreas segment, 1 intestine segment, and 505 liver segments).[4]

For the donor, there is little danger in living with one kidney; the remaining kidney enlarges to do the work that both kidneys shared. The liver has the ability to regenerate the segment that was donated. Lung lobes do not regenerate.

5. Are organ transplants successful?

Yes, organ transplants are very successful and save the lives or improve the quality of life for more than 20,000 people each year. The table below demonstrates the excellent survival rates among individuals undergoing transplantation procedures. These rates continue to improve because of advances in technology, immunosuppressive therapy, and organ preservation techniques.

One-Year Graft and Patient Survival Rates by Organ:
January 1994–January 2001

ORGAN	% 1-YEAR GRAFT SURVIVAL RATE	% 1-YEAR PATIENT SURVIVAL RATE
Kidney (cadaveric)	87.2	94.4
Kidney (Living)	93.9	97.7
Heart	84.4	84.8
Liver	78.2	84.7
Lung	74.8	75.4
Heart-Lung	64.2	65.6
Pancreas	72.9	94.0

OPTN UNOS data as of May 3, 2002.

6. How long can a patient live after receiving a transplant?

Patients can live a long life after receiving a transplant as is demonstrated by the reported longest-living, continuously functioning transplants in the table below.

Longest Survival of Functioning Transplants

TYPE OF ORGAN TRANSPLANT	LONGEST REPORTED SURVIVAL OF FUNCTIONING TRANSPLANT
Kidney (living-related)	41 years, 2 months
Kidney (cadaveric)	34 years, 9 months
Kidney/Pancreas	19 years, 8 months
Pancreas	17 years, 7 months
Liver	30 years, 11 months
Heart	23 years, 11 months
Lung (single)	13 years, 3 months
Lung (double)	14 years, 1 month
Heart-lung	17 years, 1 month
Intestine	11 years, 9 months
Cluster transplant (liver, pancreas, duodenum and partial stomach)	12 years, 2 months

Data from Cecka JM,Terasaki PI: World transplant records. In Checka JM, Terasaki PI (eds): Clinical Transplants. Los Angeles, UCLA Immunogenetics Center, 2000, pp 515–547.

7. What is the government's role in organ transplantation?

The 1984 National Organ Transplant Act (NOTA) mandated the establishment of a national Organ Procurement and Transplantation Network (OPTN) and the Scientific Registry of Organ Transplant Recipients (SRTR) in the United States. Under the U.S. Department of Health and Human Services, Health Resources and Services Administration, the Division of Transplantation administers both the OPTN and the SRTR contracts.

The Division of Transplantation (DoT) provides federal oversight and funding support for the nation's organ procurement, allocation, and transplantation system; coordinates national organ and tissue donation activities; funds research to learn more about what works to increase donation; and administers the national bone marrow donor registry program.

8. How is transplantation organized in the United States?

The following chart demonstrates the organizational structure of the transplantation system in the United States. It includes government agencies as well as private contractors.

U.S. Organ Transplantation Organizational Structure

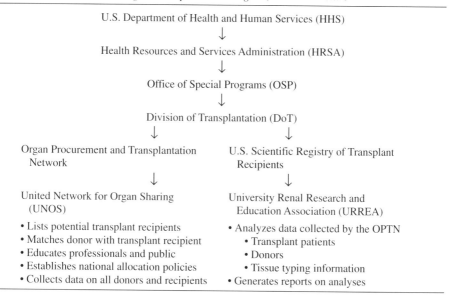

U.S. Department of Health and Human Services (HHS)
↓
Health Resources and Services Administration (HRSA)
↓
Office of Special Programs (OSP)
↓
Division of Transplantation (DoT)
↓   ↓

Organ Procurement and Transplantation Network	U.S. Scientific Registry of Transplant Recipients
↓	↓
United Network for Organ Sharing (UNOS)	University Renal Research and Education Association (URREA)

• Lists potential transplant recipients
• Matches donor with transplant recipient
• Educates professionals and public
• Establishes national allocation policies
• Collects data on all donors and recipients
	• Analyzes data collected by the OPTN
	  • Transplant patients
	  • Donors
	  • Tissue typing information
	• Generates reports on analyses

9. What is the Organ Procurement and Transplantation Network?

Under the National Organ Transplant Act of 1984, the U.S. Congress established the Organ Procurement and Transplantation Network (OPTN). The act called for a unified transplant network to be operated by a private, nonprofit organization under federal contract. The OPTN is a unique public–private partnership linking all of the professionals involved in the donation and transplantation system.

To help ensure the success and efficiency of the U.S. organ transplant system, the OPTN fulfills the following responsibilities:

- Developing consensus-based policies and procedures for organ recovery, distribution (allocation), and transportation
- Collecting and managing scientific data about organ donation and transplantation
- Providing data to the government, the public, students, researchers, and to the U.S. Scientific Registry of Transplant Recipients for use in the ongoing quest for improvement in the field of solid organ allocation and transplantation
- Developing and maintaining a secure web-based computer system, which maintains the nation's organ transplant waiting list and recipient/donor organ characteristics
- Facilitating the organ matching and placement process through the use of the computer system and a fully staffed organ center operating 24 hours a day, 7 days a week.
- Providing professional and public education about donation and transplantation, the activities of the OPTN, and the critical need for donation.

Under federal law, all U.S. transplant centers and organ procurement organizations must be members of the OPTN to receive any funds through Medicare. Other members of the OPTN include independent histocompatibility laboratories involved in organ transplantation; relevant medical, scientific and professional organizations; relevant voluntary health and patient advocacy organizations; and members of the general public with a particular interest in donation and/or transplantation.

10. What is the United Network for Organ Sharing?

The United Network for Organ Sharing (UNOS) is a private, nonprofit corporation organized to improve the effectiveness of human organ donation, procurement, distribution, and transplantation. UNOS works under contract to HHS to maintain, promote, and scientifically advance organ procurement and transplantation on a national scale. As the federal government's contractor to operate the national OPTN, UNOS coordinates the matching and placement of donor organs, policy development, and education. UNOS also collects, validates, and maintains data on all organ donors and solid organ transplant recipients. UNOS maintains the most comprehensive data available in any single field of medicine.

Additionally, UNOS is a membership organization made up of OPOs, transplant centers, histocompatibility laboratories, health organizations, ethicists, patients, donor families, and public members. UNOS is divided into eleven regions, each of which holds meetings, deliberates on issues that affect transplantation, and advises the OPTN/UNOS Board of Directors.

11. Is there a central place that maintains the list of patients who need an organ?

Yes, the national computer-based waiting list of patients in need of an organ for transplant is maintained by UNOS in its Richmond, Virginia, office. OPOs and transplant centers access the waiting list to add or delete patient names, or to run a list to match an organ with potential recipients.

12. Who is responsible for the recovery of organs and tissues?

The OPO and tissue recovery agencies that provide services to the donor hospital are responsible for the recovery of organs and tissues. Responsibilities include offering donation as an option to the family; securing consent from the next-of-kin, if necessary; coordinating donor management; mobilizing surgical teams and supervising organ recovery; coordinating the distribution of organs; and facilitating the recovery, preservation, and distribution of tissues.

13. Who pays for the cost of organ recovery?

The OPO reimburses the donor hospital for all costs related to organ recovery. No charges related to organ donation should appear on the donor's hospital bill. In turn, the OPO is reimbursed mainly through patient insurance by the recipient's hospital where the organ is transplanted. Most transplant costs are covered by third-party payers (i.e., the recipient's private insurance, Medicare, or Medicaid).

14. What is the Scientific Registry of Organ Transplant Recipients?

The Scientific Registry of Organ Transplant Recipients (SRTR) was created by NOTA to maintain data for continuous evaluation of the clinical status and outcome of transplant recipients in the United States. The SRTR provides analytic support to the OPTN/UNOS Board and Committees in their efforts to develop and perform ongoing evaluations of organ allocation policy and study the clinical status of organ procurement and transplantation. The SRTR's goals include the following:

- Operating a secure computer system to support the research and analysis of pre- and post-transplant data collected by the OPTN.
- Providing ongoing research and analytic support to the OPTN and to the Secretary of HHS's Advisory Committee on Transplantation.
- Conducting ongoing analyses of pre- and post-transplant data.
- Developing an annual report containing information on the scientific and clinical status of solid organ transplantation in the United States.

15. What is the University Renal Research and Education Association?

The University Renal Research and Education Association (URREA) is a nonprofit health research foundation that works in collaboration with the University of Michigan. URREA, under contract with the HHS, maintains the SRTR. The SRTR supports the ongoing evaluation of the scientific and clinical status of solid organ transplantation in the United States.

16. Who decides how organs are allocated to recipients?

Organ allocation policies are developed by the OPTN/UNOS membership through a series of regional meetings, national committee deliberations, public comment periods, and a final vote by the OPTN/UNOS Board of Directors. The Board of Directors is composed of OPTN/UNOS members, healthcare professionals, patients, and public members. The Secretary of HHS reviews all allocation policies and renders ultimate approval. Member compliance with all approved allocation policies is supported through a stringent review process.

17. What are the HHS Hospital Conditions of Participation for organ donation?

The 1998 Conditions of Participation (CoP) was modeled after legislation first initiated in 1986 under the Omnibus Budget Reconciliation Act that required hospitals to establish procedures for identifying potential organ donors and make their families aware of the option to donate as a condition of Medicare participation. This condition was known as required request, which evolved into routine referral whereby all acute care hospitals were to notify their designated OPO of all deaths. However, even with these regulations in place, many hospitals continued to consistently fail to report potential donors to OPOs. Therefore, the CoP was designed with more rigorous provisions to make organ donation more effective with an anticipated result of an increase in the number of organ and tissue donors in the United States.

Components include the following:
- Hospitals must contact the OPO in a timely manner regarding all patients who have died or whose death is imminent.
- The OPO, in collaboration with local tissue and eye banks, determines if the patient is a medically suitable donor.
- Hospitals must work in collaboration with the OPO to ensure that families of suitable donors are offered the opportunity to donate by using designated requestors that have participated in an OPO-approved training program or who are employees of procurement organizations.

18. How are organs allocated?

National organ allocation policies governing the transplantation system are based on medical and scientific criteria and do not permit favoritism based on political influence or discrimination on the basis of race, gender, or financial status. Information from each cadaveric organ donor is entered into the national computer located at UNOS and compared against the list of recipients waiting nationally to determine priority for organ allocation.

As outlined in OPTN/UNOS policy, a unique algorithm is applied for each organ system to eliminate waiting patients that are incompatible with an available donor. The computer then assigns a point score to every compatible patient based on medical urgency, blood group compatibility, tissue typing (kidney and/or pancreas), location of recipient and donor, and age. The organ is then offered to the patient with the highest score. Acceptance of the organ is left to the discretion of the transplant surgeon who takes into consideration the medical status of the candidate at that time and the medical characteristics of the donor.

19. Can someone who needs an organ buy one?

No, the National Organ Transplant Act of 1984 prohibits the buying or selling of human organs in the United States. One of the reasons for establishing this law is to help ensure that all individuals in need of a transplant have equal access.

20. Do organs have to "match" in order to be transplanted?

There are many factors taken into consideration when "matching" donated organs with potential recipients. The factors employed depend on the organ being offered. Some of these factors include the following considerations:
- Blood type
- Size of the organ

• Histocompatibilty matching (tests to determine the likelihood that the recipient's body will accept the organ). This matching is used most frequently in renal transplantation.
• Prospective crossmatch

21. If a person indicates the desire to be an organ donor on his or her driver's license, is that enough?

No, there is another important step the potential donors need to take. To ensure that their wishes to donate will be honored, they must talk to their family and have them witness the signing of a donor card. When someone dies, the next-of-kin are usually offered the option to donate. A living will and/or durable power of attorney also allows a patient's wishes to be indicated. Some states are now using donor registries as a means to authorize organ and tissue donation procedures.

22. Can diseases be transmitted when an organ is transplanted?

Yes, diseases can be transmitted via transplanted organs. To prevent the possible transmission of disease, OPTN/UNOS policy requires that the evaluation of a potential donor include the following:

• Extensive medical and social histories, including possible presence of malignant tumors or sepsis
• Physical examination
• Pertinent tests to screen for hepatitis, syphilis, cytomegalovirus (CMV), and human immunodeficiency virus (HIV).

23. Are brain death criteria legally accepted in the United States?

Yes, the criteria for determining brain death are well established in the United States. There are two recognized methods to pronounce death. An individual can be pronounced dead if there is 1) an irreversible cessation of circulatory and respiratory functions (death declared by cardiopulmonary criteria) or 2) an irreversible cessation of all functions of the entire brain, including the brain stem (death declared by neurological criteria). There are four elements in diagnosing brain death: absence of neurological function, apnea, irreversibility, and additional physiological confirmatory tests.

24. How does the non-heartbeating donor differ from the brain-dead donor?

Historically, most organ donors are patients who have suffered an irreversible and catastrophic brain insult and have total cessation of brain function. Although these individuals are declared brain dead, the they remain on the ventilator and the heart continues to beat until the organs are recovered.

In contrast to the cadaveric donor, the non-heartbeating donor is an individual who has suffered a catastrophic brain injury that is not anticipated to progress to brain death. When a family has chosen to remove the patient from ventilatory support in order to allow the person to die, there are situations when the patient may be an appropriate organ donor. Separate from and following the decision to withdraw ventilatory support, the family is offered the option of organ donation if it is determined that the patient will reach cardiorespiratory cessation within approximately 1 hour following withdrawal of ventilatory support. Once the family has consented to donation, the patient is removed from ventilatory support, and, following declaration of death, the organs are recovered.

25. Can an organ donor have an open casket viewing?

Yes, organ donation does not disfigure the body and does not interfere with having an open casket viewing.

26. Is it true that people have awakened on park benches or in bathtubs surrounded by ice with notes that have said they have had a kidney removed?

No, these urban legends have circulated for years, but there is no valid basis for them.

27. What is the nurse's responsibility regarding organ and tissue donation?
The nurse plays a significant role in the donation process by providing timely notification of death to the OPO, supportive care to the donor family, and ongoing patient care to the organ donor until the patient is taken to the operating room for the recovery of organs. The nurse should recognize that every person in the United States has the legal right to donate any part, or all, of his or her body. Therefore, each person's right to donate should be safeguarded. Throughout the process, the nurse remains the donor and family's advocate.

INTERNET RESOURCES

For more information, visit the following Web sites or call your local OPO.
www.hrsa.gov/osp/dot
www.organdonor.gov
www.optn.org
www.unos.org
www.urrea.org
www.ustransplant.org

BIBLIOGRAPHY

1. 2000 Annual Report: The U.S. Scientific Registry of Transplant Recipients and the Organ Procurement and Transplantation Network. Transplant Data 1990–1999. Richmond, VA, UNOS, 2000.
2. Cecka JM, Terasaki PI: World transplant records. In Cecka JM, Terasaki PI (eds): Clinical Transplants. Los Angeles, UCLA Immunogenetics Center, 2000, pp 515–547.
3. Center for Organ Recovery and Education: The organization and its mission. Available at: www.transweb.org/reference/maps/opo_image_map/corepa.htm. Accessed August 23, 2001.
4. Critical Data. Available at: www.unos.org. Accessed May 15, 2002.
5. Diringer MN, Wijdicks FM: Brain death in historical perspective. In Wijdicks FM (ed): Brain Death. Philadelpia, Lippincott Williams & Wilkins, 2001, pp 5–27.
6. Gaedeke MK: The National Transplant System. In Chabalewski F (ed): Donation and Transplantation: Nursing Curriculum. Richmond, VA, UNOS, 1996, pp 27–41.
7. Holmquist M, Chabalewski FL, Blount T, et al: A critical pathway: Guiding care for organ donors. Crit Care Nurs 19(2):84–100, 1999.
8. McCoy J, Argue P: The role of the critical care nurse in the donation process: A case study. Crit Care Nurs 19(2):48–52, 1999.
9. Pierce GA, McDonald JC: UNOS history. In Phillips MG (ed): UNOS Organ Procurement, Preservation and Distribution in Transplantation, 2nd ed. Richmond, VA, UNOS, 1996, pp 1–7.
10. Sullivan J, Seem DL, Chabalewski, FL: Determining brain death. Crit Care Nurs 19(2):37–45, 1999.
11. In Symphony...What We Play Is Life [booklet]. Richmond, VA, UNOS, 1999.
12. Transplant Statistics. Available at: www.ustransplant.org. Accessed May 15, 2002.

2. IMMUNOLOGY

Linda Ohler, MSN, RN, CCTC, FAAN, *and*
Robert A. Bray, PhD, Diplomate (ABHI)

1. What is human leukocyte antigen?

Human leukocyte antigens (HLA) are a set of proteins (markers) present on the surface of most cells of the body. These markers (antigens) are involved in immune recognition, which is the discrimination of **self** from **non-self**. HLA testing (tissue typing) is the process of identifying, characterizing, and matching these antigens and is usually performed by testing white blood cells from patients and donors. The white blood cells are the body's line of defense against infection and cancer. HLA antigens are the markers that the white blood cells use to determine if tissues or cells are normal or abnormal, infected or malignant. The genetic material inside each cell (deoxyribonucleic acid [DNA]) carries the information that determines which HLA antigens (proteins) are expressed on the outer surfaces of cells. Through matching of HLA antigens between donor and recipient, transplant specialists attempt to trick the immune system into believing that the transplanted organ is self-tissue and not abnormal tissue.

2. How are human leukocyte antigens identified?

Identification of an individual's HLA antigens or tissue type can be done by measuring the proteins on the cell surface or by examining the DNA directly. Because the protein is a direct product of the DNA, DNA-based tissue typing can identify an individual's HLA type. Although the HLA system has six major loci, the most commonly identified HLA antigens in solid organ transplantation are HLA-A, HLA-B, and HLA-DR. HLA antigens are inherited in a Mendelian fashion and are expressed in a codominant manner. Codominance means that for each locus (A, B or DR), one HLA antigen from each inherited chromosome is expressed equally. There are no dominant or recessive HLA genes. Thus, in HLA-A, HLA-B and HLA-DR typing, a total of six antigens, two from each locus, are measured. In other words, the individual inherits two sets of A, B and DR antigens, one set from each parent. Each locus (A, B or DR) can carry different alleles (different antigens), which further identify the individual.

The table demonstrates HLA typing for a child with both parents represented. The child has inherited a set of HLA-A, HLA-B and HLA-DR alleles from each parent. An inherited set of HLA antigens is referred to as a **haplotype**. Each person inherits two haplotypes, one from each parent, which in combination form a complete genotype. Identification of a **genotype** means that both sets of inherited parental haplotypes have been identified. In the past, HLA typing was used as a means of determining relationships in cases of disputed paternity.

HLA Typing for a Family

	A	B	DR	HAPLOTYPE CODE		A	B	DR	HAPLOTYPE CODE
Father	1	8	3	a	Sibling 1	1	8	3	a
	2	7	4	b	(HLA-identical match)	3	14	2	c
Mother	3	14	2	c	Sibling 2	1	8	3	a
	24	51	11	d	(Haplotype match)	24	51	11	d
Patient	1	8	3	a	Sibling 3	2	7	4	b
	3	14	2	c	(Haplotype match)	3	14	2	c
					Sibling 4	2	7	4	b
					(Complete mismatch)	24	51	11	d

The table illustrates that within a family, a patient has a 1-in-4 (25%) chance of having a perfect match with any of his or her siblings (see sibling 1). There is a 2-in-4 (50%) chance that the patient will have a sibling who shares at least one haplotype (see siblings 2 and 3). Finally, there is a 1-in-4 (25%) chance that a sibling will be a complete mismatch to the patient (see sibling 4).

If a family study is not performed, it is not possible to determine haplotypes. Thus, two unrelated individuals who are HLA-identical are said to be phenotypically identical; i.e., they share the same HLA antigens only.

3. What is the importance of the different methods for human leukocyte antigen typing?

In the early days of transplantation, tissue typing was performed using serology testing. This test required living cells and attempted to measure the HLA proteins that are expressed on the surface of the cell. However, this method of typing was often incomplete. Today, a more specific test directly measures the DNA sequence that codes for the specific HLA protein. The test can be performed on small amounts of blood or on any material from the patient that contains nucleated cells (e.g., buccal swabs, hair follicles, or skin). DNA-based HLA typing has identified hundreds of new alleles not previously recognized. The findings have enabled scientists to note very subtle differences in the proteins, which are extremely important in stem cell transplantation but do not seem to be as critical in solid organ transplantation. However, new studies are showing that the immune system can recognize subtle differences and make antibodies specific for apparently minor differences. Whether these antibodies will be of significance in solid organ transplantation is not yet known.

4. What is a panel-reactive antibody?

Panel-reactive antibody (PRA) assessment is one of the first tests done on transplant candidates. The test detects preformed HLA antibodies that may have developed as a result of previous blood transfusions, pregnancies, or transplantations. The presence of HLA antibodies can restrict a patient's access to transplantation. PRA analysis is performed by mixing serum from the transplant candidate with lymphocytes from a selected group of panel donors whose HLA antigens are known. If the patient does not possess any HLA antibody, none of the panel donors' lymphocytes will react and the PRA value will be reported as 0%. If, however, there is reactivity with some or all of the panel cells, the PRA is the percentage of panel donors who have positive reactions with the patient's serum. For example, if the patient's serum reacts with one-half of the donors in the panel, the PRA is reported as 50%. If the patient's serum reacts with all of the panel cells, the PRA is reported as 99%. There will always be a chance, however slight, that a random person may have the same HLA type as the patient; therefore, PRAs are never reported as 100%.

5. Why is panel-reactive antibody testing important in transplantation?

PRA testing serves two important functions. First, the %PRA is used as an index of a patient's probability of having a negative crossmatch (discussed below) with any given donor. Low PRA values are good because they indicate that a patient has a high likelihood of a negative crossmatch (therefore, of getting a transplant). By contrast, high PRA values (i.e., >30) can mean that a patient will wait longer to find an appropriate donor. According to United Network for Organ Sharing (UNOS) data, on average, only approximately 12% of cadaveric renal transplants occur in patients with antibodies > 20%. Such patients may wait 2–4 times as long for a transplant as patients with a 0% PRA. On average, approximately 30% of transplant candidates listed with UNOS have a PRA > 20%.

For patients with an HLA antibody, PRA testing also determines the specificity of that antibody. Consequently, the laboratory knows which HLA antigens the patient has made antibodies against. With this information, the laboratory can then list the antigens as unacceptable for the UNOS match run. When a donor is available, the HLA type of the donor is entered into the UNOS computer with the intent of identifying appropriate HLA-matched transplant candidates. If a patient possesses antibodies against any HLA antigen of the donor, the patient is excluded from the match run under the assumption that he or she will have a positive crossmatch with the donor. The listing of all the possible unacceptable antigens for a given patient helps to ensure that when the patient does show up on the UNOS match run, he or she has a reasonable likelihood of having a negative crossmatch. This process significantly expedites the selection of an appropriate recipient.

Many transplant centers test patients for PRA activity on a regular basis (most often monthly) according to the center's standard practice. However, patients who receive blood transfusions or blood components of any type should be tested more frequently because transfusions may result in an increase in current PRA values. In cardiac transplant patients, the increased use of the left ventricular assist device (LVAD) as a bridge to transplantation has been reported to increase PRA within a short period after implantation. LVAD patients may also be tested more frequently for changes in their antibody levels. It is important to impress upon patients the significance of notifying their transplant center if they have a received *any* blood products while awaiting a suitable donor organ. The transfusion of any blood product, not just whole blood, can increase a patient's PRA. It should also be noted that even leukocyte-filtered blood is not without risk of increasing a patient's PRA percent, particularly if the patient already has a PRA.

6. Is there an association between panel-reactive antibody and rejection?

Associations have been drawn between the incidence and severity of rejection and the PRA value prior to transplantation. In other words, the higher the PRA, the greater the risk for rejection even if the crossmatch is negative. A fresh serum sample is drawn weekly in many instances to have the most recent specimen to test against potential donors in the crossmatch.

7. What is a crossmatch?

The crossmatch is generally the final test performed immediately before the transplantation. Even though the laboratory has performed PRA testing and is knowledgeable of a patient's sensitization history and unacceptable antigens, PRA testing may not identify all of the HLA antibodies present. Therefore, the crossmatch evaluates reactivity between the serum of a potential organ recipient and lymphocytes from the organ donor. A positive crossmatch indicates that the patient possesses HLA antibody directed against the donor that could result in early graft rejection. Crossmatching is performed prospectively on all renal allograft recipients. Heart, lung, and pancreas transplant candidates usually have testing done retrospectively, unless the PRA is > 10–15%, in which case the crossmatch may be performed prospectively. For liver transplantation, crossmatching is performed retrospectively.

In most instances of renal or cardiac transplantation, the transplant would not be performed across a positive crossmatch. However, newer techniques such as plasmapheresis and intravenous immunoglobulin administration may permit some patients to be transplanted across a positive crossmatch. Nevertheless, because the long-term effects of such treatments are not yet known, only a few centers are using this procedure at this time.

8. How is the crossmatch performed?

Briefly, lymphocytes are obtained from the organ donor's peripheral blood, lymph node, or spleen and are mixed with the potential recipient's serum. If the recipient has antibodies directed against the donor's HLA type, the antibodies will bind to the donor's cells. Antibody binding is detected either by a complement-dependent cytotoxicity test (increased cell death) or flow cytometry (increased fluorescence). The demonstration that a recipient HLA antibody has bound to donor white cells indicates a positive crossmatch and may be a contraindication for transplantation. The laboratory may also do other testing to determine the class of antibody: IgG or IgM. In general, IgG antibodies appear to be the most harmful to transplanted organs.

9. Why do most solid organ transplants use retrospective crossmatching?

In cardiac, lung, liver, pancreas or islet cell transplantation, time is the most crucial element. If not transplanted quickly, these organs can be lost once they are removed. The time during which an organ is physically out of the donor's body is called **ischemic time**. Cardiac and lung tissues have an ischemic time limit of about 4–5 hours. The longer these organs are without blood flow, the greater the risk for graft dysfunction. Because the crossmatch process requires a sample of the donor's white blood cells and can take several hours to complete, it may not be logistically possible to perform the crossmatch before the transplantation. This is especially true if the donor is in another city or state because donor cells for crossmatch may not be available before organ recovery.

If a patient has a negative PRA, the risks for hyperacute rejection are small, and the crossmatch may be performed retrospectively. If, however, a patient has a PRA of > 10%, a prospective crossmatch must be done before transplantation. To facilitate this process, many transplant centers and Organ Procurement Organizations (OPOs) have begun obtaining donor material before the actual organ recovery. Depending on the cause of death, peripheral blood may be used to obtain sufficient white blood cells for testing. Alternatively, through a minor surgical procedure, an inguinal lymph node may be obtained that will provide sufficient lymphocytes for testing. Inguinal nodes are generally preferred, particularly if the donor has received multiple blood transfusions or certain types of medications (steroids) before becoming an organ donor. Multiple transfusions and/or medications can result in a false negative crossmatch.

10. What is dithiotreitol?

Dithiothreitol (DTT) is a chemical that can destroy IgM antibodies but not IgG antibodies. DTT treatment of a patient's serum can be used in PRA testing as well as in the crossmatch to determine whether the sensitized patient has IgM antibodies. Many non-HLA antibodies tend to be IgM and can result in false-positive or false-negative crossmatches. Antibodies that are non-HLA are of no consequence for the transplant. Hence, failure to perform such testing may result in some patients being inappropriately denied access to a transplant.

11. Describe the methods used to test for crossmatch results.

In most centers, crossmatch results are reported by the method used and the cells tested. For example, a laboratory may perform both cytotoxicity crossmatches and flow cytometric crossmatches and test both T-cells and B-cells. Why are such discriminators important? The difference in the methods is mostly a matter of sensitivity. In other words, the crossmatch methods can tell the clinical laboratory how much antibody (i.e., quantity of IgG) a patient possesses. The type of cells that are reactive can help to determine the specificity of the antibody. Whether the antibody is directed against class I HLA antigens (HLA-A, HLA-B or HLA-C) or class II antigens (HLA-DR, HLA-DQ or HLA-DP) can sometimes be determined by the cells that are reactive.

Class I antibodies generally produce crossmatches that are T- and B-cell–positive because class I antigens are present on all nucleated cells in the body. Class II antigens, which are expressed only on B-cells, produce a positive result only for B-cells. Understanding a positive crossmatch depends on whether the reactivity is against T-cells and B-cells or just B-cells. High titer, class I antibodies (T- and B-cell–positive) tend to be more harmful than class II antibodies, although high-titer class II antibodies have been shown to produce hyperacute rejection. It is important to note here that the above description is a general one. As with most aspects of biology, there are exceptions. The HLA laboratory will be knowledgeable about the exceptions.

12. What happens if the crossmatch is positive?

A positive crossmatch is an indication that the potential recipient has been sensitized to the HLA antigens of the donor, usually as a result of transfusion, pregnancy, or previous transplant. As such, transplants are seldom performed across a positive crossmatch because of the high risk for hyperacute or early accelerated rejection. Occasionally, a patient with a history of a 0% PRA may have an unanticipated positive crossmatch, retrospective or prospective. It is the role of the HLA laboratory to determine the significance of the positive crossmatch; i.e, although the test may produce a positive result, only antibodies directed against HLA antigens are considered detrimental to the allograft.

Therefore, most laboratories perform additional tests to determine if the positive crossmatch is truly the result of HLA-specific antibodies. For example, patients with systemic lupus may possess autoantibodies that produce a positive crossmatch against donor cells. These antibodies are directed, non-HLA proteins and will not damage the graft. The laboratory may also do tests to determine the class of the antibody, IgG or IgM. IgG antibodies have been shown to be more detrimental to allografts than IgM antibodies. The presence of IgG anti-HLA antibodies also indicates that the recipient has developed a significant immune response to these HLA antigens and may also possess cytotoxic T-cells directed against the donor HLA type. Poor outcomes have been reported in patients who have a positive crossmatch due to IgG antibodies against donor lymphocytes.

13. Describe clinical interventions for a positive crossmatch.

How the clinician deals with a positive crossmatch varies depending on the type of transplant, the type of positive crossmatch as well as patient history. For renal transplantation, a truly positive crossmatch is generally a contraindication for transplantation. The high incidence of hyperacute and accelerated rejections makes this a risky transplant. However, methods have been used recently to circumvent the positive crossmatch in selected patients. Clinicians can now use high-dose intravenous immunoglobulin (IVIg) preparations or a combination of IVIg and plasmapheresis to reduce the amount of HLA antibody present in a patient, thereby permitting a successful transplant. First of all, although this procedure has been quite successful, it is not appropriate for all patients, and the long-term results are not known. Nonetheless, patients with high-titer HLA antibody who are in need of a transplant can benefit from these procedures. Furthermore, this procedure is very expensive. Plasmapheresis can cost $2,000 per treatment, and IVIg treatment can cost $4,000–$10,000 per dose. The pretransplant costs for such treatments can exceed $100,000. Unfortunately, Medicare and private insurance do not cover this treatment because of its experimental nature and the lack of long-term outcomes.

14. What causes rejection in a transplanted organ?

Rejection is a complex biological process whereby the body's immune system perceives the transplanted organ as foreign (i.e., non-self) or abnormal and mounts a defensive response. In general, this response is no different from the body's response to an invading bacteria or virus. Because this response is directed at a tissue, however, the result is the rejection and destruction of the tissue. Good HLA matching helps to reduce the incidence of rejection; nevertheless, not all recipients receive a well-matched graft. Thus, preventing and treating graft rejection has kept physician-scientists studying methods to manipulate the immune system. The long-term goal is to create an environment of immune tolerance (i.e., a state in which the graft is accepted by the recipient with minimal or no use of immunosuppressive drugs).

15. Does rejection always destroy the transplanted organ?

Not necessarily. Several types of rejection episodes cause various types of damage to the cells of the transplanted organ. If identified early enough, antirejection therapy can be successful in reversing the process and preserving graft function. **Hyperacute rejection** is the most destructive and is caused by a high concentration of donor-specific antibody present in the recipient's body. This presensitization is identified through the PRA and crossmatch tests. Hyperacute rejection develops during the first minutes to hours after the new organ is transplanted into a recipient and usually results in immediate graft loss. With the sophisticated testing available today, hyperacute rejection is a rare entity. In addition to HLA antibodies, a major ABO mismatch can also cause hyperacute rejection. Verification of ABO type and crossmatch results or specificities can prevent this devastating form of rejection.

16. What other forms of rejection can occur in a transplanted organ?

If the transplant is not subject to hyperacute rejection, the next immediate concern is **early accelerated rejection**. This form of rejection can occur within hours (usually > 24 hr) to days posttransplant. It usually occurs in patients who have a history of sensitizing events (pregnancy, transfusion, or previous transplant). Accelerated rejection can be caused by a low concentration of HLA antibody or may be caused by activated immune cells.

The next worry for the transplant recipient is **acute rejection**, which can occur anytime from days to months posttransplant. This form of rejection is usually mediated by immune cells and can be treated successfully with immunosuppression in most cases.

The last form of rejection, **chronic rejection**, is an insidious process that develops over time, usually > 1 year posttransplant. Once initiated, most current immunosuppression is *not* successful in reversing the effects, and the graft ultimately will be lost. Chronic rejection is the most difficult to diagnose and treat.

17. Describe the events in an acute rejection episode.

Transplantation rejection involves the lymphocytes or white blood cells of the body. T-lymphocytes are the white blood cells that initiate the immune response based upon recognition of the transplanted organ as foreign. Initiation of the immune response is a form of cell-to-cell communication. Donor tissue is recognized as foreign first by circulating T- cells (direct recognition) and later by antigen-presenting cells (APCs) such as macrophages (indirect recognition). The APCs produce many different types of cytokines in response to the foreign antigens, which then alert the T-cells. One group of T-cells, the helper T-cells, then activates the effector arms of the immune system, which include cytotoxic T-cells (T-cells designed to damage the graft) and B-cells (cells that produce antibody). Together, both the cellular attack and antibody-mediated processes cause damage to the endothelial layers of the graft, which leads to thrombosis and ultimately graft dysfunction. Unless the immune system is suppressed, the graft will be destroyed. Chapter 7 describes drugs used to suppress the immune response and to treat or prevent rejection.

18. Why does a transplanted organ cause an immune response?

The immune system reacts to the transplanted organ for several reasons. For the most part, the grafted organ is viewed as foreign by the immune system, whose function is to protect the body from infection. Unfortunately, immune cells cannot tell the difference between an invading organism and life-saving transplanted tissue. A second factor is the postischemic reperfusion injury and surgical trauma that can also impact the immune system's response. Reperfusion injury and surgical trauma can cause the organ to express markers that are not normally present, which can include HLA proteins. This fact contributes to the immune system's recognition of the transplant graft as foreign. Of interest, transplantations performed between unrelated individuals who are HLA-nonidentical appear to enjoy good graft survival, perhaps because there is virtually no trauma or ischemic time for these transplants. As a result, in 2001, slightly more renal transplants were performed from living donors than were performed from cadaveric donors.

19. What is tolerance?

Tolerance is considered the "Holy Grail" of immunology. Tolerance is the process that allows organs to be transplanted across HLA boundaries yet be accepted as self. For example, one's own immune cells are tolerant of one's own tissues. When this self-tolerance fails, the result is autoimmune disease. For the transplanted organ, successful tolerance may mean that the immune system does not respond to the allograft, and immunosuppressive drugs may not be required. Immune tolerance has been achieved in experimental settings using nonhuman primates. Scientists are working hard to bring tolerance induction into the clinical arena.

20. How is tolerance achieved?

The exact mechanisms for inducing tolerance are not completely known or understood. Several approaches that have been used have shown some success in inducing tolerance to transplanted organs. One approach, T-cell ablation, has been studied in several institutions. In this model, potent immunosuppression that removes T-lymphocytes is used a day or two before transplantation and for several days after the new organ is implanted. It is believed that removing mature T-cells at the time of transplantation may permit new T-cells to become tolerant to the transplanted organ. However, administration of immunosuppression for several days before surgery is possible only in living donor transplants.

21. What is costimulation?

Another approach under evaluation for achieving tolerance involves blocking of costimulation. In this regimen, communication between APCs and T-helper cells is disrupted in such a way that an "incomplete" activation of the immune cells occurs. Once the cells have been incompletely activated, it is not possible to reactivate them to mount a functional immune response. In essence, incomplete activation renders the cell nonresponsive to subsequent immune challenge. The approach is very appealing because it can be tailored in a way that only responses to the transplanted organ are affected. A patient still maintains complete immune-responsiveness to other entities such as bacteria and viruses. This approach holds the most promise for inducing long-lasting and specific immune tolerance.

BIBLIOGRAPHY

1. Cosimi AB: Clinical application of tolerance induction in solid organ transplantation. Transplant Proc 31:1803–1805, 1999.
2. Gebel HM, Bray RA: Sensitization and sensitivity: Defining the unsensitized patient. Transplantation 69:1370–1374, 2000.
3. Harlan DM, Kirk AD: The future of organ and tissue transplantation: Can T-cell co-stimulatory pathways revolutionize the prevention of graft rejection. JAMA 282:1076–1082, 1999.
4. Itescu S, Burke E, Lietz K, et al: Intravenous pulse administration of cyclophosphamide is an effective and safe treatment for sensitized cardiac allograft recipients. Circulation 105:1214–1219, 2002.
5. John R, Lietz K, Burke E, et al: Intravenous immunoglobulin therapy in highly sensitized cardiac allograft recipients facilitates transplantation across donor specific IGG positive cross matches. J Heart Lung Transplant 20:213, 2001.
6. Rodey GE: HLA Beyond Tears. Introduction to Histocompatibility, 2nd ed. Durango, CO, De Novo Press, 2001.
7. Schuster M, Kocher AA, John R, et al: Allosensitization following left ventricular assist device (LVAD) implantation is dependent on CD40–CD40 ligand interactions. J Heart Lung Transplant 20:211–212, 2001.
8. Schweitzer EJ, Wilson JS, Fenandez-Vina M, et al: A high panel-reactive antibody rescue protocol for crossmatch positive live donor kidney transplants. Transplantation 70:1531–1536, 2000.
9. Stringham JC, Bull DA, Fuller TC, et al: Avoidance of cellular blood product transfusions in LVAD recipients does not prevent HLA allosensitization. J Heart Lung Transplant 18:160–165, 1999.
10. Szeto WY, Rosengard BR: Basic concepts in transplantation immunology and pharmacologic immunosuppression. In Baumgartner B, Reitz B, Kasper E, Theodor J (eds): Heart and Lung Transplantation, 2nd ed. Philadelphia, W.B. Saunders, 2002.
11. Wrenshall L: Determinants of antigen presentation. Graft 2:28–30. 1999.
12. Zachary AA, Hart JM: Relevance of antibody screening and crossmatching in solid organ transplantation. In Leffel MS, Donnenberg AD, Rose NR (eds): Handbook of Human Immunology. Boca Raton, FL, CRC Press, 1997.

3. THE ROLE OF THE TRANSPLANT COORDINATOR

Terri Allison Donaldson, RN, MN, ACNP

1. What is the transplant team?

The transplant team is a multidisciplinary group composed of transplant surgeons, transplant medical specialists, transplant coordinators, social workers, research nurses, ethicists, rehabilitation personnel, and financial counselors. Members of the team often collaborate with other specialists (e.g., endocrinologists, infectious disease physicians, psychiatrists, and psychologists) who are integral to clinical decision making. The transplant coordinator typically is the individual who coordinates the interactions among team members and between the transplant team and other specialists.

2. What is the role of a transplant coordinator?

By definition, *coordination* means to work together harmoniously, to act together in a smooth, concerted manner. A transplant coordinator is a person who facilitates the transplant process. Implementation of the role varies among transplant programs and geographical areas; however, certain commonalties are shared by most transplant coordinators.

Historically, transplant coordinators have been involved in the entire transplant continuum, from donor identification and organ retrieval to long-term postoperative management of the recipient. Initially, the transplant coordinator's responsibilities encompassed both organ procurement and care of transplant candidates and recipients. Over the years, as technology became more complex and transplant volume increased, the transplant coordinator's responsibilities expanded. Eventually, this single role evolved into two separate roles. Donor coordinators assumed responsibility for donor management and the procurement and placement of organs. Clinical coordinators assumed responsibility for the evaluation of patients referred for transplantation and the care of transplant candidates and recipients. This chapter focuses on the role of the clinical transplant coordinator.

3. What factors determine the clinical transplant coordinator's responsibilities?

As the field of transplantation became more complex, clinical transplant coordination became a specialized field in nursing. Today, clinical transplant coordinators are involved in the care of candidates and recipients of heart, lung, heart-lung, liver, pancreas, kidney, intestinal and islet cell transplants. The clinical transplant coordinator's responsibilities may be based on a number of factors:

- Types of organs transplanted at the institution
- Size of the transplant program
- Types of patients (adult and/or pediatric)
- Transplant phase (pre- or posttransplant)

A large transplant center that transplants all organs likely has at least one, if not several, transplant coordinators for each specific organ. If both adult and pediatric patients are involved, there may be separate coordinators for each age group. On the other hand, smaller transplant centers may have one transplant coordinator who covers several organs and types of transplant procedures, for example, heart, lung, and heart-lung. In kidney and pancreas transplant programs, clinical coordinators commonly manage the care of both single- and multiple-organ recipients.

Some larger transplant centers divide the clinical coordinator's responsibilities according to the transplant phase. For example, there may be a pretransplant coordinator, who is typically responsible for new referrals and transplant candidates, and a posttransplant coordinator, who covers all transplant recipients. At smaller programs, one individual is responsible for both phases. Regardless of how the clinical coordinator's responsibilities are delineated, the number of transplant coordinators is directly proportional to the number of transplant procedures performed and the number of patients managed by the program.

4. How is coordination of the multiple-organ transplant recipient managed?

Multiorgan transplantation requires collaboration between the individual organ programs involved. A combined heart-kidney transplantation procedure, for example, requires frequent communication between the heart and kidney transplant coordinators for management of all aspects of transplant care. Close collaboration is especially important in long-term outpatient care when antirejection medications must be adjusted to meet the needs of each organ.

5. What is the educational background of most transplant coordinators?

Transplant coordinators are usually registered nurses, although some may be physician assistants. Educational preparation may be at the diploma undergraduate or graduate level. There are a few doctorally prepared transplant coordinators. Many coordinators are advanced practice nurses. Transplant candidates and recipients require expert and specialized nursing care. Care of this patient population can be complex and challenging. The transplant coordinator must have the education, knowledge, and clinical experience to function in an expanded role and ensure the continuity of care of the transplant recipient.

6. What clinical experience should the transplant coordinator have?

Experience in transplantation per se is not always a prerequisite for the entry-level transplant coordinator. It is helpful, however, if the transplant coordinator has clinical expertise in a transplant-related field. For instance, renal transplant coordinators may have experience in the care of dialysis patients or other end-stage renal disease (ESRD) patients. Heart transplant coordinators are often nurses with expertise in caring for cardiology or cardiac surgery patients. Liver transplant coordinators may have general surgery or medical-surgical experience in the intensive care unit.

In light of Benner's novice-to-expert model,[2] new transplant coordinators are likely to be most successful if they have nursing skills at the competent level. Competent nurses see their interventions in terms of long-range patient goals. The competent nurse is able to distinguish between information that is important to a given clinical situation and that which is not. Because of the complexity of transplant patient care, the transplant coordinator should be able to function at least at the competent level on Benner's continuum.

7. In which practice settings might a transplant coordinator function?

Transplant coordination involves the care of both hospitalized patients and outpatients. In smaller transplant programs, these two practice areas may be covered by the same individual. For larger programs with more than one coordinator, the inpatient and outpatient responsibilities may be divided. Key aspects of the inpatient transplant coordinator's role might include
  • Attending rounds on pre- and posttransplant patients.
  • Facilitating communication between and among the transplant team, the patient/family, and other healthcare providers involved in the patient's care (for example, physician house staff, social workers, case managers, consulting physicians, staff nurses, and physical therapists).
  • Evaluating acutely ill patients for transplantation.
  • Teaching patients and families.
  • Discharge planning.
The role of the outpatient transplant coordinator is varied and typically includes
  • Evaluating outpatients referred for transplantation.
  • Assessing patients in transplant clinic, planning and evaluating interventions.
  • Coordinating the multidisciplinary care of transplant candidates and recipients.
  • Teaching patients and families.

Regardless of the practice setting, it is imperative that transplant coordinators communicate with one another and with all other members of the healthcare team to ensure continuity of care for this complex patient population.

8. What areas of expertise should the transplant coordinator develop?

The transplant coordinator should develop a comprehensive knowledge base to manage the complex issues involved in the care of transplant candidates and recipients. These issues include, but are not limited to, the following:

- Signs and symptoms of the absolute and relative contraindications to transplantation
- Transplant medications (indications, dose ranges, therapeutic levels, side effects, food-drug and drug-drug interactions)
- Signs and symptoms of and treatment options for allograft rejection
- Signs and symptoms of and treatment options for the major complications associated with transplantation (infection, hypertension, renal insufficiency/failure, vasculopathy, metabolic disorders, malignancy)

In addition to clinical proficiency, the transplant coordinator should develop the following skills:

Assessment skills	Signs and symptoms of rejection Signs and symptoms of infection Complications associated with transplantation Drug interactions
Communication skills	With patients, families, team members, hospital staff, referring and community physicians With departments within the hospital setting Documentation
Teaching skills	Learning theory (adult and/or pediatric) Use of audiovisual materials Use of the internet for patient education materials Development of alternative teaching strategies for patients/families with barriers to learning
Organizational skills	Maintaining accurate, organized records Ability to manage many varied tasks at one time Time management skills
Triaging skills	Assessment of patient problems by telephone Managing concurrent patient problems
Administrative skills	Managing office staff Developing budgets Managing data bases
Problem-solving skills	Managing competing priorities Tailoring solutions to individual situations

9. What type of orientation is recommended for the new transplant coordinator?

In addition to the time required to cover the organizational structure of the transplant program itself, the length of the orientation period typically depends on several factors including the coordinator's educational background, advanced degrees (if any), and prior clinical experience. The orientation program is individualized to the novice's needs and typically lasts 3–6 months.

If the individual has no prior transplant experience, during the first 3 months of the orientation period the orientee becomes acquainted with the transplant program's patients (candidates and recipients) and learns about transplant protocols, procedures, medications, and therapeutic goals. During the following 3–6 months, the orientee continues to develop clinical expertise and may begin to take call. Given the complexity of the field, it is important that a preceptor, senior transplant coordinator or physician be available to the orientee during and after the orientation period.

Twice yearly, the North American Transplant Coordinators' Organization (NATCO) offers a week-long introductory course for new transplant coordinators. Information about this course can be found at www.natco1.org.

10. What role does the transplant coordinator play in the transplant evaluation process?

The goal of the transplant evaluation process is to identify patients who have the greatest need for and will receive the greatest benefit from transplantation in terms of survival and quality of life. Through this comprehensive process, a determination is made regarding the indications for transplantation, the severity of the illness, the patient's prognosis, and any physiological or psychosocial contraindications to transplantation.

The role of the transplant coordinator is multifaceted and varies among transplant centers. In general, however, during the evaluation process the transplant coordinator typically

- Schedules, coordinates, and expedites required diagnostic tests.
- Obtains test results in a timely manner so that the transplant team can make a decision regarding an individual's candidacy for transplantation.
- Functions as a liaison between the transplant center and referring physicians, consultants, and third-party payers.
- Educates the patient and family about all aspects of the transplant process so that the eligible transplant candidate can make an informed decision about whether to be placed on the waiting list (see chapter 4).

11. Describe the transplant coordinator's role in patient education.

The transplant coordinator plays an important role in patient education. This role often begins with the initial referral conversation and may continue throughout the patient's life. During the evaluation process, the goal is to provide patients with essential information so that they can make an informed decision about transplantation. Patients often think of transplantation as a magic cure. Realistically, however, transplantation often involves trading a diseased organ for a healthy organ, but one that requires frequent follow-up care, multiple medications, and treatment for potentially life-threatening complications.

For discussion purposes, patient education topics may be divided according to transplant phase. However, there is much overlap and many topics are discussed in both phases. The major patient education topics are listed below.

PRETRANSPLANT EDUCATION	POSTTRANSPLANT EDUCATION
Evaluation process (rationale for evaluation process; specific tests and procedures)	Anticipated length of stay
Indications for transplantation	Medications (purpose, dose, frequency, side effects)
Contraindications to transplantation	Drug-drug and food-drug interactions
Alternatives to transplantation	Monitoring activities at home (e.g., blood pressure, weight)
Listing process	Follow-up (short- and long-term)
Allocation system	Rejection surveillance (biopsy schedule)
Role of transplant team members	Rejection (signs and symptoms, diagnosis and treatment)
Waiting list	Potential complications
Responsibilities while on waiting list	Infection prevention and prophylaxis
Surgical procedure	Cancer prevention
Posttransplant hospitalization	Medications prescribed by other healthcare providers
Follow-up (short- and long-term)	Over-the-counter medications and supplements
Rejection (signs and symptoms, diagnosis and treatment)	When to call the transplant team
Medications (purpose, dose, frequency, side effects)	Communication between the transplant team and other healthcare providers
Potential complications	

12. Does the transplant coordinator have other teaching opportunities?

Because transplantation is a specialized body of knowledge, the transplant coordinator is often requested to participate in the formal and informal education of physician fellows, residents, and nursing staff. Coordinators may be invited to lecture about organ donation and transplantation in nursing school classrooms or in community settings. The transplant coordinator may also participate in the evaluation of nursing staff competency relative to transplantation.

13. What is the coordinator's role in the decision-making process to list patients?

At most transplant centers, patients who have completed the evaluation process are presented to the multidisciplinary transplant team for a decision regarding placement on the waiting list. Typically, the transplant coordinator or attending physician presents the patient to the team. All of the medical and psychosocial data obtained during the evaluation process are reviewed and discussed by team members, and a consensus is reached regarding the patient's eligibility for transplantation. Patients who meet eligibility criteria are then placed on the waiting list. The transplant coordinator's role in this process typically includes

- Gathering and organizing all test results and consultation reports.
- Providing input into the discussion (given the degree of interaction with the patient/family during the evaluation process, the coordinator's insight and perspective are highly valued).
- Placing the eligible patient on the United Network for Organ Sharing (UNOS) waiting list.
- Updating the patient's original listing information in the UNOS database, as necessary (for example, changes in patient's weight or UNOS status).

14. Are there other ancillary roles that a transplant coordinator may assume?

Transplant coordinators may have additional responsibilities in caring for patients along the transplant continuum. Major patient populations cared for by various types of transplant coordinators are listed below.

TYPE OF COORDINATOR	PATIENT POPULATION
Heart	Patients with congestive heart failure or cardiogenic shock Patients on ventricular assist devices
Kidney	Patients with acute or chronic renal failure Patients on dialysis Patients with diabetes mellitus
Liver	Patients with fulminant hepatic failure Patients on liver assist devices
Lung	Patients with adult respiratory distress syndrome, end-stage pulmonary fibrosis, chronic obstructive pulmonary disease, cystic fibrosis

15. What are the on-call responsibilities of a transplant coordinator?

On-call responsibilities differ among transplant centers. Transplant call (24 hours/day, 7 days/week) is typically shared by all coordinators. If there is only one coordinator for a given program, on-call responsibilities may be shared with transplant fellows or attending physicians.

Basically, there are two types of on-call responsibilities—donor call and medical-surgical call. Donor call involves coordination of a potential transplant procedure. It begins with the transplant coordinator receiving the initial call from the organ procurement (OP) coordinator. The OP coordinator provides information about the potential donor. The transplant coordinator typically relays this information to the attending physician, and a decision is made whether to accept or reject the organ offer. If the organ offer is accepted, the transplant coordinator then

- Contacts the intended candidate.
- Notifies the organ retrieval and implant teams.
- Arranges transportation for the retrieval team, if necessary.

- Schedules the surgery in the operating room and notifies the appropriate personnel.
- Facilitates communication among all personnel involved.

Medical-surgical call involves triaging phone calls from transplant candidates and recipients. These calls vary in importance and urgency (for example, from requests for prescription refills to truly emergent situations such as troubleshooting a ventricular assist device alarm). An attending physician typically is available to assist the transplant coordinator (see chapter 24).

16. Describe the transplant coordinator's role in managing the recipient's medications.

The transplant coordinator's precise role in managing recipients' immunosuppressants and other medications is based on state practice guidelines, the coordinator's credentials, and the institution's privileging policies. Essential components of this role may include

- Adjusting immunosuppression doses according to therapeutic goals, treatment protocols, biopsy results, laboratory test results, and the patient's clinical status (in consultation with the attending physician).
- Monitoring patients for signs and symptoms of medication side effects.
- Monitoring serum drug levels and other laboratory tests.
- Educating patients and families about medications.
- Obtaining waivers from third-party payers for nonformulary medications.
- Identifying alternative sources of medications for patients—for example, state pharmacy assistance programs or indigent drug programs (often in consultation with the social worker).

17. What are the major psychological stressors that confront transplant coordinators?

For the most part, the role of a transplant coordinator is professionally and personally rewarding. As with any multifaceted role in the current healthcare environment, however, there are several potential sources of psychological stress, some examples of which are provided in the following table:

TYPE OF STRESSOR	EXAMPLE
Interpersonal conflicts	Conflicts with physicians, hospital and administrators
Patient morbidity and mortality	Death of candidates (10 to 30% die while on the waiting list) Death of recipients Serious transplant-related complications
Inadequate staffing	Increase in coordinator-to-patient ratio Delivering consistent level of care with fewer resources
Moral/ethical dilemmas	Selection of transplant candidates Use of marginal or high-risk donors Listing recipients for re-transplantation Living unrelated organ donation End-of-life issues

18. Why is the transplant coordinator's job physically demanding?

Transplant coordinators often work long hours. In most instances, organ donation is unpredictable, and transplant procedures take place at any hour of the day or night. A transplant coordinator who is on-call may experience sleep deprivation. In addition, the same coordinator may be required to report to work at 7 AM after a night of interrupted sleep. The consequences of chronic sleep deprivation are well-documented and can result in ineffective coping and job burnout.

19. What is *burnout*? What strategies can the transplant coordinator use to avoid it?

Maslach defined *burnout* as "a syndrome of emotional exhaustion, depersonalization, and reduced personal accomplishment among individuals who do 'people work' of some kind. It is a response to the chronic emotional strain of dealing extensively with other human beings, particularly when they are troubled or having problems"[5] (p. 3). Both work environment and personal charac-teristics can contribute to burnout. The burnout syndrome affects both the quality of patient care and the caregiver's quality of life.

Because of the intense nature of the job, a transplant coordinator can easily develop burnout, unless he or she uses restorative practices to disengage from the stressors of the day. The first step in avoiding burnout is to take care of oneself. Specific self-care strategies are listed below.

- Assess your coping style.
- Set realistic goals.
- Develop self-knowledge.
- Use meditation.
- Listen to music.
- Exercise regularly.
- Take a course in conflict resolution.
- Learn assertiveness techniques.
- Practice relaxation techniques.
- Accentuate the positive.
- Develop a life away from work.
- Develop coworker relationships.
- Seek professional help.

20. How can the expansion of a successful transplant program be a source of stress?

As a transplant center grows in size and volume, the coordinator-to-patient ratio gradually increases. Job stress may occur as coordinators attempt to deliver the same level of care with fewer resources and support. Strategies to deal with the increasing workload of an expanding transplant program include use of ancillary personnel for non-nursing tasks, job sharing, and flexible schedules.

Patients accustomed to a lower coordinator-to-patient ratio may also feel frustrated as the program expands. Frequent verbal (e.g., during support group meetings) or written (via newslet-ters) updates to patients about the program may prove useful. These updates can include actions that patients can take to expedite their care (e.g., requesting written prescriptions in advance of clinic appointments).

21. How can a transplant coordinator maintain balance between professional demands and personal needs?

It may be difficult for the transplant coordinator to balance the demands his or her profession with a personal life. Sometimes the job seems as if it is more than full-time work. To maintain balance, he or she must separate from work when off-duty. Work-related issues should not im-pinge on time off or vacation. Vacation time should be used to restore the body and soul—not to catch up on paperwork or projects. When overly fatigued or sleep deprived, the coordinator must be able to recognize the risk for emotional and physical decompensation. In this situation, he or she may be able to negotiate with coworkers and supervisors for an unscheduled day off for recu-peration. This strategy can prove beneficial for all concerned—the transplant coordinator, col-leagues, and patients.

Overwhelming stress in any job is inevitable from time to time. It is essential that the trans-plant coordinator recognize when stress is occurring, devote energy to identifying its sources, and implement measures to reduce stress to a more manageable level.

22. How does a transplant coordinator deal with patients who demonstrate negative coping behaviors?

Patients who are critically ill often have limited coping abilities. Occasionally patients and families will demonstrate maladaptive behavior patterns such as the following:

- Dependency
- Anger
- Controlling behavior
- Apathy
- Denial
- Manipulation

The transplant coordinator must understand that patients' prior life experiences and well-es-tablished patterns of behavior influence their ability to cope with current stressors. Any attempts to change patients' behavior or belief systems may be met with resistance and are likely to be un-successful. The transplant coordinator must meet the patient and family "where they are" to indi-vidualize and optimize patient care. Specifically, the transplant coordinator can

- Help the patient/family to identify current stressors.
- Introduce the patient/family to other transplant candidates and recipients.
- Conduct support group meetings for patients/families.
- Reward positive coping behaviors.
- Refer the patient/family to a social worker, psychiatrist, or psychologist.

23. Does the transplant coordinator have any opportunities to participate in research?

Transplant coordinators have a range of opportunities to participate in research. Many coordinators serve as research coordinators for national drug or device trials or for center-specific investigations.

Transplant coordinators also participate in nursing research as principal investigators, co-investigators, or site study coordinators. Given the relatively small number of transplant patients at any one institution, transplant centers often collaborate on nursing research studies. Several professional organizations (e.g., NATCO) offer research grants for transplant professionals.

24. How does the transplant coordinator interact with third-party payers?

Given the high costs associated with transplantation, many third-party payers (private and governmental) assign a case manager to patients referred for transplantation. Transplant coordinators, financial counselors, and social workers may all interact with this case manager. However, the transplant coordinator is typically responsible for

- Providing clinical data supporting the medical necessity for transplantation.
- Obtaining preauthorization for the transplant procedure.
- Providing periodic clinical updates while the candidate is on the waiting list.
- Notifying the third-party payer when the transplant procedure occurs.
- Providing clinical information about the postoperative course.
- Providing clinical information for referrals for follow-up care.

The transplant coordinator may also collaborate with the financial counselor and social worker in identifying the patient's transplant and prescription benefits. It is essential that the parameters of these benefits be assessed early in the transplant evaluation process so that any gaps in coverage can be identified and resolved.

Even patients with fairly substantial insurance benefits may exceed their life-time maximum coverage. Therefore, it is important that the transplant coordinator continue to collaborate with the financial counselor and social worker to ensure that the transplant patient does not experience any discontinuity in care due to the lack of appropriate resources.

25. Does the transplant coordinator have any role in hospital case management?

Case management focuses on identifying the discharge needs of patients to streamline services and decrease length of stay. The hospital case manager facilitates communication between the hospital and the third-party payer and provides information about the patient's clinical status, estimated length of stay, complications, and anticipated discharge needs. In some institutions, the transplant coordinator assumes the role of the hospital case manager.

26. Describe the transplant coordinator's involvement with clinical pathways.

Clinical pathways use best-practice standards to guide patient care. The clinical pathway outlines the timing for all aspects of patient care, including laboratory tests, procedures, activity, diet, medications, and patient education. The transplant coordinator, often in collaboration with clinical nurse specialists, staff nurses, and other hospital personnel, develops the initial drafts of the clinical pathway. The multidisciplinary transplant team approves the pathway before it is implemented.

27. Name some transplant journals that may be of interest to transplant coordinators.

Many general and specialty journals publish articles about transplantation. The following list exemplifies the variety of journals that are of interest to transplant coordinators:

Advances in Renal Replacement Therapy
ANNA Journal/American Nephrology Nurses Association
Chest
Gastroenterology
Journal of Heart and Lung Transplantation
Liver Transplantation
Nephrology Dialysis Transplantation
Progress in Transplantation (formerly, The Journal of Transplant Coordination)
Transplantation
Transplantation Proceedings

28. What professional organizations are of particular interest to transplant coordinators?
There are a number of transplant specialty organizations that may be of interest to transplant coordinators. The following organizations may be accessed directly through their Web addresses or through links on the United Network for Organ Sharing Web site. Many of the specialty organizations publish journals that contain valuable information for the transplant coordinator.

American Board of Transplant Coordinators: www.abtc.net
American Nephrology Nurses Association (ANNA): http://anna.inurse.com
American Society of Transplantation (AST): www.a-s-t.org
American Society of Minority Health and Transplant Professionals:
    www.lifegift.org/mi_asm.htm
European Transplant Coordinators Organization: www.etco.org
International Society for Heart and Lung Transplantation (ISHLT): www.ishlt.org
International Transplant Coordinators Society (ITCS):
    www.med.kuleuven.ac.be/itcs/Home/html
International Transplant Nurses Society (ITNS): www.itns.org
North American Transplant Coordinators Organization (NATCO): www.natco1.org
United Network for Organ Sharing (UNOS): www.unos.org

29. Is there a certification examination for transplant coordinators?
The American Board of Transplant Coordinators (ABTC) offers a certification examination for clinical and procurement coordinators. Professionals who sit for this examination must meet certification standards established by the ABTC. The test is computer-based and may be taken at approximately 100 sites throughout the country. It is offered periodically throughout the year. The certification is for 3 years. Recertification may be obtained either by meeting educational requirements or taking the examination again.

Practitioners who pass the examinations meet the competency and certification standards established by ABTC and become members of the American Registry of Transplant Coordinators. Certification is available to both clinical and procurement coordinators who have worked in the transplantation field for a minimum of 1 year. The two certifications that are available are

CCTC: Certified Clinical Transplant Coordinator
CPTC: Certified Procurement Transplant Coordinator

ACKNOWLEDGMENT

The author thanks Elizabeth Towery Davidson, R.N., M.S.N., ACNP for her editorial assistance with this paper.

BIBLIOGRAPHY

1. Benner, P: From Novice to Expert. Upper Saddle River, NJ, Prentice Hall Health, 2001.
2. Chapman JR, Deierhoi M, Wight C (eds): Organ and Tissue Donation for Transplantation. New York, Oxford University Press, 1997.
3. Cupples SA, Spruill LC: Evaluation criteria for the pretransplant patient. Crit Care Nurs Clin North Am 12:35–45, 2000.

4. Lin EM: A combined role of clinical nurse specialist and coordinator: Optimizing continuity of care in an autologous bone marrow transplant program. Clin Nurse Specialist 8:48–55, 1994.
5. Maslach C: Burnout—The Cost of Caring. Englewood Cliffs, NJ, Prentice Hall, 1982.
6. Morse CJ: Advance practice nursing in heart transplantation. Prog Cardiovasc Nurs 16:21–24,38, 2001.
7. Nason M: Psychosocial needs of critical care staff. In Clochesy JM, Breu C, Cardin S, et al (eds): Critical Care Nursing. Philadelphia, W.B. Saunders, 1993, pp 102–113.
8. Penson RT, Dignan FL, Canellos GP, et al: Burnout: Caring for the caregivers. Oncologist 5:425–434, 2000.
9. Smith S (ed): Tissue and Organ Transplantation. St. Louis, Mosby, 1990.
10. Taormina RJ, Law CM: Approaches to preventing burnout: The effects of personal stress management and organizational socialization. J Nurs Manage 8:89–99, 2000.
11. Williams BAH, Sandiford-Guttenbeil DM (eds): Trends in Organ Transplantation. New York, Springer, 1996.

4. EVALUATION OF PATIENTS FOR SOLID ORGAN TRANSPLANTATION

Jacqueline M. Corsini, MS, ANP, CCRN,
Connie White-Williams RN, MSN, FNP, and
Sandra A.Cupples, DNSc, RN

1. How does the transplant referral process work?

The potential transplant recipient is usually referred by a primary care physician or specialist. The referring physician has often cared for the patient for many years and sends clinical information to the transplant center for review. After the transplant team has reviewed the information, the patient is scheduled for a pre-evaluation visit, the purpose of which is to determine whether the patient has end-stage disease and to ensure that all available medical and/or surgical treatment options have been exhausted. If the patient has comorbid conditions that may preclude transplantation, the patient and referring physician are informed, and the initial visit may be deferred until these issues are resolved. One exception occurs in the setting of kidney transplantation. Preemptive transplantation may be performed in select patients approaching end-stage renal disease before the initiation of dialysis.

The most essential factor in patient referral is timing. The referral should occur early, before the patient is too ill to be considered a viable candidate for transplantation or to survive the increasingly long wait for a donor organ. All too often, organs are not available in time because of the limited pool of solid organ donors.

2. What is the purpose of a transplant evaluation?

The potential transplant candidate is thoroughly evaluated to ascertain the cause of end-organ disease, determine the indications and contraindications for transplantation, and address the clinical conditions that require further work-up and management before transplantation. The timing of the evaluation is determined by the patient's need for transplantation and the availability of a living donor, if applicable. The patient and family also have an opportunity to gather information and make an informed decision about their desire to proceed with transplantation.

3. How long does it take to complete a transplant evaluation?

The length of time for completion of a pretransplant evaluation is variable and depends on the following factors:

- The transplant center's selection criteria and evaluation requirements
- The presence of significant comorbidities in the potential transplant candidate that require further work-up and management before placement on the waiting list
- Any preauthorization for evaluation tests as required by third-party payers

The evaluation may take place in the hospital or outpatient setting. If a living donor is available, evaluation for both the potential candidate and the donor may take several months to complete.

4. What are the indications for transplantation?

Transplantation is indicated for individuals experiencing end-stage failure of the organ(s) to be transplanted. End-stage organ failure results from complications of disease processes that are no longer manageable, even with maximal medical and/or surgical intervention. It is the complications of disease processes that result in most indications for solid organ transplantation.

Requirements regarding posttransplant life expectancy in patients with comorbid conditions vary among transplant centers and the types of organs transplanted.

Kidney transplantation. Not all patients with end-stage renal disease are kidney transplant candidates. The risks and benefits of dialysis versus transplantation are carefully reviewed to determine which type of renal replacement therapy is most appropriate for each individual patient. The decision to proceed with transplantation should be driven by medical need and patient preference. In contrast to other types of organ transplantation, kidney transplantation can be delayed, if clinically appropriate, while the patient is maintained on either hemodialysis or peritoneal dialysis. Kidney transplantation may be considered in some patients approaching end-stage renal disease with a creatinine clearance < 20 ml/min before the initiation of dialysis. This preemptive transplantation is usually possible when a living donor is available.

Kidney-pancreas transplantation is typically indicated for patients with insulin dependent diabetes mellitus with end-stage diabetic nephropathy, who
- Are less than 50 years of age.
- Have minimal, repairable, or no atherosclerotic vascular disease.
- Have no history of congestive heart failure.
- Meet the indications for kidney and pancreas transplantation.

Pancreas transplantation may be indicated in patients who require a kidney transplant (i.e., simultaneous pancreas-kidney) or who have undergone a previous transplant (i.e., sequential pancreas transplantation after kidney transplantation) for treatment of type I diabetes mellitus in the setting of minimal or no secondary diabetic complications. Some transplant centers perform pancreas transplants alone in patients with brittle or labile type 1 diabetes mellitus, who experience significant hypoglycemia unawareness, have no evidence of advanced diabetic nephropathy, and/or experience failure of exogenous insulin to achieve glycemic control.

Liver transplantation usually is indicated in the setting of acute or chronic liver disease associated with complications due to portal hypertension and/or reduced liver mass. Signs and symptoms of these complications include
- Bleeding from esophageal varices
- Coagulopathy
- Hepatic encephalopathy
- Spontaneous bacterial peritonitis
- Refractory ascites, unresponsive to diuretic therapy

Some patients with unusual conditions related to cholestatic disease that significantly impair quality of life, such as pruritus unresponsive to medical therapy, metabolic bone disease, or xanthomatous neuropathy, may be considered for liver transplantation. Liver transplantation may also be a treatment option for the correction of genetic diseases involving the liver, with an extrahepatic presentation, such as Crigler-Najjar syndrome.

Intestinal transplantation primarily refers to transplantation of the small bowel. This type of solid organ transplant is indicated in the setting of structural or functional failure of the intestine associated with a deterioration in the candidate's condition despite optimal therapy with total parenteral nutrition. Structural failure is characterized by a reduction in the intestinal mass. Functional failure involves deficient nutrient absorption or severe dysmotility of the gut. Intestinal failure can occur at any age.

Heart transplantation is indicated in patients with
- End-stage heart disease not correctable by medical or surgical intervention.
- Congestive heart failure, New York Heart Association (NYHA) Class III–IV symptoms on maximal treatment. Most patients suffer from systolic failure. In most instances, the patient must also demonstrate a reduced exercise capacity on a metabolic stress test, with a maximal oxygen uptake of < 14 ml/kg/min.
- Refractory angina despite optimal therapy.
- Life-threatening ventricular dysrhythmias.

Lung transplantation is indicated in patients with irreversible end-stage lung disease who are
- Less than 65 years of age.
- Dependent on supplemental oxygen.
- Significantly affected by a poor quality of life.

The following table summarizes the most common disease indications for each specific type of organ transplant.

TYPE OF TRANSPLANT	MOST COMMON DISEASE INDICATIONS
Heart	Cardiac tumors (myxomas) Congenital heart disease Ischemic cardiomyopathy Dilated cardiomyopathy (idiopathic, postpartum, viral) Hypertrophic cardiomyopathy Restrictive cardiomyopathy Myocarditis Valvular heart disease
Heart-lung	Eisenmenger's syndrome with cardiac repair Primary pulmonary hypertension

Kidney	Genetic diseases
	  Polycystic kidney disease
	Primary glomerulonephritis
	Systemic diseases
	  Diabetic nephropathy
	  Focal segmental glomerulonephrosclerosis
	  Glomerulonephritis
	  Hepatitis C
	  Human immunodeficiency virus-associated nephropathy
	  Hypertension
	  Systemic lupus erythematosus

Kidney-pancreas	End-stage diabetic nephropathy Type 1 diabetes mellitus with life-threatening hyperglycemia and/or hypoglycemic unawareness despite optimal medical therapy No significant secondary complications due to diabetes mellitus

Liver	Alcoholic liver disease
	Cholestatic disease
	  Primary biliary cirrhosis
	  Primary sclerosing cholangitis
	Chronic hepatitis
	  Autoimmune hepatitis
	  Hepatitis B or C
	Genetic diseases
	  Crigler-Najjar syndrome
	  Familial hypercholesterolemia
	  Hereditary hemochromatosis, in select cases
	  Hereditary oxalosis
	Hepatocellular carcinoma < 5 cm in size in the presence of cirrhosis
	Metabolic diseases
	  Wilson's disease

Single lung	Chronic obstructive pulmonary disease
	  Emphysema
	Interstitial lung diseases
	  Eosinophilic granuloma
	  Idiopathic pulmonary fibrosis
	  Lymphangioleiomyomatosis
	  Sarcoidosis
	Pulmonary vascular diseases
	  Eisenmenger's syndrome with cardiac repair
	  Primary pulmonary hypertension

(Cont'd. on next page.)

TYPE OF TRANSPLANT	MOST COMMON DISEASE INDICATIONS

Bilateral sequential lung	Chronic obstructive pulmonary disease
	    Emphysema
	Infectious lung diseases
	    Bronchiectasis
	    Cystic fibrosis
	Pulmonary vascular diseases
	    Eisenmenger's syndrome with cardiac repair
	    Primary pulmonary hypertension

Pancreas	Brittle or labile type 1 diabetes mellitus without advanced diabetic nephropathy

Intestine	Structural disease processes:
	    Necrotizing enterocolitis
	    Midgut volvulus secondary to malrotation
	    Gastroschisis
	    Atresias/stenosis of small bowel
	    Crohn's disease
	    Vascular accidents/mesenteric thrombosis/trauma
	    Familial adenomatous polyposis
	Functional problems:
	    Chronic intestinal pseudo obstruction syndrome
	    Congenital enteritis
	    Total intestinal aganglionosis
	    Radiation enteritis

5. In general, what are the contraindications to solid organ transplantation?

The following table summarizes the typical contraindications to all types of solid organ transplantation that are applicable at most, but not all, transplant centers. Absolute contraindications refer to clinical situations in which the outcome of transplantation is so poor that this therapeutic option should not be offered. Relative contraindications include those conditions that may have a negative impact on patient survival, but not to the extent that transplantation should not be considered.

ABSOLUTE CONTRAINDICATIONS
Active drug, tobacco, or alcohol abuse
Active infection
Active peptic ulcer disease
Acute pulmonary embolism
Bleeding diathesis
Acquired immune deficiency syndrome
Diverticulitis
Evidence of psychopathology
Inability to comply with the therapeutic regimen
Inability to understand the procedure or the risks involved
Recent malignancy
Severe, irreversible organ system damage other than organ(s) to be transplanted

RELATIVE CONTRAINDICATIONS
Cachexia (80% predicted weight)
Human immunodeficiency virus infection
Lack of financial resources to pay for surgery, hospitalizations, medications, and follow-up care
Lack of functional psychosocial support system
Morbid obesity (> 140% predicted weight)
Severe osteoporosis

6. What are the major organ-specific physiologic contraindications to transplantation that are applicable at most transplant centers?

The following table summarizes the organ-specific contraindications to transplantation that are applicable at most, but not all, transplant centers.

ORGAN	CONTRAINDICATIONS
Heart	Autoimmune disorders
	Cerebrovascular accident
	Diabetes mellitus with end-organ damage
	Peripheral vascular disease
	Pulmonary hypertension with elevated pulmonary vascular resistance > 5 Wood units or a transpulmonary gradient > 15 mmHg unresponsive to treatment
	Pulmonary infarction
	Significant kidney disease (serum creatinine > 2 mg/dl or creatinine clearance < 50 ml/min)
	Significant liver or pulmonary disease
Heart-lung	Autoimmune disorders
	Cerebrovascular accident
	Deformity in thoracic anatomy
	Diabetes with end-organ damage
	Pulmonary infarction
	Significant kidney or liver disease
	Severe deconditioning (not able to walk 500 feet in a 6-min walk test)
Kidney	Advanced cardiopulmonary disease
	Hepatitis C-positive status with cirrhosis noted on liver biopsy
	Potential risks of immunosuppressive therapy outweigh the risks of dialysis
	Significant abnormality of the urinary tract
	Severe peripheral vascular disease
Kidney-pancreas	Advanced cardiovascular disease not amenable to surgical intervention
	Severe end-organ damage associated with diabetes mellitus
	Severe peripheral vascular disease
Liver	Advanced cardiopulmonary disease
	Active extrahepatic infection
	Current alcohol or substance abuse
	Extrahepatic malignancy
	Multisystem organ failure—3 or more organ system involvement
	Severe pulmonary hypertension
Lung	Age > 65 years for single-lung, > 55 years for bilateral lung, > 45 years for heart-lung
	Active systemic collagen vascular disease
	Cardiac insufficiency—right or left ejection fraction < 20%
	Complicated or uncontrolled diabetes mellitus
	Corticosteroid dependency >20 mg of prednisone or equivalent per day
	Creatinine clearance < 50 ml/min
	Dependent on mechanical ventilation and clinically unstable
	Hepatitis B virus surface antigen-positive
	Hepatitis C virus infection with biopsy-proven evidence of liver involvement
	Nonrehabilitative pulmonary disability
	Significant infection present outside the lungs and upper respiratory tract
	Significant, untreatable coronary artery disease—more than 1 vessel disease
	Surgically uncorrectable chronic thromboembolic disease

(Cont'd. on next page.)

ORGAN	CONTRAINDICATIONS
Pancreas	Age > 60 years
	Diabetic complications are not clearly defined
	Severe peripheral vascular disease
	Significant, uncorrectable cardiovascular disease (ejection fraction <30%)
Intestine	Multisystem organ failure
	Uncontrolled sepsis
	Human immunodeficiency virus infection
	Malignancy outside of intestines with metastasis
	Severe, unresolvable cardiac, respiratory, or cerebral complications

7. Can patients who are human immunodeficiency virus-positive undergo transplantation?

There have been several reports of patients undergoing cardiac, liver, kidney, and pancreas transplantation in the setting of human immunodeficiency virus (HIV) infection. Chronic renal and liver disease are often associated with HIV infection. HIV-associated nephropathy (HIVAN) may develop in patients who are HIV-positive and precipitate end-stage renal disease.

Hepatitis C is a common cause of liver failure and is also often associated with HIV infection.

The survival of patients with HIV infection has improved considerably with the development of highly active antiretroviral therapy (HAART). This treatment has been shown to reduce the viral load significantly, increase CD4 count, and improve survival in HIV-positive patients. In the past, patients would die of acquired immunodeficiency syndrome (AIDS) before dying of end-stage organ disease. Now, however, because these patients are living longer, some are experiencing end-organ disease and may require transplantation for survival.[8]

It has been suggested that HIV infection should be considered to be like any other comorbid condition.[15] Some transplant centers, after consultation with infectious disease specialists, may consider transplanting patients who meet the following criteria:

- The CD4 count is > 200 cells/mm^3 for more than 6 months.
- The patient has been maintained on stable antiretroviral therapy for more than 3 months.
- There is no diagnosis of AIDS.
- There are no opportunistic infections or other complications commonly associated with AIDS.
- HIV-1 RNA levels are undetectable.[21]

Transplantation in the setting of HIV infection is not considered a standard of care at this time but is an area of continued research. Patients who are HIV-positive and require a transplant should understand that this treatment is still considered experimental. Such patients should also be informed of the risks and benefits associated with the entire transplant process, including the surgical procedure, immunosuppressive therapy, and posttransplant complications.

8. Can patients who are hepatitis C virus-positive undergo transplantation ?

This controversial clinical issue is addressed by each transplant center's policy, patient selection criteria, and type of organ transplant. Hepatitis C virus (HCV) infection is a common indication for liver transplantation in the setting of decompensated cirrhosis. HCV infection has a high rate of recurrence in the transplanted liver and may progress to cirrhosis in the graft; however, survival in this subgroup of patients after liver transplantation is considered excellent when compared with transplantation for other clinical conditions.

In renal transplantation, liver failure from chronic HCV infection is a leading cause of death in patients who are long-term transplant survivors. The presence of HCV infection can also be associated with the development of membranoproliferative glomerulonephritis, a condition that may result in graft loss. If cirrhosis is found on liver biopsy, renal transplantation is not recommended. The use of interferon-α therapy for the treatment of chronic HCV infection in transplant patients is not recommended because of the increased risk of graft dysfunction and low efficacy in this clinical setting.

9. What are the key aspects of the pretransplant evaluation process?

Before transplantation, the patient undergoes a comprehensive medical-surgical and psychosocial assessment. The evaluation is best completed by using a multidisciplinary approach. Key aspects of the evaluation process include the following:

- Determination of the cause of end-organ disease
- Assessment of the indications for transplantation
- Identification of the contraindications to transplantation (for example, advanced cardiopulmonary disease, malignancy, infection, severe systemic disease, current alcohol or substance abuse, or lack of adherence with medical therapy)
- Estimation of the patient's risk for development of recurrent disease in the allograft
- Estimation of the patient's risk for undergoing transplant surgery
- Identification of any comorbidities that may affect the postoperative course
- Evaluation of the patient's ability to tolerate immunosuppressant therapy
- Identification of potential living donor(s), if applicable

The following table summarizes the essential components of the evaluation history and physical examination for the potential transplant candidate.

PARAMETER		SPECIFIC CONSIDERATIONS
History of present illness		Cause of end-stage organ disease
		Biopsy results
		Prior treatment of end-stage organ disease
		Signs and symptoms of end-stage organ disease
		Requirement for life-sustaining therapies such as dialysis and assist devices
		Requirement for assistance with activities of daily living
		Impact of end-stage disease on the patient's quality of life
Past medical history	Cardiovascular	Ischemic heart disease
		Myocardial infarction
		Congestive heart failure
		Congenital anomalies
	Endocrine	Diabetes mellitus
		Hyperlipidemia
		Hyperparathyroidism
	Infection	Recurrent infections (e.g., pneumonia, bronchitis, sinusitis, osteomyelitis)
		Sexually transmitted diseases
		Risk for cytomegalovirus infection, tuberculosis, hepatitis B or C, *Strongyloides stercoralis*
		Prior residence in geographic areas known for endemic mycoses
		Recent travel history
		Previous or current exposure to birds, cats, mice, or rabbits
	Malignancy	Breast, cervical, colon, or skin (basal cell or malignant melanoma) carcinoma
	Neurologic	Cerebrovascular accident
		Transient ischemic attacks
		Seizures
	Pulmonary	Use of tobacco products
		Smoking history (number of pack years)
		Chronic obstructive pulmonary disease
	Renal	Nephrolithiasis
		Renal insufficiency
		Urinary tract infections
		Childhood pyelonephritis or reflux

(*Cont'd. on next page.*)

PARAMETER		SPECIFIC CONSIDERATIONS
Past medical history (*cont'd.*)	Vascular	Intermittent claudication Venous ulcers
	Psychiatric	Depression Anxiety disorders
	Immunizations	List of immunizations and dates given
	Sensitization	Number of previous blood product transfusions Females: number of pregnancies; date of last pregnancy
Past surgical history	Previous surgery (including transplant procedures)	
Review of systems	Signs or symptoms of organ dysfunction or conditions that would contraindicate transplant surgery or immunosuppressant therapy Unstable comorbid conditions that require further evaluation	
Family history	Genetic disorders Malignancies Other major diseases (e.g., coronary artery disease, diabetes mellitus, hypertension, renal disease)	
Medications	Current medications Current use of corticosteroids, chemotherapeutic agents, immunosuppressant agents Medication allergies	
Psychosocial history	Occupation Living environment Social support Neurocognitive deficits Level of education; reading ability Prior and/or current substance abuse (e.g., alcohol, drugs) Prior and/or current noncompliance with medical therapy	
Physical examination	Assess patient for physical evidence of infection, malignancies, systemic disease, or organ dysfunction, such as cardiovascular disease.	

10. What are the rationale for and the essential components of the psychosocial evaluation of the potential transplant candidate?

Psychosocial factors have a significant impact on the outcome of transplantation. When the patient has a commitment to and positive attitude toward the transplant procedure and follow-up care, the individual is more likely to achieve better clinical outcomes.

A transplant social worker often performs this part of the pretransplant evaluation. The components of a transplant psychosocial assessment include the following:

COMPONENT	EXAMPLE
Demographics	Age, marital status, number of children
Emotional and tangible support	Number and location of individuals in support network; type of support individuals can provide
Commitment to transplant process	Patient's versus family's desire for transplantation
Emotional status	History of or current depression, mental illness
Health maintenance behaviors (prior and current)	Compliance history; routine dental and eye examinations, routine cancer screening, current medical requirements (e.g., oxygen, dialysis)
Home environment	Type of dwelling (single family, apartment, trailer), telephone, running water, heat and air conditioning, stairs

(Cont'd. on next page.)

COMPONENT	EXAMPLE
Social habits	Substance abuse (alcohol, tobacco, drugs)
Coping skills	Preferred coping strategies
Neurocognitive issues	Educational level, reading/comprehension ability; ability to understand the risks and benefits of transplantation and give informed consent; ability to follow a complex posttransplant regimen
Transportation	Ability to travel to the transplant center for scheduled and unscheduled appointments and follow-up care
Financial issues	Health insurance, savings, income, actual and potential resources (personal, community, governmental)

11. What consultations are typically obtained during the transplant evaluation process?

At some point during the evaluation process, the patient and family or significant other meets with the transplant coordinator, transplant physician (e.g., cardiologist, nephrologist, pulmonologist), transplant surgeon, social worker, and financial counselor, if available. Additional consultations are obtained as indicated by the patient's medical history and clinical status (e.g., dentist, gynecologist, dietician, ophthalmologist, psychiatrist, oncologist).

12. What diagnostic tests are typically obtained for patients undergoing transplant evaluation?

Routine screening tests are obtained to evaluate patients for active or latent infections, malignancies, and evidence of organ dysfunction. Evaluation protocols vary among transplant centers. The following table summarizes the tests that are typically obtained for patients undergoing transplant evaluation.

Tests Commonly Obtained for Patients Undergoing Transplant Evaluation

Laboratory studies	Histocompatibility testing
	Blood type
	Tissue typing (human leukocyte antigens) of both the recipient and donor (if available)
	Panel reactive antibody screen
	Serologies/infectious disease
	Cytomegalovirus: IgG and IgM antibodies
	Epstein-Barr virus: IgG and IgM antibodies
	Hepatitis B: surface antigen, surface antibody, core antibody
	Hepatitis C antibody
	Human immunodeficiency virus antibody
	Rapid plasma reagin
	Herpes simplex virus
	Varicella-zoster virus
	Toxoplasmosis titers*
	Serum chemistries including calcium and phosphorus levels
	Liver function tests
	Thyroid function tests
	Lipid profile
	Complete blood cell count with differential
	Prothrombin time, partial thromboplastin time, International Normalized Ratio
	C-peptide level and hemoglobin A1-C[†]
	Intact parathyroid hormone[‡]
	Prostate specific antigen level (males older than 40 years)
	Urinalysis and urine culture
	24-hour urine for creatinine clearance and protein excretion

(Cont'd. on next page.)

Tests Commonly Obtained for Patients Undergoing Transplant Evaluation (Continued)

Laboratory studies (*cont'd.*)	Serum β-HCG level (females of childbearing age) Stool for occult blood Stool for ova and parasites (if indicated)
Diagnostic tests	Abdominal ultrasound Papanicolaou test Chest radiograph Pulmonary function tests Electrocardiogram Purified protein derivative Mammogram (as indicated)

* Indicated for potential heart transplant candidates
† In patients with diabetes mellitus
‡ Indicated for potential kidney or kidney-pancreas transplant candidates

13. What diagnostic tests are obtained as indicated?

Diagnostic Tests Obtained as Indicated

SELECT DIAGNOSTIC TESTS	INDICATION(S)
Bone density*	History of osteoporosis Substantial smoking history Osteopenia
Cardiac catheterization	Positive stress test
Carotid duplex studies	Suspected cerebrovascular disease
Colonoscopy	Patients older than 50 years Positive stool guaiac History of primary sclerosing cholangitis or ulcerative colitis with abnormal lesions on biopsy
Computed tomography scan of abdomen or pelvis	Abnormal abdominal or pelvic ultrasound
Computed tomography scan of chest	Abnormal chest radiograph
Doppler studies or angiography	Suspected peripheral vascular disease
Drug and alcohol testing	Current or previous history of substance abuse
Echocardiography	Abnormal cardiac examination Patients older than 40 years History of myocardial infarction, valvular disease or congestive heart failure (to assess left ventricular function) History of hypertension (to assess left ventricular hypertrophy)
Liver biopsy	History of cirrhosis Hepatitis C, if enzyme-linked immunoabsorbent assay-3 and recombinant immunoblot assay-3 are positive and confirmed viral load by polymerase chain reaction
Mammography	Women older than 50 years Women older than 40 years in potential recipients at high risk for breast cancer
Pelvic examination with Papanicolaou test	All women of child-bearing years
Stress testing	Patients older than 50 years Diabetes mellitus Abnormal electrocardiogram Hypertension

* Given the significant risk of bone loss in first 6 months posttransplant, some transplant centers now obtain bone density scans routinely on all patients.

14. What organ-specific diagnostic tests are performed during the evaluation period?

Organ-Specific Diagnostic Tests

Heart	Left and right heart catheterization Echocardiogram Metabolic exercise test 24-hour Holter monitoring
Kidney	β-2 microglobulin C-Reactive Protein (predicts risk for acute rejection) Renal ultrasound Voiding cystourethrogram, particularly in the setting of difficult voiding or genitourinary dysfunction or to measure bladder capacity in anuric patients
Liver	α-fetoprotein Antimitochondrial antibodies Antinuclear antibodies Ferritin Pao_2 testing ($Pao_2 < 70$ mmHg requires pulmonary function tests and bubble-contrast echocardiography to assess for intrapulmonary right to left shunting)
Lung	Computed tomography of chest with high-resolution images Pulmonary function tests 6-min walk or other test to evaluate exercise capacity Quantitative ventilation/perfusion scans, if indicated
Pancreas	Comprehensive cardiovascular evaluation C-peptide level Hemoglobin A-1C
Intestine	Depending upon underlying disease process: Plain abdominal radiography — Angiography of mesenteric vessels Upper and lower gastrointestinal series — Upper and lower GI tract endoscopy, with biopsy as indicated Abdominal ultrasonography Computed tomography of abdomen — Genetic testing

15. If any of the following conditions are found during the evaluation process, how are they usually managed during the pretransplant period?

During the transplant evaluation process, unexpected comorbid conditions may be found incidentally. The following table summarizes several conditions that require further evaluation and management before the patient's placement on the transplant waiting list.

CONDITION	RATIONALE FOR TREATMENT BEFORE TRANSPLANTATION	DIAGNOSTIC AND TREATMENT OPTIONS
Cardiovascular disease	Cardiovascular events are a major cause of posttransplant morbidity and mortality.	Cardiology consultation Advanced disease may preclude transplantation. Patients with diabetes mellitus, positive smoking history, or age older than 45 years should undergo a complete cardiac work-up.
Conditions requiring surgical intervention	Increased surgical risk after transplantation Increased risk of infection associated with immunosuppressant therapy Potential life-threatening emergencies	Significant coronary artery disease may require revascularization for noncardiac transplant patients. Cholelithiasis: Cholecystectomy in specific populations, such as patients with diabetes mellitus

(Cont'd. on next page.)

CONDITION	RATIONALE FOR TREATMENT BEFORE TRANSPLANTATION	DIAGNOSTIC AND TREATMENT OPTIONS
Conditions requiring surgical intervention (*cont'd.*)		Native nephrectomy indicated in the following settings: Infected stones Significant reflux Uncontrolled hypertension Polycystic kidney disease (in the setting of significantly enlarged kidneys, recurrent infection, or bleeding) Significant peripheral vascular disease: aortoiliac or carotid disease may require revascularization.
Gastrointestinal disease: Peptic ulcer disease Gastritis Hepatobiliary disease	Posttransplant corticosteroid therapy can increase the risk of gastrointestinal bleeding. Diverticular disease increases the risk of superinfections with enteric organisms after transplantation. Peptic ulcer disease can increase the risk of gastrointestinal hemorrhage during and after surgery. Several complications associated with chronic liver dysfunction can be prevented with early treatment.	Gastroenterology consultation Additional diagnostic tests as indicated: Endoscopy Upper or lower gastrointestinal series Peptic ulcer disease or gastritis: H_2-blockers Diverticular disease: surgical intervention in select cases Esophageal varices: β-blockers or transjugular intrahepatic portosystemic shunt procedure for refractory variceal bleeding Spontaneous bacterial peritonitis: antibiotic therapy (sulfa-methoxazole/trimethoprim, norfloxacin)
Infection	Increased risk of reactivation of infection with posttransplant immunosuppressive therapy	Infectious disease consultation Treat infections with indicated antimicrobial agent. • Tuberculosis requires treatment and surveillance for at least 1 year after medical intervention. Hepatitis C infection—liver biopsy needed to assess presence of and degree of cirrhosis Ensure that immunizations are current. Treat occult infections, such as dental abscesses and those involving vascular access devices. Treat diabetic foot ulcerations.
Malignancy	Immunosuppressive medications can have a deleterious effect on the natural course of a malignancy.	Oncology consultation Assess patient for history of severe sunburn and exposure to carcinogens such as tobacco, alcohol, and occupational chemicals. Malignancies such as breast cancer and melanoma that have recurrence rates posttransplant may require a longer waiting interval before the patient can be placed on the waiting list (e.g., 5 yr).

(*Cont'd. on next page.*)

CONDITION	RATIONALE FOR TREATMENT BEFORE TRANSPLANTATION	DIAGNOSTIC AND TREATMENT OPTIONS
Malignancy (*cont'd.*)		Patients with carcinoma in situ (e.g., basal cell carcinoma) usually can be placed on the waiting list without a waiting period. Most transplant centers require at least a 2-year waiting period or "disease free interval" after treatment for a malignancy, prior to placement on the waiting list. Patient must be informed of risk for recurrence of malignancies or new (de novo) carcinomas after transplantation and required posttransplant screening. Individuals who • Are > age 45 years should be routinely screened for cancer common to the general population (per American Cancer Society guidelines) • Have a history of analgesic abuse or acquired cystic kidney disease should be screened for urinary tract or renal cancer • Have a history of ulcerative colitis should be screened for colon cancer
Pulmonary vascular hypertension	Individuals with chronic heart failure can develop irreversible pulmonry vascular hypertension. This can result in acute right heart failure of the donor heart and possible death at the time of transplantation.	• Periodic right heart catheterizations during the waiting period to monitor pulmonary pressures • If pulmonary hypertension is present, medical therapy may include vasodilators, diuretics, or inotropic support
Renal insufficiency	Increases morbidity and mortality in patients undergoing cardiac, lung, liver, or pancreas transplantation. Immunosuppressive agents may increase risk of posttransplant renal insufficiency.	Nephrology consultation Determine underlying cause of renal dysfunction and treat as indicated.
Severe systemic disease	Can increase morbidity and mortality after transplantation or decrease quality of life Immunosuppressant therapy may exacerbate the disease or facilitate disease progression. May preclude transplantation if the risks associated with general anesthesia and/or the transplant surgery itself are too high.	Disease-specific consultations as indicated Systemic disease such as lupus erythematosus should be stable, with no further progression. Some diseases may recur in the allograft. Evaluation must include the anticipated natural progression of disease posttransplantation.

(Cont'd. on next page.)

CONDITION	RATIONALE FOR TREATMENT BEFORE TRANSPLANTATION	DIAGNOSTIC AND TREATMENT OPTIONS
Substance abuse	Increases the risk of noncompliance with the posttransplant therapeutic regimen	Psychiatric consultation Offer assistance with drug rehabilitation before being listed. Consider contracting with patient for length of abstinence, as required by the transplant center. Random drug and nicotine screening Smoking cessation program

16. What happens after the transplant evaluation is completed?

When the transplant evaluation is completed, the multidisciplinary transplant team typically meets to review all patient data. During this meeting members of the transplant team also engage in anticipatory planning for patients who may have special needs before or after transplantation. Each patient's potential candidacy for transplantation is determined on an individual basis. The patient may be

- Accepted as a transplant candidate and listed on the cadaveric transplant waiting list or scheduled for living donor surgery.
- Not accepted because of contraindications.
- Deferred until a problem found during the evaluation is resolved.

The patient, family, and referring physician are informed of this decision.

17. What are the two antigen systems that have a significant effect on transplantation?

The two antigen systems that have a significant effect on transplantation are blood type (ABO) compatibility and the human leukocyte antigen (HLA) system. ABO compatibility is the major determinant of solid organ transplantation. The guidelines for ABO grouping that apply to blood transfusion therapy also apply to transplantation. The HLA system enables the immune system to differentiate self from non-self and recognizes foreign tissue introduced into the body. Rejection occurs if antigens on a donor organ are recognized as foreign tissue by the recipient's immune system.

18. Why is histocompatibility testing performed?

Histocompatibility testing is performed to predict the compatibility between a living or cadaveric donor organ and a potential recipient. Rejection and graft loss are likely to occur in the setting of preformed antibodies against the donor's antigens. Rejection of the transplanted organ may be less likely to occur when the donor and recipient tissues are closely matched. Three types of matching procedures can be performed:

- HLA typing of white blood cells
- Assessment of anti-HLA antibodies
- Crossmatch testing of the recipient and donor

19. How is a transplant candidate's panel-reactive antibody level determined?

Serum from the transplant candidate is tested against samples of pooled lymphocytes from selected donors. The percentage of samples to which the candidate's serum reacts is known as the panel reactive antibody (PRA) level. Factors associated with elevated PRA levels include exposure to blood transfusions, previous pregnancies, or prior transplants. A number of methods are in use to detect PRA, including cytotoxicity, enzyme-linked immunoabsorbent assay, and flow cytometry.

20. How is the information from the panel-reactive antibody level used?

The PRA percentage is used to predict the candidate's risk for reacting to a donor organ. Because PRA levels can change over time, the test may be repeated monthly while the candidate is on the waiting list.

In many instances, a prospective crossmatch with a potential donor is obtained before transplantation. Highly sensitized patients (e.g., those with high PRA levels) may have prolonged waiting times before a negative-crossmatch donor is available.

21. What does a positive crossmatch indicate?

The crossmatch is done to determine whether the candidate has preformed antibodies to the potential donor's lymphocytes. Donor white blood cells are mixed with recipient serum. Preformed antibodies are detected by cytotoxicity or flow cytometry. The presence of preformed antibodies increases the recipient's risk for posttransplant rejection of the allograft. A positive crossmatch contraindicates the use of the organ from that particular donor.

22. Which immunizations are typically recommended before transplantation?

Infection can be a significant cause of morbidity and mortality after solid organ transplantation. Therefore, it is important to prevent infection in the pretransplant, as well as the posttransplant, period. Moreover, because vaccines in the posttransplant period may be ineffective in the setting of immunosuppressive therapy, many transplant centers recommend that the following immunizations be given during the pretransplant period:

• Influenza
• Hepatitis B
• Pneumococcus
• Varicella vaccine (should be considered in varicella-zoster virus–seronegative patients)

If indicated, live vaccines (e.g., varicella-zoster, oral polio, and measles, mumps, and rubella [MMR]) should be administered several months before transplantation. Live vaccines are generally not recommended for transplant recipients or others occupying the same household.

Before liver transplantation, candidates should receive the hepatitis A and B vaccines. Because of the risk of recurrent hepatitis B virus (HBV) infection after liver transplantation, select patients untreated for chronic HBV infection may receive passive immunization with high-dose hepatitis B immunoglobulin (HBIG). HBIG administration decreases the risk of recurrent infection. HBIG may require lifetime administration and can be costly. Lamivudine, a nucleoside analogue, may also be given to inhibit HBV replication. Some transplant centers are using the combination of lamivudine and HBIG to further reduce the risk of HBV reinfection after liver transplantation, specifically in candidates who are HBV-positive prior to transplant.[15]

For patients with tetanus-prone wounds, tetanus toxoid may be given.

23. What information is needed to list and prioritize candidates on the waiting list?

Although general guidelines have been established by specialty committees and consensus conferences, listing criteria for solid organ transplantation may vary among transplant centers and third-party payers. The Organ Procurement and Transplantation Network (OPTN) has developed policies to guide organ allocation in the United States and ensure equitable distribution of donated organs. The following table summarizes the suggested listing and organ allocation criteria for each type of solid organ transplant.

SPECIFIC ORGAN TRANSPLANT	LISTING AND ORGAN ALLOCATION CRITERIA
Heart	Blood type Panel reactive antibody level (requirement for prior crossmatch) Height and weight Waiting time Status on waiting list
Heart-lung	Blood type Panel reactive antibody level Height and weight Waiting time

(Cont'd. on next page.)

SPECIFIC ORGAN TRANSPLANT	LISTING AND ORGAN ALLOCATION CRITERIA
Kidney	Blood type and human leukocyte antigen typing Age Creatinine clearance < 20 ml/min Initiation of dialysis, if applicable Panel reactive antibody level Previous kidney transplant Quality of antigen mismatch Waiting time
Kidney-pancreas	Blood type Creatinine clearance <20 ml/min Panel reactive antibody level Type 1 diabetes mellitus with end-stage renal disease Type 1 diabetes mellitus confirmed by a low or undetectable C-peptide level Waiting time

Liver	Blood type
	Panel reactive antibody level
	Model for End-Stage Liver Disease (MELD) Score
	   Score of 10 (less ill)—score of 40 (gravely ill)
	Status 1: For patients with fulminant hepatic failure or primary graft
	   nonfunction in ICU setting

Lung	Blood type Panel reactive antibody level Height and weight Waiting time*
Pancreas	Blood type Panel reactive antibody level Type 1 diabetes mellitus with poor glycemic control, despite optimal medical therapy Type 1 diabetes mellitus confirmed by a low or undetectable C-peptide level Waiting time
Intestine	Blood type Height and weight Waiting time Status on waiting list

* Patients with the diagnosis of idiopathic pulmonary fibrosis are assigned an additional 90 days' waiting time.

24. What happens if it is determined that an individual is not a transplant candidate?

The transplant team informs the patient and family that the patient is not a candidate. The physician explains why transplantation would not be in the patient's best interests. The referring physician is informed by written letter. Members of the transplant team may make recommendations for optimizing medical treatment options. For example, the transplant cardiologist may recommend home inotropic therapy for a patient with end-stage heart disease who has been ruled out for transplantation.

25. Name some emotional stressors that confront patients during the evaluation and waiting periods.

Both the evaluation and waiting periods can be stressful. Patients may feel anxious, depressed, or ambivalent about the evaluation process and/or the transplant procedure. Other major stressors include

- Fear that a previously undiagnosed condition will make them ineligible for transplantation
- Fear that they will not survive until a suitable donor organ becomes available
- Fear of becoming a burden to their families
- Grief when fellow transplant candidates die while on the waiting list
- Guilt about wishing that a donor organ will become available

Counseling and therapy are often required throughout the evaluation and waiting period in order to help patients and families cope with these and other stressors.

26. What resources are available to help patients and their families cope with the stressors of the evaluation and waiting periods?

A number of resources are available to patients and families. These include
- Support group meetings that provide information about all aspects of the transplant process and an opportunity for candidates and recipients to meet each other and share their concerns and coping strategies.
- Referrals to mental healthcare providers (social workers, psychologists, psychiatrists, and recreational therapists)
- Judicious use of internet web sites, such as the United Network for Organ Sharing (UNOS) patient education site, and other transplant web sites.

27. How frequently are candidates on a cadaveric transplant waiting list reevaluated?

Because transplant candidates may spend several months to years on the waiting list, they require periodic reevaluation. Semiannual or annual reevaluations are often performed in order to
- Document the continued need for transplantation.
- Determine the progression of the end-stage disease and make interim treatment modifications as necessary.
- Determine the progression of any comorbid conditions.
- Determine the development of any new disease(s).

Occasionally, candidates are removed from the transplant list because of an improvement in their end-stage disease. If potential contraindications to transplantation are identified, candidates may also be removed temporarily from the list or placed in inactive status until these issues are resolved.

28. What does the periodic reevaluation for transplant candidates typically involve?

Transplant candidates typically require an updated history and physical examination. The history should include recent blood transfusions, travel, infections, weight changes, new health problems, new allergies, current medications, and any modifications in the treatment regimen.

Periodic testing typically includes PRA levels, routine cancer screening, and organ-specific tests, which are listed in the following table.

TYPE OF TRANSPLANT	TYPE OF TESTING
Heart	Echocardiogram to reevaluate left ventricular function and ejection fraction Metabolic exercise testing Serial hemodynamic measurements to assess pulmonary vascular resistance
Kidney	Repeat noninvasive cardiac testing at least annually, particularly in patients with diabetes mellitus* Coronary angiography repeated as indicated*
Liver	Abdominal ultrasound α-fetoprotein levels at least every 6–12 months
Lung	Assessment of oxygen requirements Computed tomography scan of chest Echocardiogram at least annually Exercise capacity tests

(Cont'd. on next page.)

TYPE OF TRANSPLANT	TYPE OF TESTING
Pancreas	Repeat noninvasive cardiac testing at least annually
	Coronary angiography repeated as indicated
Intestine	Liver function tests
	Periodic weight measurement, particularly in infants and children

* Per transplant center protocol.

Demographic information is also updated, including current address, telephone, and pager numbers to contact patient at the time of transplant. If the patient has a pager, it should be tested to make certain that it is operational.

BIBLIOGRAPHY

1. American Diabetes Association: Position statement: Pancreas transplantation for patients with type 1 diabetes. Diabetes Care 23:117, 2000.
2. Bartucci MR: Kidney transplantation: State of the art. AACN Clin Issues 10:153–163, 1999.
3. Carithers RL Jr: Liver transplantation. American Association for the Study of Liver Diseases. Liver Transpl 6(1):122–135, 2000.
4. Chan PD, Winkle PJ: History and Physical Examination in Medicine, 2nd ed. Laguna Hills, CA, Current Clinical Strategies, 1997.
5. Child Pugh and Meld. Available at: http://organtx.org/tx/ctp-meld.htm. Accessed 7/29/02.
6. Cupples SA, Spruill LC: Evaluation criteria for the pretransplant patient. Crit Care Nurs Clin North Am 12(1):35–47, 2000.
7. Danovitch GM (ed): Handbook of Kidney Transplantation, 3rd ed. Philadelphia, Lippincott Williams & Wilkins, 2001.
8. Gow PJ, Pillay D, Mutimer D: Solid organ transplantation in patients with HIV infection. Transplantation 72:177–181, 2001.
9. Hanafusa T, Ichikawa Y, Kishikawa H, et al: Retrospective study on the impact of Hepatitis C virus infection on kidney transplant patients over 20 years. Transplantation 66:471–476, 1998.
10. Humar A, Leone JP, Matas AJ: Kidney transplantation: A brief review. Front Biosci 2:e41–47, 1997.
11. Kasiske BL, Ramos EL, Gaston RS, et al, for the Patient Care and Education Committee of the American Society of Transplant Physicians: The evaluation of renal transplant candidates: Clinical practice guidelines. J Am Soc Nephrol 6:1–34, 1995.
12. Kirklin JK, Young JB, McGiffin DC (eds): Heart Transplantation. New York, Churchill Livingstone, 2002.
13. Morris PJ (ed): Kidney Transplantation: Principles and Practice, 5th ed. Philadelphia, W.B. Saunders, 2001.
14. Nelson S: Listing criteria for solid organ transplantation [editorial]. Transplantation 66:946–947, 1998.
15. Norman DJ, Turka LA: Primer on Transplantation, 2nd ed. Malden, MA, Blackwell Publishers, 2001.
16. OPTN/UNOS Policy Notice Memo. Available at: www.unos.org/Newsroom/archive_policy_20010716_meld.htm. Accessed 7/29/02.
17. Parker J (ed): Contemporary Nephrology Nursing. Pitman, NJ, American Nephrology Nurses' Association, 1998.
18. Penko ME, Tirbaso D: An overview of liver transplantation. AACN Clin Issues 10:176–184, 1999.
19. Pirenne J: Conference report: Advances in intestinal transplantation: Report from the VII International Small Bowel Transplant Symposium, September 12–15, 2001, Stockholm, Sweden. Medscape Transplantation 3(1), 2002. Available at: www.medscape.com/viewarticle/415042. Accessed 7/29/02.
20. Rohrer, KS: Transplantation immunology. In Nolan MR, Augustine SM (eds): Transplantation Nursing: Acute and Long-Term Management. Norwalk, CT, Appleton & Lange, 1995.
21. Steinman TI, Becker BN, Frost AE, et al: Guidelines for the referral and management of patients eligible for solid organ transplantation. Transplantation 71:1189–1204, 2001.
22. White-Williams C: Management of clients requiring transplantation. In Black JM, Hawks JH, Keene AM (eds): Medical Surgical Nursing: Clinical Management for Positive Outcomes, 6th ed. Philadelphia, W.B. Saunders, 2001, pp 2213–-2230.
23. Williams L, Horslen SP, Langnas AN: Intestinal transplantation. In Cupples S, Ohler L (eds): Solid Organ Transplantation: A Handbook for Primary Health Care Providers. New York: Springer, 2002, pp 292–333.

5. PSYCHOSOCIAL ISSUES IN TRANSPLANTATION

Jane D. Harrison, LCSW, C-ASWCM, and
Sandra A. Cupples, DNSc, RN

1. Do all transplant centers include a psychosocial assessment as part of the transplant evaluation process?

Nearly all U.S. transplant centers (95%) include a psychosocial assessment as part of the evaluation process. The assessment can be performed by psychiatrists, psychologists, or social workers. Many transplant centers use a combination of these professionals for the psychosocial evaluation; however, social workers typically are relied upon most heavily.[17]

2. Are psychosocial criteria used for candidate selection?

A 1990 survey of cardiac, liver, and renal transplant programs indicated that 23%, 14%, and 7% of these programs used formal psychosocial criteria for candidate selection, respectively. Other programs had informal psychosocial selection criteria.[16]

3. What is the rationale for the psychosocial assessment?

The psychosocial assessment is not conducted to determine the social worth of or to order patients according to rank. Rather, the issues addressed during the psychosocial assessment (e.g., social support, psychopathology, compliance history, substance abuse) are likely to affect survival and have a bearing on the patient's and family's ability to cope with the entire transplant process. More specifically, the psychosocial assessment is conducted to
- Predict the patient's ability to cope with transplant-related stressors, screen out or intervene with patients who appear to lack effective coping skills.
- Identify any mental health comorbidities and plan appropriate interventions.
- Determine whether the patient can be taught a sufficient amount of information to give informed consent for the transplant procedure and successfully assume the roles of transplant candidate and recipient.
- Determine whether the patient will be able to work collaboratively with the transplant team and comply with all aspects of the therapeutic regimen.
- Assess the patient's history of substance abuse and recovery; predict the patient's potential for long-term abstinence.
- Increase the transplant team's knowledge of the patient to provide more effective clinical care.
- Identify the psychosocial needs of the patient and family and plan for interventions and services during each phase of the transplant process.
- Establish baseline pretransplant measures of mental functioning to identify pre- to postoperative changes.[17]

4. What are the major components of the psychosocial evaluation?

The psychosocial assessment varies among transplant programs; however, it usually includes an evaluation of the factors listed in the following table.

COMPONENTS	AREAS ADDRESSED
Psychiatric history and current status	Mood disorders, anxiety disorders, psychosis, suicidal ideation and/orattempts, evidence of personality disorder; treatment history and compliance with treatment

(Cont'd. on next page.)

45

COMPONENTS	AREAS ADDRESSED
Compliance history and current status	Adherence to current and past medical regimens with regard to medication-taking, monitoring of health (e.g., insulin and blood pressure checks), dietary and fluid restrictions, exercise, and attendance at medical appointments and treatments
Substance use history and current status	Quantity and frequency of current and heaviest use of alcohol, nicotine, and other substances; symptoms of abuse and/or dependence; treatment and rehabilitation history and compliance
Mental status	Orientation in person, time, place; appearance and affect; insight and judgment; cognitive status (e.g., attention and concentration, memory, visuospatial skills)
Social history and availability of support	Employment status, marital status, and relationship stability, living arrangements, financial status; contact, availability, and emotional supportiveness of family, friends, and community or religious organizations; religious beliefs and orientation; concurrent stressors (work-related, home-related, other)
Family social and mental health history	Stability of family system; mental health and substance use history
Perceived health, coping style, and quality of life	Perceptions of medical condition, perceptions of health-related impairments in daily life, expectations and under-standing of the transplant process, strategies typically used to cope with health-related and other life stressors

From Dew MA, Switzer GE, DiMartini AF, et al: Psychosocial assessments and outcomes in organ transplantation. Prog Transplant 10:239–259, 2000, with permission.

5. Of the 7 assessment areas, which components are used most frequently in decision-making about a patient's suitability for transplantation?

Decision-making about a patient's suitability for transplantation typically is based on information about the patient's psychiatric status, medical compliance, and substance abuse history.

6. What psychosocial factors are associated with poor transplant outcomes?

Psychosocial factors that increase the risk of poor posttransplant outcomes include
• Poor social support
• Psychiatric disorders that are likely to negatively affect posttransplant compliance (e.g., psychoses, anxiety, or affective disorders)
• Self-destructive behaviors (e.g., alcohol, tobacco, or drug abuse)
• History of poor compliance with medical treatment and a failure to comprehend the necessity for improving compliance behavior
• Intractable maladaptive personality traits (e.g., counter-dependence)[17]

7. Are there any transplant-specific instruments for psychosocial screening?

Two instruments have been reported in the literature: the Psychosocial Assessment of Candidates for Transplant (PACT) scale[20] and the Transplant Evaluation Rating Scale (TERS).[24]

8. Is psychological testing used to screen patients?

Many centers use formal psychological testing during the evaluation process. The results of this testing, however, may be influenced by the physiological and psychosocial stressors associated with end-stage organ disease and the need for transplantation (e.g., cognitive deficits secondary to inadequate perfusion of the brain). Neuropsychological testing is more likely to uncover organic brain dysfunction than clinical examination.

9. Are patients ever rejected for transplant on psychosocial grounds?
Refusal rates vary greatly, from 0 to nearly 40%. In their 1993 survey, Levenson and Olbrisch found that transplant refusal rates based on psychosocial criteria were 5.6% for cardiac transplant programs, 2.8% for liver programs, and 3.0% for renal programs.[16]

10. What accounts for the variability in refusal rates?
Levenson and Olbrisch posit that the variability may be due to differences in how selection criteria are applied, psychosocial resources available at the transplant center, and the prevalence of psychosocial problems within the transplant center's referral pool.[16]

11. Name some psychosocial reasons that patients may be rejected for transplantation.
In a landmark survey of the psychosocial evaluation of patients referred for heart, liver, or kidney transplantation, Levenson and Olbrisch noted the following social and psychopathological contraindications to transplantation. Transplant programs may consider these contraindications to be absolute, relative, or irrelevant.[16]

SOCIAL CONTRAINDICATIONS	PSYCHOPATHOLOGICAL CONTRAINDICATIONS
Patient is not a U.S. citizen	Family history of mental illness
Patient is not a resident of the state in which the transplant center is located	Active schizophrenia
	Controlled schizophrenia
Patient has no social support	Current affective disorder
Patient has experienced a recent death or loss	History of affective disorder
	Recent suicide attempt
Patient is currently a felony prisoner	Distant suicide attempt
Patient has a history of significant criminal behavior	History of multiple suicide attempts
	Current suicidal ideation
	Dementia
	Personality disorder
	Mental retardation: Intelligence quotient < 70
	Mental retardation: Intelligence quotient < 50

12. Why is social support an important consideration in solid organ transplantation?
Social support has been defined by Lewis and colleagues as "the network of relationships that provide concrete, emotional, and informational assistance to meet the perceived subjective or objective needs of the patient"[18] (p. 262). Higher levels of social support have been associated with improved health and well-being in various patient populations, including patients with chronic and end-stage diseases. Among transplant patients, higher levels of social support have been associated with better psychological adjustment, greater marital satisfaction, and lower levels of depression.

13. Are there any tools that help patients to identify their actual and potential sources of social support?
The Tracy and Whittaker Social Network Map (SNM)[23] is a proactive social assessment and intervention strategy that has been used by social workers to initiate discussions with transplant recipients about the structural and functional dimensions of their support networks. The purpose of these discussions is to help transplant recipients to
- Identify their needs.
- Ascertain available social support resources.
- Determine how these resources can meet their needs.
- Use individuals in their support networks to meet their needs.
- Strengthen the network to increase support.

14. What does the social network mapping process entail?

The SNM process involves asking the patient to (1) name individuals from 8 areas of life who have provided assistance during the last several months, (2) classify the types of support these individuals have provided (concrete, emotional or informational), and (3) identify other characteristics of these supportive relationships (e.g., reciprocity, closeness, frequency) (see table, next page).

An analysis of the structural and functional components of the 8 network areas enables the social worker to develop a practice plan that focuses on reinforcing or strengthening the patient's social support system.

15. Name some advantages of social network mapping.

Transplantation is inherently stressful and places numerous demands on both patients and family members. In this setting, SNM can be particularly advantageous because it
- Enables patients to identify both current and potential sources of support and the nature of support available from these sources.
- Facilitates discussion about stressful topics.
- Empowers patients to address problems.
- Serves as a starting point for addressing or clarifying inadequate or ambiguous support issues.
- Provides a basis for additional interventions or referrals.

16. What are some of the stressors associated with the organ waiting period?

Both candidates and family members experience many stressors while waiting for a donor organ. Major stressors include the following:
- Lack of control over the availability of a donor organ and timing of the transplant surgery
- Deterioration of health
- Worry that a donor organ will not arrive in time
- Living life on hold: not being able to travel; having to be immediately available for the transplant surgery
- Wearing a pager that may go off in error (false alarms)
- Being called into the transplant center only to have the procedure aborted

The last stressor is especially anxiety-producing. Many candidates, however, reframe this experience and refer to it as a dry run. They state that it actually was helpful because they now know what to expect when they arrive at the transplant center. Patients who have been on the waiting list for a particularly long period of time often remark that it was reassuring to know that they have not been forgotten and that they actually are on the waiting list.

17. Many transplant centers offer support groups for transplant candidates. Are there any disadvantages associated with these groups?

Support groups are advantageous in many respects. Some transplant professionals, however, cite an increased competition for organs when patients and families get to know one another better through group participation. Nevertheless, most professionals also report that the majority of patients believe the "sickest" patient should receive the next available organ and that the allocation process is the fairest and works as it was intended.

18. Are mentoring programs ever used in transplantation?

The self-help process of mentoring has been used effectively in many areas of health care, including transplantation. The process affords transplant candidates an opportunity to discuss this major life event with someone who has already coped successfully with the transplant experience. Mentoring programs are particularly beneficial in transplantation because few candidates know someone who has undergone transplantation. Although not a substitute for formal educational interventions by transplant professionals, mentoring does offer candidates an opportunity to communicate on a one-to-one basis with transplant recipients who share their individual and unique perspectives and advice.

Social Network Grid Used to Document Results of the Network Mapping Exercise

Name	AREA OF LIFE	CONCRETE SUPPORT	EMOTIONAL SUPPORT	INFORMATION/ ADVICE	CRITICAL	DIRECTION OF HELP	CLOSENESS	HOW OFTEN SEEN	HOW LONG KNOWN
	1. Household 2. Other family 3. Work/school 4. Organizations 5. Friends 6. Neighbors 7. Professionals 8. Others	1. Hardly ever 2. Sometimes 3. Almost always	1. Hardly ever 2. Sometimes 3. Almost always	1. Hardly ever 2. Sometimes 3. Almost always	1. Hardly ever 2. Sometimes 3. Almost always	1. Goes both ways 2. You to them 3. Them to you	1. Not very close 2. Sort of close 3. Very close	1. Does not see 2. Few times/yr 3. Monthly 4. Weekly 5. Daily	1. < 1 yr 2. 1–5 yr 3. > 5 yr
1									
2									
3									
4									
5									
6									
7									
8									
9									
10									
11									
12									
13									
14									

Reprinted with permission from Families International, 1170 West Lake Park Drive, Milwaukee, WI 53224.

A mentoring relationship may also be useful for patients who are overwhelmed by the prospect of transplantation and uncertain about its risks and benefits. Mentors often help patients work through ambivalent feelings and decide whether to pursue transplantation.

Many transplant centers have formalized the approach to mentorship with regularly scheduled group instruction about this role and ongoing supervision by transplant professionals.[25]

19. What qualifications should a mentor have?

Mentors are typically selected by members of the transplant team. They are transplant recipients or their partners who
- Are at least 6-months posttransplant.
- Have excellent communication and interpersonal skills.
- Have a nonjudgmental attitude.
- Have no significant emotional problem such as depression.
- Demonstrate an ability to actively listen to others.[25]

20. Discuss the controversy about transplanting patients with alcohol-induced liver disease.

Despite the fact that the prevalence of alcoholism among adults in the United States is approximately 9%, the frequency of alcohol-induced end-stage disease is relatively low.[11] However, alcohol is the most common cause of liver disease, and alcohol-induced liver disease (ALD) is the most common cause for liver transplantation. Survival rates of patients transplanted for ALD are comparable to or exceed survival rates of patients transplanted for other types of end-stage liver disease.[1] Despite these statistics, the issue of transplanting patients with alcohol-induced disease remains controversial. The pros and cons of this ethical debate about transplanting patients with ALD are summarized below:

PROS	CONS
Survival rates of patients transplanted for ALD are comparable to or exceed survival rates of patients transplanted for other types of end-stage liver disease.[1,11]	Given the shortage of donor organs, patients who have not demonstrated responsibility in maintaining their health should not be eligible for liver transplantation.
Keeping patients with ALD off the waiting list discriminates against the poor because they have less ability to pay for alcohol rehabilitation programs.	Alcoholism occurs in every socio-economic group; therefore, it is not discriminatory to keep patients with ALD off the waiting list.
Alcoholism is a medical diagnosis, and patients with ALD should receive fair treatment.	
The resource utilization (length of stay, number of days on ventilator, and number of readmissions during first posttransplant year) of alcoholic liver transplant recipients is comparable to that of nonalcoholic liver transplant recipients.[11]	Alcoholism compromises long-term survival because of recidivism and recurrence of ALD.
Patients with ALD should not be kept off the waiting list unless a certain level of moral virtue is required of all types of transplant candidates.	Alcoholics are less compliant with medical therapy.
Given the lack of prospective longitudinal studies that incorporate various alcohol-related outcome measures, there is no conclusive evidence that directly links pretransplant alcohol use to posttransplant alcohol-related morbidity and mortality.	Public awareness about the number of patients with ALD who are undergoing liver transplantation is thought to affect organ donation adversely.

21. What is the rate of recidivism among patients who undergo liver transplantation for alcohol-induced liver disease?

Overall, a number of studies have indicated a mean relapse rate of approximately 15%.[3,15] In a 1997 survey of U.S. liver transplant programs, Everhart and Beresford[13] found that the mean rate of relapse to drinking at 2 years posttransplant was 14%; however, the mean rate of relapse to uncontrolled or addictive drinking that had medical or social consequences was only 5%.

22. What are the predictors of posttransplant alcoholic recidivism?
Few investigators have prospectively studied alcohol use among patients who have undergone liver transplantation for alcoholic liver disease. In a longitudinal study, DiMartini and colleagues found that posttransplant alcohol use was significantly associated with the following factors:
- Prior nonalcohol substance abuse
- Family history of alcoholism in a first-degree relative
- Prior rehabilitation for alcoholism

Somewhat surprisingly, recidivism was not associated with psychiatric history or pretransplant sobriety less than 6 months.[10]

23. Are there any instruments that measure a patient's risk of alcohol relapse?
The High-Risk Alcoholism Relapse (HAR) scale[26] was designed to study recidivism risk among male veterans and has been used with the liver transplant population. The HAR uses information about daily alcohol consumption, duration of drinking, and previous treatment history to assess the severity of alcoholism. HAR predictive validity for relapse within the first 6 months of treatment has been established (sensitivity, 69%; specificity, 65%). However, the HAR has not been validated in terms of post–liver-transplantation relapse rates or outcome data. The HAR has not been used with women.[17]

24. How long do patients have to be drug- or alcohol-free before they can be placed on the transplant waiting list?
In 1996, the United Network for Organ Sharing (UNOS) recommended that patients with alcoholic cirrhosis complete a mandatory 6-month period of sobriety and that patients with < 6 months' demonstrated sobriety enter into and sign a behavioral contract with the transplant team. These recommendations were reviewed by the U.S. Department of Health and Human Services; however, they were not implemented.

Currently, many U.S. transplant programs require a 6-month period of abstinence from alcohol or drugs. Some centers may also require behavioral contracting, enrollment in addiction treatment programs, periodic drug or alcohol testing, or additional follow-up before placing the patient on the waiting list. Although requirements vary across the different types of organ transplantation, heart, lung, and liver transplant programs use these criteria most frequently and most stringently.

25. Discuss the manner in which transplantation affects psychosocial outcomes.
A number of theories describe the relationship between transplantation and psychosocial outcomes. One model posits that the effects of transplantation permeate all areas of the recipient's life. As depicted in the model, the effects radiate outward and lead to adjustment and changes in various domains, starting with the psychological domain and extending to the behavioral and social domains—all of which influence the recipient's overall quality of life. Examples of domain-specific outcomes are listed in the model (see figure, top of next page).

26. After transplantation, why is return to work beneficial?
Improved quality of life is one goal of transplantation. Employment offers structure, provides meaningful activity, and bestows a sense of purpose that contributes to positive self-esteem and thereby has the potential to enhance posttransplant quality of life. Individuals who are able to return to work, school, or volunteer activity are able to put the transplant in perspective and are less likely to become "professional patients." If transplant recipients cannot return to work, they are more likely to think of themselves as disabled.

27. How many transplant recipients who can return to work actually do so?
Studies conducted in the early and mid-1990s indicated that approximately 50% of transplant recipients medically assessed as capable of returning to work actually did so (kidney transplant,

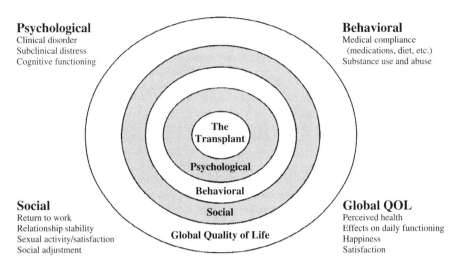

Psychological
Clinical disorder
Subclinical distress
Cognitive functioning

Behavioral
Medical compliance
  (medications, diet, etc.)
Substance use and abuse

Social
Return to work
Relationship stability
Sexual activity/satisfaction
Social adjustment

Global QOL
Perceived health
Effects on daily functioning
Happiness
Satisfaction

The Transplant — Psychological — Behavioral — Social — Global Quality of Life

Effects of transplantation on psychosocial outcomes. QOL = quality of life. (From Dew MA, Switzer GE, DiMartini AF, et al: Psychosocial assessments and outcomes in organ transplantation. Prog Transplant 10:239–259, 2000, with permission.)

41%; heart transplant, 45%; liver transplant, 57%[21]). Patients may have less incentive to return to work or more difficulty in obtaining employment if they are close to retirement age; are older; have been out of the work force for a prolonged period of time; or have health insurance benefits through disability, through private or public sources (Medicare or medical assistance), or through a spouse's employment benefits.

28. Does pretransplant alcohol/drug abuse affect posttransplant employment?

Some studies have indicated that substance abuse is not associated with the potential for employment or rehabilitation. However, the recipient's ability to obtain posttransplant employment may be influenced by a number of factors, including prior employment history and current physical capacity, cognitive functioning, and behavioral patterns. In general, the longer the period of sobriety before transplantation, the greater the likelihood of returning to work. In some instances, however, the effects of addiction may prohibit employment altogether.

29. What is the most significant barrier to returning to work?

The most difficult barrier to returning to work is the psychological component. Before patients can return to work or seek employment, they must believe that they are physically able to do so. In the early posttransplant period, patients must cope with a number of physical and emotional changes. They often do not feel well; they are adjusting to a complicated medication regimen; and they must return to the transplant center frequently for follow-up visits. Consequently, patients often consider themselves to be sick and cannot visualize themselves as being able to return to work.

30. What can be done if a transplant recipient cannot return to a physically demanding job?

Transplant recipients who previously performed physically demanding manual labor may have to find different employment. Unfortunately, it may be difficult for these recipients to translate their previous job skills into a new type of employment. Such recipients should be referred to a vocational rehabilitation counselor or employment specialist. Depending on educational level and prior skills, there are a number of employment opportunities available for transplant recipients. Telemarketing is an example of less strenuous employment that many transplant recipients could undertake.

31. When should the concept of returning to work be discussed with patients?

Many transplant centers emphasize the importance of returning to work during the initial transplant evaluation conference. By doing so, the transplant team conveys the message, early on, that the patient is expected to return to work. This strategy lets the patient know from the outset that the return to work is an important issue that must be addressed. It also helps to mitigate the element of surprise when employment and disability issues arise after transplantation. Centers that stress the importance of returning to work have higher return-to-work rates.

32. Do most transplant centers have employment specialists?

A number of large-volume transplant centers have added employment specialists to their transplant teams. Smaller transplant centers, however, may share an employment specialist to decrease personnel costs and still provide patients with this important resource.

33. What prevents transplant recipients from obtaining new employment?

There are a number of factors, but health insurance remains one of the greatest concerns, particularly when coverage is based on disability. Even though income can be greatly improved with employment, private health insurance often remains unaffordable. Smaller companies with few employees may have a difficult time offering insurance options. Job skills that are limited, even if specialized, are problematic. Patients often experience side effects from new medications that can be difficult to cope with, and starting a new job adds to the stress.

34. When and how should a patient return to work after transplantation?

Patients typically may return to work when the physician determines that they are medically stable. The return-to-work schedule is influenced by the degree of pretransplant deconditioning, type of transplant procedure, and type of employment to which the patient is returning. An example of a return-to-work time table for transplant recipients is provided below:
- 2–3 months posttransplant: The patient is referred for vocational rehabilitation assessment and training. Training and/or employment begins on a part-time basis, 2–4 hours per day for 2–4 weeks.
- Depending on the patient's tolerance, over the next 4–6 weeks the number of work hours is slowly increased.
- By 3–4 months posttransplant, the patient should be working on a full-time basis.[21]

35. Which transplant recipients are more likely to require vocational rehabilitation?

The amount of vocational rehabilitation required depends on a number of factors. In general, recipients require more extensive vocational rehabilitation if they have limited education, possess few work skills, have health perceptions that differ significantly from those of the transplant team, or believe that they are physically unable to work. On the other hand, recipients typically require little or no vocational rehabilitation if they are less than 55 years old, have at least a high school diploma, have a history of white collar employment, or believe that they are physically capable of working.

36. How often is Social Security Disability reviewed?

In the past, patients who were found to be disabled due to end-organ failure had life-long disability benefits. With the passage of the Balanced Budget Act of 1991, Social Security disability requirements are reviewed on a regular basis, usually every 3 years.

37. Immunosuppressant medications are expensive. What resources are available to transplant recipients?

Patients who do not have substantial prescription benefits as part of their health insurance plan face a significant challenge in obtaining immunosuppressant medications during post-transplant care. Patients with Medicare coverage due to disability are covered for 80% of their immunosuppressant costs for life if they were Medicare recipients at the time of the transplant procedure. Patients who have Medicare due to end-stage renal disease have this coverage for only 3 years posttransplant. For those patients who are unable to obtain insurance coverage for medications and who fall within certain income levels, most pharmaceutical manufacturers provide patient-assistance programs. A member of the transplant team, most often the social worker, obtains an application form for the patient. Pharmacy-assistance programs require constant monitoring; some require reapplication as frequently as every 45 days, which can be very labor intensive. Some transplant centers rely on volunteers to assist with this process. Other centers use software programs to track the information.

38. Why is *quality of life* an important consideration in transplantation?

The World Health Organization (WHO) defines health as a state of complete physical, mental, and social well-being. The term *quality of life* typically refers to the patient's functional status and well-being in each of the WHO dimensions of health as well as the patient's overall assessment of his or her quality of life.

Over the last 3 decades, solid organ transplantation has become an accepted treatment modality for various end-stage diseases. As the prevalence of transplantation has increased, it has become correspondingly more important to consider the costs and benefits of this therapy with respect to patients, families, and society at large. Information about quality of life has been used to guide health policy, clinical decision making, and resource allocation.

39. Does quality of life improve with transplantation?

In the most exhaustive review of the transplant quality-of-life (QOL) literature to date, Dew and colleagues[9] examined 218 independent QOL studies conducted in 23 countries between 1972 and 1996. These studies involved over 12,000 kidney, kidney/pancreas, pancreas, liver, heart, lung, and heart/lung transplant recipients. Three major conclusions emerged from the analysis:

1. Overall, QOL improves pre- to posttransplantation in the domains of physical functioning, mental health/cognitive status, social functioning, and overall perception of QOL. However, QOL does not improve in all patients, nor does it improve equally across all domains or across all types of organ transplantation.

2. QOL in transplant recipients exceeds that of similarly ill comparison groups (primarily transplant candidates), particularly with respect to the QOL domains of physical functioning and overall perception of QOL.

3. QOL of transplant recipients does not equal that of healthy nonpatient samples, particularly with respect to physical functioning, mental health, and social functioning. Across all types of transplant procedures, recipients overwhelmingly rate their global QOL as high, despite modest changes in their domain-specific ratings of QOL. The reasons for this apparent discrepancy are unclear. Perhaps transplant recipients, having been given the gift of life, redefine the term *normal life* and value life dearly in spite of the side effects and complications associated with transplantation. Thus they may reframe their standards of reference or reconfigure the value formerly placed on individual components of their lives such that their overall QOL ratings are high.[5]

40. What burdens confront the family members of transplant recipients?

Transplantation clearly affects family members' quality of life. Most of the research in this area has focused on adult family members, the majority of whom were female. The four major areas of perceived burdens in transplant families are summarized below:[5]

PERCEIVED BURDEN	EXAMPLE
Family roles and responsibilities	Changes regarding home maintenance, family finances, and household chores
	Change in major wage earner
	New, shared responsibility for maintenance of transplant recipient's health
	Unwillingness to relinquish roles that were assumed during the illness period.
Time	Time constraints on all work and leisure activities

(Cont'd. on next page.)

PERCEIVED BURDEN	EXAMPLE
Worry/concern about transplant procedure and recipient's health	Concerns about complications and need for retransplantation Fear that recipient might die Hesitancy to plan for future and to make future commitments
Finances	Concerns about medical and nonmedical expenses Feeling unprepared for the myriad posttransplant expenses

41. Summarize what is known about the quality of life of family members.

Compared with the number of studies of transplant recipients' QOL, there is relatively little research about family member's QOL. The majority of such studies have focused on the families of heart transplant recipients, although a few have examined QOL in other populations. The findings are summarized below according to domain:[5]

DOMAIN	TYPE OF TRANSPLANT	FINDINGS
Physical functioning	Heart	Of a sample of spouses, 20% had 3 or more concurrent chronic illnesses that required medical care. Improvement in pre- to posttransplant perceptions of general health. Although sleep difficulties persisted after transplantation, they were worse during the waiting period than in the posttransplant period.
Mental health	Heart	Psychiatric distress levels decreased during first posttransplant year.
	Heart Kidney	Spouses had less overall distress, lower levels of depressive and anxiety-related symptomatology, and lower rates of diagnosable psychiatric disorders than did recipients. When compared with a normative sample, spouses had higher levels of distress and higher rates of diagnosable psychiatric disorders.
	Heart Kidney Liver	After the first posttransplant year, symptoms of overall distress, depression, and anxiety were similar to those found in the normal population.
Social functioning	Heart	Spouses rated their own role performance and that of the recipient as poorer during the posttransplant period than during the pretransplant period. Negative perceptions about roles and responsibilities persisted at 5 years posttransplant. Spouses were able to carry out their home and family responsibilities adequately; their role performance did not differ from that of nontransplant spouses. Posttransplant role performance increased spouses' self-esteem (because they acquired new skills) and lowered levels of psychological distress. The transplant experience improved the spouses' perceptions of the marital relationship in terms of feelings of closeness and tenderness. Spouses' ratings of the marital relationship were poorer than those of the transplant recipient. Spouses did not perceive that transplantation had impaired their relationships with other family members or friends.
	Kidney	Recipient-spouse dyads' ratings of marital satisfaction and perceived ability to offer support to one another were similar to the ratings of nontransplant couples.
Global QOL	Heart	Spouses' overall perceptions of QOL improved pre- to posttransplant. Spouses' level of satisfaction with life remains stable over the first few years after transplantation.

42. How do children react to a family member's transplant?

Studies indicate that young children (< 5 years old) often react with prolonged symptoms of depression, withdrawal, and grief. Older children may appear confused about the experience. Adolescents may have feelings of depression, resentment, or anger over the family's preoccupation with the transplant patient. All of these reactions underscore how important it is that the well caregiver attend to the needs of the entire family in addition to those of the ill partner.[5]

The transplant team can use the following strategies to help children of transplant patients:

- Provide assistance to caregivers in identifying and solving family problems.
- Provide age-appropriate education for children (information about the underlying illness and the medical treatment plan).
- Form support groups if there are a number of children within the same age range. Support groups can provide education and peer support.
- Liaison with the school system and provide assistance with any educational problems.

43. Do caregivers to transplant recipients develop post-traumatic stress disorders?

Yes. Threats to close others can elicit a post-traumatic stress disorder (PTSD), and transplant-related anxiety can reach the traumatic levels traditionally associated with PTSD. In perhaps the only study of its kind that looked at PTSD in both patients and their caregivers, Stukas and colleagues[22] noted that

- There were similar rates of PTSD among heart transplant recipients and their caregivers.
- The specific transplant-related elements that triggered the traumatic response were learning about the need for a heart transplant and the waiting period.
- PTSD was more likely to occur in females and individuals who had less support from friends, a lower sense of mastery, and a history of either major depressive disorder or generalized anxiety disorder.
- The number of transplant-related PTSD symptoms was significantly higher in females, individuals younger than 50 years, individuals who used more avoidance coping strategies, and individuals who had less support from friends, a lower sense of mastery, lower family cohesiveness, and a personal history of psychiatric illness.

This study has important implications for transplant professionals. First, it has commonly been thought that the risk of developing PTSD increases with the intensity and proximity of the stressor. Thus, it may have been falsely assumed that only transplant recipients are at risk for PTSD. The study shows, however, that caregivers to transplant recipients are equally susceptible to PTSD. Second, interventions designed to increase caregivers' social support or bolster family cohesiveness may help ameliorate the symptoms associated with PTSD. Third, caregivers who predominantly use avoidance coping strategies may benefit from interventions designed to promote more adaptive coping strategies and increase their sense of mastery over the situation.

44. What else is known about psychological distress among caregivers?

Most studies that have examined psychological distress among caregivers have been done in the heart transplant population. In a 1996 study, Canning and colleagues[4] found the following:

- Compared with the general population, family caregivers had psychological distress levels that were significantly higher 2 months after the transplant surgery. By the seventh posttransplant month, the levels decreased and approximated the normal level. However, one-third of the caregivers demonstrated clinically significant distress levels at least once during the first posttransplant year.
- Predictors of early psychological distress included employment status, time constraints associated with caregiving, and the quality of the relationship between the caregiver and the transplant recipient. Caregivers who were at highest risk for psychological distress were those who were unemployed, who felt that caregiving infringed upon their personal time, and who perceived their relationship with the recipient to be poor.
- Predictors for late psychological distress (i.e., 12 months after transplantation) included caregiver health status, sense of control, and level of social interaction. Caregivers who had

the highest risk of psychological distress 1 year after transplantation were those who had poor initial health, had a low sense of control, and were socially withdrawn. Over the course of the first year, the context of caregiving changes from an acute, novel phase to a more chronic, routine phase. During the course of this transition, the caregiver's own personal and health concerns bubble to the surface.

These findings have implications for transplant professionals. First, caregiver employment may confer benefits in terms of self-esteem, finances, social support, and respite that are not available in the home environment. It may be beneficial for certain caregivers to return to work; the benefits of employment may offset some of the burdens associated with caregiving. Second, caregivers' personal health and psychosocial environment contribute to their distress throughout the first posttransplant year. Therefore, interventions designed to bolster caregivers' resources early on may help to minimize their psychological distress.

45. What about the posttransplant quality of life of patients bridged to heart transplantation with left ventricular assist devices?

Because of the shortage of donor hearts, more patients must be bridged to transplantation with a left ventricular assist device (LVAD). Given that the survival rates of VAD patients can equal the survival rates of non-VAD patients, it is important to consider long-term QOL in this patient population. In the first prospective, longitudinal QOL study of VAD versus non-VAD transplant recipients during the first posttransplant year, Dew and colleagues[6] found that

- Both VAD and non-VAD recipients improved in physical functional status.
- VAD patients had more rapid improvement in global functioning than non-VAD patients.
- VAD patients had fewer somatic complaints than non-VAD patients.
- The emotional well-being of VAD patients was similar to that of non-VAD patients, even with respect to transplant-related post-traumatic stress disorder.
- VAD patients showed significantly higher rates of mild cognitive impairment than non-VAD patients
- VAD patients were significantly less likely to return to work than non-VAD patients; the inability to work appeared to be associated with enduring cognitive impairment.
- Interpersonal withdrawal worsened significantly in VAD patients during the first posttransplant year.
- Duration of VAD support was not associated with any posttransplant QOL variables.
- There were no significant differences in QOL variables between VAD patients who were discharged home to wait for a donor heart and patients who remained hospitalized until the time of transplant.

46. Is there any way to predict which patients are more likely to be noncompliant after transplantation?

Somewhat surprisingly, background health-related and sociodemographic factors do not predict posttransplant compliance (e.g., factors such as indication for transplant, age, gender, or education). On the other hand, psychosocial factors in the early posttransplant period are important predictors of compliance. For example, Dew and colleagues, along with many other investigators, found that the environment to which the patient returns plays a significant role in either facilitating or impeding compliance. Specific predictors of noncompliance included the following:[7]

- Low levels of social support (Few family members or friends to motivate the patient and provide continued attention to the medical regimen)
- Increased anxiety
- Use of avoidant coping behaviors
- Too strong a sense of personal mastery

47. Discuss some tips for dealing with noncompliant patients.

The Mid-Atlantic Renal Coalition[19] recommends the following strategies for dealing with noncompliant patients:

- Listen to patients' stories and try to understand their perspectives.
- Ascertain patients' goals for therapy.
- Allow patients to assume control and responsibility for their treatment by educating them so that they can make informed decisions, and involve them in the treatment plan as much as possible.
- When necessary, consult with a psychiatrist or psychologist for assistance in determining patients' decision-making abilities or in managing patients.
- Remain patient and persistent.

Patients usually have a reason for not being compliant with the therapeutic regimen. It is important to talk with patients and family members in an attempt to determine the reasons for noncompliance. In many instances, the problems associated with noncompliance are resolvable. The use of patient/family care conferences early in the treatment, when compliance issues are first identified, can be most beneficial in engaging the patient in the therapeutic process and supporting both caregivers and staff.[12]

BIBLIOGRAPHY

1. Belle SH, Beringer KC, Detre KM: Liver transplantation for alcoholic liver disease in the U.S.: 1988–1995. Liver Transplant Surg 3:212–219, 1997.
2. Berlakovich GA, Steininger R, Herbst F, et al: Efficacy of liver transplantation for alcoholic cirrhosis with respect to recidivism and compliance. Transplantation, 58:560–565, 1994.
3. Bunzel B, Laederach-Hofmann K: Solid organ transplantation: Are their predictors for posttransplant noncompliance? A literature review. Transplantation 70:711–716, 2000.
4. Canning RD, Dew MA, Davidson S: Psychological distress among caregivers to heart recipients. Soc Sci Med 42:599–608, 1996.
5. Dew MA, Goycoolea JM, Switzer GE, et al: Quality of life in organ transplantation: Effects on adult recipients and their families. In Trzepacz PT, DiMartini AF (eds): The Transplant Patient: Biological, Psychiatric and Ethical Issues in Organ Transplantation. Cambridge, Cambridge University Press, 2000, pp 67–145.
6. Dew MA, Kormos RL, Winowich S, et al: Quality of life outcomes after heart transplantation in individuals bridged to transplant with ventricular assist devices. J Heart Lung Transplant 20:1199–1212, 2001.
7. Dew MA, Roth LH, Thompson ME, et al: Medical compliance and its predictors in the first year after heart transplantation. J Heart Lung Transplant 15:631–645, 1996.
8. Dew MA, Switzer GE, DiMartini AF, et al: Psychosocial assessments and outcomes in organ transplantation. Prog Transplant 10:239–259, 2000.
9. Dew MA, Switzer GE, Goycoolea JM, et al: Does transplantation produce quality of life benefits? Transplantation, 64:1261–1273, 1997.
10. DiMartini A, Day N, Dew MA, et al: Alcohol use following liver transplantation: A comparison of follow-up methods. Psychosomatics 42:55–62, 2001.
11. DiMartini A, Trzepacz P: Alcoholism and organ transplantation. In Trzepacz PT, DiMartini AF (eds): The Transplant Patient: Biological, Psychiatric and Ethical Issues in Organ Transplantation. Cambridge, Cambridge University Press, 2000, pp 214–238.
12. Edwards SS: The "noncompliant" transplant patient: A persistent ethical dilemma. Prog Transplant 9:202–208, 1999.
13. Everhart JE, Beresford TP: Liver transplantation for alcoholic liver disease: A survey of transplantation programs in the United States. Liver Transplant Surg 3:220–226, 1997.
14. Grant BF: Alcohol abuse, alcohol consumption and alcohol dependence. The United States as an example. Addictions 89:1357–1365, 1994.
15. Keeffe EB: Liver transplantation: Current status and novel approaches to liver replacement, Gastroenterology 120:749–762, 2001.
16. Levenson JL, Olbrisch ME: Psychosocial evaluation of organ transplant candidates: A comparative survey of process, criteria, and outcomes in heart, liver, and kidney transplantation. Psychosomatics, 34:314–323, 1993.
17. Levenson JL, Olbrisch ME: Psychosocial screening and selection of candidates for organ transplantation. In Trzepacz PT, DiMartini AF (eds): The Transplant Patient: Biological, Psychiatric and Ethical Issues in Organ Transplantation. Cambridge, Cambridge University Press, 2000, pp 21–41.
18. Lewis K, Winsett RP, Cetingok M, et al: Social network mapping with transplant recipients. Prog Transplant 10:262–266, 2000.
19. Mid-Atlantic Renal Coalition: Working with Noncompliant and Abusive Patients Midlothian, VA, Mid-Atlantic Renal Coalition, 1994.

20. Olbrisch ME, Levenson JL, Hamer R: The PACT: A rating scale for the study of clinical decision making in psychosocial screening of organ transplant candidates. Clin Transplant 3:164–169, 1989.

21. Paris WD, Calhoun-Wilson G, Slentz B, et al: Employment and the transplant patient. J Rehabil 63:10–16, 1997.

22. Stukas AA, Dew MA, Switzer GE, et al: PTSD in heart transplant recipients and their primary family caregivers. Psychosomatics 40:212–221, 1999.

23. Tracy EM, Whittaker JK: The social network map: Assessing social support in clinical practice. Fam Soc J Contemp Hum Serv 71:461–470, 1990.

24. Twillman RK, Manetto C, Wellisch DK, et al: The Transplant Evaluation Rating Scale: A revision of the psychosocial levels system for evaluating organ transplant candidates. Psychosomatics 34:144–153, 1993.

25. Wright L: Mentorship programs for transplant patients. Prog Transplant 10:267–272, 2000.

26. Yates WM, Booth MB, Reed DA, et al: Descriptive and predictive validity of a high-risk alcoholism relapse model. J Stud Alcohol 54:645–651, 1993.

6. FINANCIAL ISSUES IN TRANSPLANTATION

Jade K. Perdue, MPA

1. Are solid organ transplant procedures covered by most third-party payers?

Many health insurance plans include benefits for solid organ transplantation. However, the terms and extent of these benefits vary greatly. Some insurers only cover the transplant procedure if it is performed at a facility with whom the insurer has a prearranged contract.

2. What happens if the patient prefers to go to a transplant center other than the facility with whom the insurer has a contract for transplantation?

Most private insurers have contracts with a few particular transplant facilities; therefore, insured members may be required to go to one of those facilities for transplantation. Patients who do not want to be treated at the contracted facility may apply for an exception with their insurer. Occasionally, exceptions are made based on such factors as continuity of care, distance between the patient's home and the transplant center, and expertise of the surgical staff. Ultimately, the patient must follow the insurer's procedure for filing an exception. The transplant center's finance office and the attending physician can assist with filing for an exception by providing the patient with information about their disease and treatment options. Without an exception, the patient must go to the facility where the insurer provides the authorization for the transplant.

3. Does Medicare cover transplantation?

Medicare currently covers kidney, liver, heart, lung, kidney–pancreas, pancreas after kidney, heart–lung, intestinal, and multivisceral transplants. Medicare Part A covers all inpatient medical costs with the exception of a benefit period deductible, which is $812.00 for 2002. This figure generally increases yearly. Medicare Part B covers outpatient testing, physician services, and a portion of immunosuppressant medications. Patients who qualify for Medicare automatically receive Part A if they have worked 40 or more quarters of Medicare-covered employment. However, all patients must pay a monthly premium for Part B. For 2002, the premium is $54.00 a month with a $100.00 per year deductible. If patients do not enroll in Part B at the time that they become eligible for Medicare, their premiums may increase by 10% for every 12 months that they could have been enrolled. To obtain updated premium amounts, please visit www.medicare.gov.

4. Do state medical assistance (Medicaid) programs cover transplantation?

There is great variability among state medical assistance programs with respect to coverage for transplant procedures. Some states cover only certain transplant procedures. If a patient has medical assistance, it is important to contact the state to determine the patient's eligibility and whether his or her particular surgery is covered. The Centers for Medicare and Medicaid (CMS) has a web site that lists the 800 numbers of each Medicaid office in the United States. This information can be found at http://www.hcfa.gov/medicaid/obs5.htm.

5. How much does a transplant procedure cost?

Transplant costs vary greatly from patient to patient. Some differences in costs can be attributed to factors such as the condition of the recipient at time of transplant, length of hospital stay, or location of the transplant facility.

The following chart depicts estimated U.S. average billed charges for one year following transplantation.

ORGAN	EVALUATION	SURGERY*	FOLLOW-UP	IMMUNO-SUPPRESSANTS	TOTAL
Heart	$16,800.00	$292,300.00	$44,800.00	$12,900.00	$366,800.00
Liver	$17,200.00	$221,800.00	$51,800.00	$13,300.00	$304,100.00
Kidney	$11,500.00	$ 90,300.00	$23,000.00	$14,300.00	$139,100.00
Kidney–pancreas	$11,500.00	$139,100.00	$23,000.00	$14,300.00	$187,900.00
Pancreas	$11,300.00	$94,200.00	$8,400.00	$14,300.00	$128,200.00
Heart–lung	$17,100.00	$398,700.00	$45,800.00	$12,500.00	$474,100.00
Lung	$17,400.00	$246,900.00	$46,600.00	$13,300.00	$324,200.00
Intestine	$31,000.00	$434,400.00	$51,800.00	$10,000.00	$527,200.00

* Surgery charges represent the average procurement, hospital, and physician charges for the first year of billed charges.
From Hauboldt RH, Milliman, U.S.A. 2002 Preliminary Update,[2] April 3, 2002.

6. What are the hidden costs associated with solid organ transplantation?

In addition to the costs associated with hospitalization and the surgical procedure, transplantation also involves such hidden costs as copayments for office visits, travel to and from the transplant center, childcare, pet boarding, pretransplant lodging for patients and pretransplant and posttransplant lodging for companions, meals, lost wages, and medications not covered by a prescription plan.

7. Are patients turned down for transplantation if they have no insurance or inadequate transplant benefits?

Given the scarcity of donor organs, most transplant centers are concerned about transplanting patients who do not have the resources to care for the donated organ, both in terms of lifetime immunosuppressant medications and the requisite follow-up care. However, most transplant centers have social workers and financial counselors who work with patients to find the necessary financial resources. Potential options include Medicare, state medical assistance programs, the Veterans Administration system, fundraising, and, in rare instances, hospital charity care.

8. What specific information should patients know about their transplant benefits?

It is important for patients to obtain answers to the following questions:
- What specific types of transplant procedures are covered by the plan (e.g., liver, intestine, heart, heart-lung)?
- Is there a maximum amount that the insurer will pay for a particular transplant procedure?
- Is there an out-of-pocket maximum, the amount the patient must pay before the insurer will cover the procedure at 100%?
- Is there a lifetime maximum benefit, and, if so, what is this amount?
- Is the organ acquisition fee included in the benefit package, and, if so, what is the maximum amount that is covered?
- Does the insurance company have a managed care contract with the transplant center?
- Is there a benefit for home healthcare, and, if so, what is the level of this benefit?
- Does the policy include a prescription plan, and does it specifically cover immunosuppressant medications such as cyclosporine, mycophenolate mofetil, or tacrolimus? If so, is there a cap on the amount of prescription benefits?
- If there is a prescription plan, what are the copayments for brand and generic medications?
- Is there a mail order pharmacy with whom the insurance company has a contract?
- Does the patient's medical care have to be coordinated through the primary care physician?

9. Under what circumstances does the patient's care have to be coordinated with the primary care physician?

In most instances, patients who are enrolled in a health maintenance organization must either have written referrals for diagnostic tests to be done at the transplant center or the tests must be done through the primary care physician's (PCP) office. Failure to comply with these insurance regulations might result in greater out-of-pocket expenses for the patient. PCPs are generally more willing to provide the necessary referrals if they have been kept informed of the patient's clinical status. One way of keeping the PCP informed is to periodically fax test results and progress notes to the PCP's office.

10. Will an insurer pay for a patient to be placed on the waiting list at more than one transplant center?

Many insurers allow patients to be placed on the waiting list at more than one transplant center. However, insurers may not necessarily pay for multiple transplant evaluations. In that case, the results of the evaluation at one transplant center may need to be shared with the second transplant center. As a general rule, transplant centers will accept most of the evaluation results of another facility if they have been performed recently. However, many transplant programs require that certain tests, such as tissue typing, be done at their facility. Patients should be informed that they may be responsible for costs associated with duplicate testing.

11. What happens when all of the evaluation tests have been completed?

After the transplant evaluation process has been completed and the patient has been deemed eligible for transplantation, the results of the evaluation tests are forwarded to the patient's insurance company, along with a letter of medical necessity that explains the need for transplantation. This information is then reviewed by the medical director or other authorized individual. If the insurance company concurs with the transplant center's recommendation that the patient is an appropriate transplant candidate, a letter authorizing the transplant procedure is typically sent to the transplant center and the patient. This letter generally includes any contract or plan limitations with regard to the transplantation procedure.

12. What can be done if the letter of authorization is not forthcoming?

Under some circumstances it may be necessary to contact the case manager at the patient's insurance company. Generally, the case manager is responsible for either authorizing the transplant procedure or providing the medical director with a recommendation on whether to give authorization. It is essential that the transplant center provide the case manager with detailed clinical information and address any outstanding issues or concerns. Some cases may prove to be more difficult because of financial, legal, or clinical constraints. Individuals or organizations that may provide assistance in this regard include the transplant financial coordinator, the employer's benefit administrator, the state insurance commissioner, or local patient advocacy groups.

13. Once the insurer authorizes the transplant procedure, is the authorization valid until the time of transplant?

The length of the authorization period varies among insurers. Many insurers require updated clinical information every 6–12 months. The update typically includes a recent history and physical examination and laboratory tests. If the transplant team has not seen the patient for an extended period, the insurer may require a total reevaluation to determine if the patient is still medically suitable for transplantation. If the patient has been hospitalized for an extended period, the concurrent review nurse assigned to the patient may also provide updated clinical information to the medical director and, in some cases, may reauthorize the transplant.

If the transplant authorization has expired and the patient undergoes transplantation, the insurer could deny the hospital payment for the transplant. Therefore, it is important for both the patient and the transplant team to be aware of the insurer's policies regarding authorization for transplantation.

Medicare does not require submission of clinical information from the initial transplant evaluation or any updates while the patient is on the waiting list. Medicare will cover the transplant procedure at a Medicare-approved transplant center so long as the patient has Medicare days available.

14. What are Medicare days?

A patient who has Medicare is entitled to 60 inpatient hospital days, 30 coinsurance days, and 60 lifetime reserve days. For the first 60 days that a patient is hospitalized, he or she is responsible for an inpatient deductible ($812.00 in 2002). On the 61st inpatient day, the patient becomes responsible for a coinsurance amount ($203.00/day in 2002). If the patient is still hospitalized on the 91st day, the patient begins to use his or her lifetime reserve days (60 days) and is responsible for $406.00 a day (in 2002). After the lifetime reserve days are exhausted, the patient no longer has Medicare benefits.

Lifetime reserve days are nonrenewable. However, inpatient and coinsurance days are renewable if a patient is out of the hospital for 60 consecutive days from the day of his or her most recent hospital discharge. If the patient was hospitalized and released and then rehospitalized within the first 60 days, the patient is responsible only for one inpatient deductible. An easy way to remember the number of Medicare days available to a patient is to remember 60/30/60. The hospital's finance office should be able to query the Medicare system to check the patient's available Medicare days.[1]

15. What is the organ acquisition fee?

The organ acquisition fee is the charge for such services as procuring the organ, preparing the organ for surgery, travel costs, and preserving the organ. Many private insurers have an organ acquisition capitation written into the policy that the patient may not be aware of. If the organ acquisition cost is $40,000 and the patient has a $10,000 capitation, any amount not covered by the insurer is passed on to the patient. Ideally, it is best to have a policy that does not have an organ acquisition capitation.

16. Does Medicare cover immunosuppressant medications?

Yes, Medicare partially covers the cost of immunosuppressant medications:
- If a patient is eligible to receive Medicare because of age or disability and receives a transplant that is paid for by Medicare, then Medicare covers 80% of the costs of immunosuppressant medications indefinitely.
- If the patient has Medicare benefits because of end-stage renal disease (ESRD), Medicare covers 80% of the cost of immunosuppressant medications for 36 months.

It is important to note that Medicare coverage of immunosuppressant medications is contingent on the patient meeting Medicare eligibility requirements.[1]

17. What resources are available for patients who have lost their prescription benefits and cannot afford to purchase immunosuppressant medications?

Patients who have lost their coverage for expensive immunosuppressant medications have few options. Hopefully, this situation is temporary, and the patient will be able to resume coverage shortly. In the meantime, many pharmaceutical companies have temporary assistance or indigent programs for which patients can apply. These programs are not meant for long-term use; therefore, patients should either resume their insurance coverage or apply to other sources such as state pharmacy assistance programs. Patients must be well educated on the importance of maintaining their immunosuppressive coverage. One suggestion is to have the patient and his or her primary caregiver sign an agreement that documents their understanding of the importance of maintaining medication coverage. Ideally, this can be done during the informed consent process.

18. Do transplant patients need periodic insurance check-ups?

It is important to periodically check with candidates and recipients to determine if there have been any changes in their health insurance plan(s). Examples of changes that may occur include the following:
- The patient may change insurance plans, particularly during open season.
- The patient may become eligible for Medicare.
- The patient's primary and secondary insurances may change positions.
- The patient may lose insurance coverage because of nonpayment of premiums.

Regardless of the type of change, it is important to have current and accurate information so that the correct insurer(s) can be billed and the patient does not incur any unexpected expenses. If a transplant candidate's insurance changes, authorization for the transplant procedure must be obtained from the new insurer.

19. If the patient has a living donor, will the donor's insurance cover the medical expenses?

There is a type of insurance known as *donor's insurance*. However, it is extremely rare. Donor-related expenses are typically covered by the recipient's insurance. Living donors should not provide their own personal insurance information to the transplant facility so that charges do not accrue against the donor's lifetime maximum. Medicare also covers expenses related to living donation for surgeries that the CMS does not consider experimental.

20. What is COBRA?

The Consolidated Omnibus Budget Reconciliation Act (COBRA), enacted in 1986, requires employers of twenty or more people to offer continued health insurance coverage at group rates to people who would no longer be eligible to receive insurance benefits because of a "qualifying event," such as a reduction in number of hours worked, termination for reasons other than "gross misconduct," or divorce. A person meeting the qualifying event criteria must sign up for COBRA benefits within 60 days from the date of offer or lose the opportunity to have these extended benefits. The benefit extension period is generally 18 months; however, this period can be extended up to 29 months if the person has a disability. This is an important consideration for patients who become ill quickly. The U.S. Department of Labor Pension and Welfare Benefits Administration at http://www.dol.gov is a user-friendly Web site where patients can obtain valuable information that will assist them in determining if they are eligible to receive these benefits.

21. What is HIPAA?

The Health Insurance Portability and Accountability Act (HIPAA) of 1996 protects the health insurance benefits of workers when they change or lose their jobs. The CMS notes that "In short, HIPAA may lower your chance of losing existing coverage, ease your ability to switch health plans and/or help you buy coverage on your own if you lose your employer's plan and have no other coverage available." (Centers for Medicare and Medicaid Services, http://www.hcfa.gov/medicaid/hipaa/content/more.asp.)

HIPAA is of particular importance to transplant patients because it may assist them in avoiding a preexisting clause with the next employer. A preexisting clause may limit the amount of care that a patient can receive for a long-standing medical condition when changing insurers. To reduce the likelihood that they will become subject to a preexisting clause, patients should

• Obtain a certificate of credible coverage from their previous employer.
• Ensure that there is not a break in health coverage of 63 or more full days.
• Consider accepting COBRA, Temporary Continuation of Coverage, or State continuation coverage.

If patients have questions concerning their rights and protections under HIPAA, the Centers for Medicare and Medicaid (formerly the Health Care Finance Administration) has an informative interactive Web site that allows patients to enter their insurance information and receive guidance on how HIPAA pertains to their specific situation. For CMS's HIPAA Online, please visit http://www.hcfa.gov/medicaid/hipaa/default.asp.

22. Transplant patients often are inundated with medical bills. What can be done to help them organize these bills?

Depending on the hospital's billing structure, patients may receive multiple bills from different sources, for example, inpatient care, outpatient care, and physician services. Often these bills are difficult to interpret, and patients cannot determine what portion of the bill is their responsibility and what portion is the responsibility of the insurer. It is helpful if patients are aware of their health benefits or at least have a copy of their benefits booklet.

It also may be helpful if patients carry a small notebook in which they can document the date, name, and specialty of their treating physician, and whether or not any tests were done at a particular visit. An example of this simple spreadsheet is provided below.

APPOINTMENT DATE	REFERRAL NUMBER	DOCTOR(S)	SPECIALTY	LABS OR OTHER TESTS	AMOUNT PAID BY INSURER	PATIENT OWES
1/1/02	8492727	Dr. Smith	Surgeon	Yes	500.00	200.00
2/11/02	9302837	Dr. Smith Dr. Allan	Nephrologist Psychologist	No		

ACKNOWLEDGEMENT

The author acknowledges the assistance of Richard Hauboldt of Milliman, U.S.A., who provided preliminary 2002 data regarding the costs associated with solid organ transplantation.

BIBLIOGRAPHY

1. Centers for Medicare and Medicaid. Available at: http://www.hcfa.gov/medicaid/hipaa, http://www.cms.gov, or http://www.medicare.gov. Accessed April 3, 2002.
2. Hauboldt RH, Milliman, U.S.A., April 3, 2002.
3. Jaklevic MC: Top billing. Mod Healthc 30(38):50, 2000.
4. Kasiske BL, Cohen D, Lucey M, Neylan JF: Payment for immunosuppression after organ transplantation. JAMA 283:2445–2450, 2000.
5. Newhouse JP: Switching health plans to obtain drug coverage. JAMA 283:2161–2162, 2000.
6. Soumerai SB, Ross-Degnan D: Inadequate prescription drug coverage for Medicare enrollees: A call for action. N Engl J Med 340:722–728, 1999.
7. United Network for Organ Sharing. Transplant 101. Available at: http://www.unos.org. Accessed March 29, 2002.
8. United States Department of Labor Pension and Welfare Benefits Administration: Health Benefits Under the Consolidated Omnibus Budget Reconciliation Act (COBRA). U.S. Department of Labor Pension and Welfare Benefits Administration. Revised July 1999. Available at: http://www/dol.gov/pwba/. Accessed April 3, 2002.

7. IMMUNOSUPPRESSION

Debi H. Dumas-Hicks, RN, BS, CCTC

1. What is immunosuppression?

For organ transplant recipients, the term *immunosuppression* refers to the pharmacologic alterations of immune system functions to prevent rejection of the allograft while maintaining sufficient immunity to prevent infection.

2. Describe the difference between induction therapy and initial immunosuppression.

Induction therapy is any immunosuppressive agent administered pretransplant or posttransplant over 1–2 weeks. Some transplant centers have standardized orders for induction therapy for all transplant recipients. Other transplant centers administer induction therapy only to transplant recipients whose risk of acute rejection is high (e.g., multiparous women) or in the setting of posttransplant tubular necrosis to delay the administration full-dose calcineurin inhibitors. Examples of agents used for induction therapy are monoclonal anti-CD3 antibodies (Muromonab-CD3) and polyclonal antilymphocyte antibodies (antithymocyte globulin).

Initial immunosuppression refers to the higher doses of posttransplant immunosuppression used in maintenance therapy immediately after transplantation.

3. List the most common immunosuppressive medications.

GENERIC NAME (MANUFACTURER)	BRAND (TRADE NAME)	METHOD OF ADMINISTRATION
Calcineurin inhibitors		
Cyclosporine USP (Novartis)	Sandimmune	IV, oral
Cyclosporine USP (modified) (Novartis)	Neoral	Oral
Cyclosporine capsules USP (modified) (Abbott)	Gengraf	Oral
Cyclosporine soft gelatin capsules USP (modified) (Sidmak)		Oral
Cyclosporine USP (modified) (Eon)		Oral
Tacrolimus, FK506 (Fujisawa)	Prograf	IV, oral
Sirolimus (Wyeth-Ayerst)	Rapamune	Oral
Corticosteroids		
Prednisone (Pharmacia & Upjohn)	Deltasone	Oral
Methylprednisolone (Pharmacia & Upjohn)	Solu-Medrol	IV
Antimetabolites		
Azathioprine (Prometheus)	Imuran	IV, oral
Mycophenolate mofetil (Roche)	Cellcept	IV, oral
Cyclophosphamide (Bristol-Myers Squibb)	Cytoxan	IV, oral
Antibody products		
Muromonab CD3 (Ortho Biotech)	Orthoclone OKT3	IV
Antithymocyte globulin (Pharmacia & Upjohn)	Atgam	IV
Antithymocyte globulin (SangStat)	Thymoglobulin	IV
Daclizumab (Roche)	Zenapax	IV
Basiliximab (Novartis)	Simulect	IV

IV = intravenous.

4. Are the methods of administration, various formulations, and brands of cyclosporine interchangeable?

Cyclosporine is given intravenously or orally (as liquid or in gelcaps). There are two formulations—the standard oil-based formulation and the modified formulations. Several brands are currently available.

Method of administration: During the immediate posttransplant period, the intravenous preparation may be administered until the recipient can tolerate oral medications. Later in the posttransplant period, some situations may require that the intravenous preparation be substituted for the oral preparation (e.g., if the recipient is experiencing prolonged vomiting).

Formulations: Cyclosporine USP (Sandimmune) and cyclosporine USP (modified) (Neoral) are not interchangeable because they are not bioequivalent. Transplant recipients who are converted from cyclosporine USP to cyclosporine USP (modified) using a 1:1 ratio (mg/kg/day) may have lower cyclosporine blood concentrations. During the conversion process, more frequent monitoring of cyclosporine levels is required to avoid underdosing.

Brand versus generic preparations: If a patient's pharmacy dispenses a preparation of cyclosporine that differs from that which the patient had previously been taking, it is important to monitor the patient's cyclosporine levels and adjust the dose accordingly.

5. Which combination of immunosuppressive agents is the most universally accepted for maintenance therapy?

Immunosuppressive medication protocols vary among different transplant centers, depending on clinical experience, patient population, and the type of solid organ transplanted. To date, the most common protocol has been the use of three immunosuppressive medications concomitantly. This triple-therapy regimen typically includes a calcineurin inhibitor (e.g., cyclosporine or tacrolimus), corticosteroids, and an antimetabolite agent (e.g., azathioprine or mycophenolate mofetil).

6. Is the choice of immunosuppressive agents influenced by specific factors?

Yes. As new immunosuppressive agents have been introduced, immunosuppressive therapy has become more individualized. The mnemonic **GRAPH** describes the factors that are considered in determining an immunosuppressive regimen:

G   Gender
R   Race
A   Age
P   Protocols of transplant centers
H   Human leukocyte antigen (HLA) incompatibility

7. How is the dosing of immunosuppression therapy determined?

The challenge of immunosuppressive therapy is to achieve a balance between efficacy and safety. There can be serious clinical consequences with over-and underdosing. Therapeutic drug monitoring of blood levels has proven to be the most widely used method for determining individual patient dosing of these critical-dose drugs.

Therapeutic Drug Monitoring

DRUG	MONITOR
Cyclosporine	12-hour trough blood level
Tacrolimus	12-hour trough blood level
Mycophenolate mofetil	12-hour trough blood level; WBC counts; platelet count
Sirolimus	22–24-hour trough blood level
Azathioprine	WBC counts; platelets

WBC = white blood cell.

8. **List some factors that can alter the blood levels of immunosuppressive agents.**

Several factors can affect the blood concentration levels of immunosuppressive agents. The mnemonic **CAMP** may aid memory of these factors:

C Coadministration of multiple drugs or foods with synergistic or antagonistic reactions

A Assay used in determining trough blood levels, particularly cyclosporine levels (high-performance liquid chromatography versus fluorescent polarization immune assay)

M Medication noncompliance (skipping doses or taking the drug incorrectly)

P Pathophysiologic dysfunction: cardiac, liver, renal, gastrointestinal dysfunction

9. **Name a specific food product that affects the absorption of the calcineurin inhibitors.**

At first, there was much excitement among transplant specialists when studies suggested that grapefruit juice increased the blood levels of calcineurin inhibitors. A group of molecules called flavinoids, which are a component of grapefruit, was found to inhibit the cytochrome P450 3A enzymes, thus decreasing the metabolism of the calcineurin inhibitors. It was believed initially that consumption of grapefruit products would be an inexpensive way to increase drug blood levels, while decreasing the amount of drug needed. Further studies, however, failed to identify a standardized "dose" of grapefruit juice that would increase serum levels of the calcineurin inhibitors. Therefore, it is recommended that transplant recipients who take a calcineurin inhibitor do not consume grapefruit or grapefruit juice because it affects the absorption of this immunosuppressant.

10. **List the drugs that interact with the calcineurin inhibitors in a synergistic or antagonistic manner.**

Concentrations of calcineurin inhibitors are influenced by drugs that affect microsomal enzymes, particularly the cytochrome P450 3A enzyme. Drugs that inhibit this enzyme can increase calcineurin inhibitor concentrations. Conversely, drugs that are inducers of cytochrome P450 3A activity can increase drug metabolism and thereby decrease calcineurin inhibitor concentrations. Close monitoring of trough blood levels and appropriate dosage adjustments are essential if these drugs are used concomitantly.

Drugs that Increase Calcineurin Inhibitor Concentrations

FUNCTIONAL CLASSIFICATION	DRUG
Calcium channel blockers	Diltiazem, nicardipine, nifedipine, verapamil
Antifungal agents	Fluconazole, itraconazole, ketoconazole
Antibiotics	Clarithromycin, erythromycin
Antigout agent	Allopurinol, colchicine
Antidysrhythmic	Amiodarone
Dopamine receptor agonist	Bromocriptine
Histamine H_2-receptor antagonist	Cimetidine
Androgen	Danazol
Cholinergic	Metoclopramide
Other	Oral contraceptive agents

Drugs that Decrease Calcineurin Inhibitor Concentrations

FUNCTIONAL CLASSIFICATION	DRUG
Antibiotics	Nafcillin, rifampin, trimethoprim/sulfamethoxazole
Anticonvulsants	Carbamazepine, phenobarbital, phenytoin

11. Which drugs induce synergistic nephrotoxicity when used with calcineurin inhibitors?

FUNCTIONAL CLASSIFICATION	DRUG
Antibiotics	Gentamicin, tobramycin, trimethoprim/sulfa-methoxazole, vancomycin
Antifungal agents	Amphotericin B, ketoconazole
Histamine H_2-receptor antagonists	Cimetidine, ranitidine
Antineoplastic agents	Melphalan

12. What are the potential drug interactions among herbal remedies, dietary supplements, and other medications frequently taken by transplant recipients?

Transplant recipients are instructed not to take any over-the-counter herbal remedies or dietary supplements without first consulting the transplant team. The potential drug interactions and physiologic consequences associated with use of these remedies and supplements are listed below:

HERBAL REMEDY OR SUPPLEMENT	DRUG INTERACTIONS	PHYSIOLOGIC CONSEQUENCES
Dong quai	Warfarin	Increased bleeding
Echinacea	Immunosuppressants	Activation of cell-mediated immunity May induce rejection
Garlic *Allium sativum*	Anticoagulants, aspirin	Increased bleeding
Ginkgo biloba	Anticoagulants, aspirin	Increased bleeding
Ginseng *Panax ginseng*	Steroids, estrogen Antidepressants Warfarin Digoxin	Potentiation of effects Induction of mania Increased clotting, thrombosis False increase in digoxin levels
Kava *Peper methysticum*	Benzodiazepines	Oversedation Coma
Licorice *Glycyrrhiza glabra*	Diuretics Corticosteroids Antiarrhythmics	Hypokalemia, hypertension Potentiation of steroid effects Dysrhythmias
Ephedra (Ma huang) *Ephedra sinica*	Caffeine, theophylline Antihypertensive agents Monoamine oxidase inhibitors Hypoglycemic agents	Toxicity, arrhythmias Hypertension Hypertensive crisis Hyperglycemia
St. John's Wort *Hypericum perforatum*	Cyclosporine Digoxin Theophylline Antidepressants (selective serotonin reuptake inhibitors)	Decreased bioavailability Increased congestive heart failure symptoms Subtherapeutic levels Serotonin syndrome
Valerian root *Valeriana officinalis*	Barbiturates Benzodiazepines, alcohol	Enhanced sedation Coma
Zinc	Cyclosporine Corticosteroids	Stimulation of immune system May induce rejection

13. Name two widely used pain medications that are not generally recommended for use by transplant recipients.

Transplant recipients are generally advised to avoid nonsteroidal anti-inflammatory drugs (NSAIDs). These products, when taken in conjunction with calcineurin inhibitors, are an additional cause of renal impairment. NSAIDs can also exacerbate steroid-induced gastrointestinal distress or bleeding. The recently developed cyclooxygenase-2 (COX-2) inhibitors may also cause renal impairment and therefore should be used with caution. Transplant recipients are instructed to call their transplant center before taking any over-the-counter product (including supplements or herbal products) or medication prescribed by healthcare providers other than the transplant team.

14. List the most prevalent side effects of immunosuppressive agents.

AGENT	ADVERSE SIDE EFFECTS
Corticosteroids	Cushingoid syndrome (adiposity, moon face, fat deposits in neck) mood alterations, dyslipidemia, hypertension, acne, myopathy, aseptic necrosis, gastrointestinal bleeding, hyperglycemia, osteoporosis, infection
Cyclosporine	Tremors, hirsutism, gingival hyperplasia, hypertension, nephrotoxicity, seizures, lymphomas, dyslipidemia, infection, headache
Tacrolimus	Hyperglycemia, tremors, neurotoxicity, alopecia, nephrotoxicity, headache, dyslipidemia, infection
Azathioprine	Bone marrow suppression (leukopenia, thrombocytopenia), alopecia, pancreatitis
Mycophenolate mofetil	Gastrointestinal disorders (nausea, vomiting, diarrhea)
Sirolimus	Dyslipidemia, gastrointestinal disorders (nausea, vomiting, diarrhea)
Muromonab-CD3	Tachycardia, fever, chills, muscle pain, hypertension, aseptic meningitis, infection
Daclizumab	Gastrointestinal disorders (nausea, vomiting, diarrhea)
Basiliximab	Gastrointestinal disorders (nausea, vomiting, diarrhea)

15. Given the chronic side effects of calcineurin inhibitors, can transplant patients be maintained on what is considered nontherapeutic levels of these drugs?

Decreasing the calcineurin inhibitors to low doses or stopping them entirely depends on the individual's rejection profile and the risk-to-benefit ratio of allograft rejection versus other organ failure. Some patients have been weaned successfully from all immunosuppression.

Note: Some patients have taken themselves off all immunosuppressive agents because of financial constraints or noncompliance. In rare instances, these patients have survived. It is extremely important that transplant team members monitor patient compliance and intervene as necessary. Many state governments and pharmaceutical companies have special programs for patients who cannot afford their medications.

16. Is there a way to minimize gingival hyperplasia in transplant recipients?

Severe gingival hyperplasia can be a side effect of cyclosporine. Mouth-breathing and local irritants such as dental plaque and dental calculus can exacerbate the condition. Decreasing these irritants with good periodontal care and lowering the cyclosporine dose, if possible, may help to reduce gingival hyperplasia. Use of gelcaps instead of the liquid cyclosporine preparation may also help to minimize this side effect. Dental surgery may be recommended if the problem is not solved. For some patients, tacrolimus is substituted for cyclosporine.

17. Why do many transplant patients have low magnesium levels?

Calcineurin inhibitors seem to be associated with lower total and ionized magnesium levels. The higher the serum concentration of the calcineurin inhibitor, the lower the blood level of magnesium. Hypomagnesemia may be exacerbated in recipients who are diabetic, pregnant, or taking diuretics. Magnesium replacement therapy is a recommended part of most transplant recipients' medication regimens. However, over-the-counter magnesium supplements are expensive and not always covered by prescription drug plans.

18. Transplant patients often take 10 to 15 medications per day. Are there any recommendations regarding how these medications should be taken?

- Food, antacids, and calcineurin inhibitors inhibit the absorption of mycophenolate mofetil. Therefore, mycophenolate mofetil should be taken 1 hour before or 2 hours after eating or taking antacids or a calcineurin inhibitor.
- Cyclosporine capsules USP (modified) and tacrolimus should be taken on a consistent schedule with regard to time of day and meals. They may be taken with or without food so long as the regimen is consistent.
- Neoral oral solution (cyclosporine USP [modified]) should be diluted, preferably with orange or apple juice served at room temperature. The combination of Neoral with milk can be unpalatable.
- Magnesium supplements should not be taken at the same time as calcineurin inhibitors or mycophenolate mofetil.
- Recipients who are on high doses of corticosteroid therapy should take this medication in divided doses (e.g., twice a day) to minimize abdominal discomfort and insomnia.
- Separate sirolimus and cyclosporine doses by 4 hours.

19. Are there any precautions for the medications that many transplant recipients take for gout?

Certain calcineurin inhibitors and diuretics may precipitate hyperuricemia and gout. Allopurinol, a xanthine oxidase inhibitor, is commonly prescribed for patients with gout because it reduces production of uric acid. Although not absolutely contraindicated, allopurinol should be used with extreme caution in patients who are taking azathioprine. This combination of drugs can lead to severe bone marrow suppression. Allopurinol and mycophenolate mofetil should also be used with caution.

20. How is acute rejection of an allograft treated?

The treatment of allograft rejection depends on several factors, such as the time interval since transplantation, the severity of the rejection episode, and the recipient's current physiologic status and immunosuppressant regimen. Therapeutic options include the following:

- Increasing the dose of the recipient's current maintenance drugs
- Administering a pulse dose of steroids:
    Moderate rejection: oral pulse of steroids (e.g., 2 mg/kg/day × 3 days) with tapering doses over a 2–4 week period or an immediate return to the previous prednisone dose.
    Severe rejection: intravenous methylprednisolone (Solu-Medrol, 1 gm IV × 3 days, and/or monoclonal antibodies [Orthoclone OKT3, 5 mg IV × 7–10 days], lymphocyte immune globulin [Atgam], or polyclonal antibodies).

21. Which test determines whether monoclonal antibodies can be administered a second time?

Muromonab CD3 (Orthoclone OKT3) has the potential to stimulate the production of antibodies when administered to humans. Therefore, antimurine antibody titers in the blood should be monitored after the initial administration of muromonab-CD3. If antibodies are present, muromonab CD3 is generally not given again.

22. Why do some transplant centers attempt to wean patients from steroids?

Most transplant immunosuppression maintenance protocols have included high doses of corticosteroids. At one time, it was not considered safe to withdraw steroid therapy. However, many transplant centers are now attempting to wean patients from steroids during the first 6–12 months posttransplant because of the serious long-term side effects associated with steroid therapy and the availability of more selective and potent immunosuppressive medication combinations (e.g, tacrolimus and mycophenolate mofetil).

Not all patients can be weaned successfully from corticosteroids because acute rejection may ensue. However, the goal remains to decrease the steroid dose to the lowest possible level.

Whether steroid withdrawal has a deleterious effect on long-term graft function has yet to be determined and requires further study.

23. With more potent immunosuppressive agents and increased posttransplant longevity, the risk of developing de novo malignancies has increased. In terms of immunosuppressive therapy, what is the approach for treating these malignancies?

In general, the goal is to keep the doses of immunosuppressive agents relatively low so that the immune system may recover from its compromised state and aid in neoplastic destruction while at the same time maintaining adequate protection against allograft rejection. Because of the possibility of severe myelosuppression associated with azathioprine, mycophenolate mofetil, and cyclophosphamide, these agents are typically the first to be decreased or discontinued. In highly malignant and advanced cancers, all immunosuppression may potentially be discontinued except for minimal doses of prednisone, which actually is a component of many chemotherapy protocols. If a renal allograft is rejected, the recipient can return to dialysis. Unfortunately, heart, liver, and lung transplant recipients do not have a similar option.

24. How is posttransplant lymphoproliferative disease treated?

In the immunosuppressed host, Epstein-Barr virus (EBV)-induced lymphoproliferative disorders may result from uncontrolled proliferation of EBV-infected B cells. The most severe pattern of posttransplant lymphoproliferative disease (PTLD) is a truly monoclonal, malignant lesion that is rapidly progressive and is associated with significant patient mortality. An important initial treatment strategy is the reduction or temporary discontinuation of immunosuppressive therapy. Other treatment options include chemotherapy, radiation therapy, and surgical resection.

25. List some tips for educating patients about their immunosuppressant medications.

Educating transplant patients about their immunosuppression medications is an ongoing process that begins in the pretransplant phase and continues throughout the posttransplant period. The mnemonic **TRANSPLANT** is a useful guide to key points for patient education:

T   Teaching tools: Develop a basic teaching plan and educational materials.

R   Records: Emphasize the importance of maintaining a current medication list.

A   Assess: Pretest patients to determine their initial knowledge base.

N   Noncompliance issues: Identify and remove barriers to compliance.

S   Support systems: Include family members and significant others in the educational process.

P   Prescription plans: Discuss patients' prescription drug benefits; if necessary, identify alternative sources of prescription coverage (e.g., state pharmacy assistance programs, indigent drug programs).

L   Labeling: Emphasize the importance of correct labeling of medicines; use pill identification stickers or color-coding strategies if patient is illiterate or visually impaired.

A   Analysis of patient education: Evaluate the effectiveness of patient education by occasionally quizzing patients about their immunosuppressive medications.

N   Numbers: The dose of immunosuppressive agents may change frequently, particularly in the early posttransplant period. Obtain several telephone numbers at which patients can be reached so that dose changes can be communicated in a timely manner. Obtain telephone numbers of patients' local and mail order pharmacies. Make certain that patients and family members have telephone numbers (office and emergency) of transplant team members.

T   Teach, teach, teach: Use all patient/family contact opportunities for teaching.

BIBLIOGRAPHY

1. Bartucci MR: Issues in cyclosporine drug substitution: Implications for patient management. J Transpl Coord 9(3):137–142, 1999.
2. Cecka JM, Terasaki PI: Clinical Transplants. Los Angeles, UCLA Immunogenetics Center, 1998.

3. Denton MD, Magee CC, Sayegh MH: Immunosuppressive strategies in transplantation. Lancet 353(9158):1083–1091, 1999.
4. Little BB: Immunosuppressant therapy during gestation. Semin Perinatol 21:143–148, 1997.
5. Makowka L, Sher L (eds): Handbook of Organ Transplantation. Austin, TX, Landes Bioscience, 1995.
6. McAlister VC, Gao Z, Peltekian K, et al: Sirolimus-tacrolimus combination immunosuppression. Lancet 355(9201):376–377, 2000.
7. Nolan MT, Augustine SA (eds): Transplantation Nursing: Acute and Long-term Management. Norwalk, CT, Appleton & Lange, 1995.
8. Peakman M, Vergani D: Basic and Clinical Immunology. New York, Churchill-Livingstone, 1997.
9. Physicians' Desk Reference, 55th ed. Montvale, NJ, Medical Economics Company, 2001.
10. Sollinger H, Pirsch J: Transplantation Drug Pocket Reference Guide, 2nd ed. Austin, TX, Landes Bioscience, 1996.

8. LUNG TRANSPLANTATION

Jan D. Manzetti, RN, PhD, CCTC, and Ann Lee, RN, CRNP, MSN, CCTC

LUNG TRANSPLANTATION

1. Is lung transplantation a widely available procedure?

Lung transplantation has become the treatment choice for selected patients with end-stage pulmonary tissue or vascular disease. In lungs, once the diagnosis of end-stage disease has been documented, there is often little to no medical treatment for patients other than supportive care. Lung candidates come to transplant according to the time they have accumulated on the national waiting list. There is no advancement with exacerbations of the underlying disease process. However, the United Network for Organ Sharing (UNOS) Thoracic Committee is considering a system of prioritization that would be similar to those used in liver and heart transplantation.

In lung transplantation the supply and demand for organs has become increasingly scarce. According to the 2000 Annual UNOS Report, 1057 lung and 91 heart-lung transplants were performed this year as compared with 1385 lung and 103 heart-lung transplants performed in 1999. The Registry of the International Society of Heart and Lung Transplantation reported that the number of heart transplant centers has declined as well as the number of heart-lung transplant centers, although the number of lung transplant centers has increased. Yet, during 1998–1999, only 3673 thoracic organ recipients were added to the national database, the smallest number over the past 5 years. Of these cases, approximately 600 were single-lung transplants and 467 were bilateral sequential/en bloc double-lung transplants.

2. Which lung diseases are considered for a lung transplant?

The following disease processes may be referred for lung transplantation:
- **Airway disease** including emphysema, bronchiectasis, cystic fibrosis, chronic bronchitis
- **Pulmonary hypertension**, including primary hypertension (unknown reason) and secondary hypertension (due to another heart or lung disease)
- **Interstitial lung disease**, including pulmonary fibrosis, sarcoidosis, silicosis, pneumoconiosis, scleroderma, **CREST** (**c**alcinosis cutis, **R**aynaud phenomenon, **e**sophageal dysmotility, **s**clerodactyly, **t**elangiectasias), eosinophilic granuloma, idiopathic pulmonary fibrosis, hemosiderosis, and Goodpasture syndrome,
- **Retransplantation** due to chronic rejection or obliterative bronchiolitis (OB)

3. When is a patient referred for lung transplantation?

The timing of referral for lung transplantation should be based on objective and subjective factors and differs for each disease process. However, in general, these include the following:
- Life expectancy of less than 24–36 months
- Consequences of the lung disease on other organ systems
- The patient's estimation of the effects of the disease process on his or her quality of life.

These factors must be balanced against the surgical risk of the procedure and the potential for functional recovery. In addition, one must consider the supply of organs, which has become increasingly scarce. The waiting time for lungs must also be factored into the decision of when to list a patient for a lung transplant. The format for allocation of donor lungs dictates that priority of transplantation be based solely on the waiting time accrued on the national list. There is no prioritization based on the severity of the lung disease. This system differs from that used for the allocation of donor hearts and livers, in which a priority status is given to a transplant based on the severity of illness. Consequently, at large centers candidates can expect to wait for extended periods of time. Unfortunately, few objective data exist to clarify this issue.

4. What are the indications for single-lung and double-lung transplantation?

The most common indications for single-lung transplantation include:

- Chronic obstructive pulmonary disease (COPD)/emphysema (45%) caused by smoking
- Idiopathic pulmonary fibrosis (IPF) (22%), unknown cause
- Alpha$_1$ Antitrypsin Deficiency (11%) enzyme deficiency - related to smoking
* Primary pulmonary hypertension (PPH) (5%), unknown cause.

For double-lung transplantation, the most common diagnosis is cystic fibrosis (33%) an inherited genetic defect. However, many centers are now performing double-lung transplants in candidates with primary pulmonary hypertension and alpha$_1$ antitrypsin deficiency.

5. What are the selection criteria for lung transplantation?

In general, most transplant centers' criteria are in accordance with the *International Guidelines for the Selection of Lung Transplant Candidates*, which were established at a Lung Transplant Consensus Conference in 1997. The purpose of this conference was to standardize practice surrounding criteria for patient selection through a joint effort by physicians representing professional transplantation societies (i.e., American Thoracic Society [ATS], the International Society for Heart and Lung Transplantation [ISHLT], the European Respiratory Society [ERS], and the American Society of Transplant Physicians [ASTP]) . The criteria included the following:

1. New York Heart Association (NYHA) 3 or 4
   - Patient able to walk 100–1500 feet
   - If > 1500 feet, the patient may be too healthy for transplantation; reevaluate at a later date.
   - If < 100 feet, the patient may be too sick for transplant.
2. Weight contraindications for lung transplantation
   - Ideal body weight (IBW) < 70%
   - IBW > 130%
3. Upper age limits
   - Single-lung transplant, patient < 65 years old
   - Double-lung transplant, patient < 60 years old
   - Heart-lung transplant, patient < 55 years old
4. Smoking/substance abuse
   - Patient must be abstinent more than 6 months as documented by nicotine free specimens of urine/blood
5. Adequate renal reserve with no active progressive parenchymal dysfunction
   - Ideal 24-hr creatinine clearance > 100 mg/ml/min
   - Unacceptable creatinine clearance < 50 mg/ml/min
6. Osteoporosis
   - Symptomatic osteoporosis requiring pain management
7. Bacterial infection/resistance(s) (excluding mycobacteria)
8. Severe musculoskeletal disease affecting the thorax
   - Kyphoscoliosis
   - Progressive neuromuscular disease
9. Elevated panel-reactive antibody testing (see Chapter 2)
10. Mechanical ventilation
11. HIV-positive, hepatitis B antigen–positive, or hepatitis C-positive; biopsy-proven histologic evidence of liver diseases
12. Active malignancy within the past 2 years with the exception of basal cell and squamous cell carcinoma.
    - Recent data on recurrence of tumors after transplant suggest that a waiting period of at least 5 years is prudent for extracapsular renal cell tumors, breast cancer stage 2 or greater, colon cancer staged > Dukes A, and melanoma level III or greater.
13. No evidence of severe cardiovascular disease
    - Greater than 1 vessel coronary artery disease
    - Left ventricular ejection fraction less than 40%

14. Psychosocial issues: Centers must remember that compliance and psychological problems are not cured with transplant. Issues that are unable to be resolved or have a high likelihood of impacting negatively on the patient's outcome, including poorly controlled major psychoaffective disorders, the inability to comply with a complex medication regimen, a documented history of noncompliance with medical care,or treatment plans even in the absence of documented psychiatric problems, are considered an absolute contraindication.
15. Adequate financial resources
16. Adequate cognitive functioning to understand the procedure and the risks, and the ability to comply with follow-up care

6. How is a patient referred for lung transplantation?

The lung transplant referral process may begin with a phone call from the patient, family, or referring physician to the transplant center. If it is not known which transplant center to contact, the UNOS Website (www.unos.org) can be of help. Following the initial telephone contact, a letter of introduction from the patient's physician is sent to the lung transplant coordinator addressing the chronological sequence of the patient's illness and providing rebuttals to all of the potential contraindications just listed. Copies of all reports that document the lung disease and the patient's clinical findings are also pertinent. If the patient appears to meet the requirements of the program, the attending physician and the patient will be notified to obtain insurance verification and financial approval for a transplant evaluation. After this clearance has been obtained, the patient is contacted and a date is selected for the evaluation. The purpose of this meeting is not only for the team to evaluate the patient's possible candidacy, but also for the patient and family to become acquainted with the transplant team. The candidate's welfare and maintenance of current quality of life are the team's goals.

7. Describe a lung transplant evaluation.

The transplant evaluation consists of various medical tests and consultations with team specialists who will assess the candidate as a whole being, made up of the physical, emotional, and social self. The experienced team has learned through many clinical examples that the greatest chance for a successful transplant outcome comes when all three aspects of the self are well cared for. The results of the evaluation give the team a clearer picture of the candidate's overall health and facilitate determination of the type of lung transplant that will be best for him or her. The evaluation may also reveal certain conditions that need to be corrected or checked carefully before the transplant surgery. In each case, the physician and coordinators will outline the treatment plan for the candidate. The transplant evaluation may be as short as 1 day or as long as a week.

8. Which tests are recommended for a lung transplant evaluation?

Depending upon the diagnosis, physical findings, and previous studies obtained, the testing should include some of the following:
- **Chest radiograph**
- **Quantitative ventilation-perfusion scan (VQ scan):** This study is divided into two portions. In the first, a very small amount of contrast material is injected into a vein, which lights up the arteries of the lung and tells the team which lung is getting the most blood flow. The second portion involves breathing in some contrast material to measure which lung receives the most air during respiration. This tests provides information that helps the surgeons to decide if one lung is significantly more affected and should be the side of choice for a single-lung procedure or helps them to designate the lung to be removed first for a double-lung procedure
- **12-lead electrocardiogram (ECG or EKG)**
- **Transthoracic echocardiogram** or **transesophageal echocardiogram (TEE):** The transesophageal echocardiogram's method of analyzing sound waves differs from the transthoracic echocardiogram because the patient receives medication to make him or her drowsy and swallows a small electrode (about the size of a large pill). The electrode is positioned in the esophagus where it can convey a more accurate picture of the structures of the heart and the vessels

surrounding it. **Not everyone undergoes this test.** The test is usually completed when the patient is diagnosed with pulmonary hypertension or congenital heart disease with secondary pulmonary hypertension.

• **Cardiac catheterization (coronary angiogram)**, which includes right heart pressures and resistance. If the candidate is older than 40 years or has a history of cardiac risk factors, a left ventriculogram and coronary angiogram are completed

• **Pulmonary function tests (PFTs):** This series of breathing tests conducted in the pulmonary laboratory measures the current function of the lungs' and the chest's ability to expand and contract to bring oxygen and remove carbon dioxide from the body. It also helps to confirm evidence of disease, detect airway hyper-reactivity, determine the degree of respiratory impairment, define the overall progression of disease, and determine the course of therapy.

• **Arterial blood gases (ABGs)**

• **Oxygen desaturation study:** This test is performed in the pulmonary function laboratory at the same time as the PFTs. It is done by placing a small device called an oximeter on the tip of the finger, which externally monitors the oxygen content of the candidate's arterial blood. It helps to establish how much, if any, supplemental oxygen the candidate needs while sitting, exercising, and sleeping.

• **Six-minute walk distance:** A specially trained physical therapist or nurse conducts this test by walking alongside the candidate (with supplemental oxygen if the candidate is prescribed or demonstrates a need for it) while continuously monitoring pulse rate and oxygen saturation levels for 6 minutes. The candidate is asked to walk as fast and as far as he or she can in that 6-minute period. If the patient gets tired, he or she can stop. If the patient feels that he or she cannot go any further because of leg pain, chest pain, or fatigue, the patient stops. The results give the team some indication that the candidate is physically strong enough to withstand the physical demands of a lung transplant as well as serve as baseline information for future comparisons.

• **Dual-energy x-ray absorptiometry (DEXA) scan:** This bone mineral density test is an x-ray that measures bone mass in the bones of the lumbar spine and hip to diagnose osteoporosis, even in its earliest stages. Most generally osteoporosis is associated with postmenopausal women because the female hormone estrogen, which maintains the normal bone cycle, decreases after menopause, and bone is lost. Similarly, osteoporosis can occur in men when the male hormone testosterone level is low. Patients with long-standing end-stage organ disease who may or may not require steroid therapy also represent a group at risk because of the manner in which this medication breaks down bones and interrupts rebuilding. However, research has demonstrated that lung transplant recipients are at great risk of developing osteoporosis within the first 6 months after the transplant because of the effects of the disease process itself in combination with the use of prednisone as an antirejection agent, immunosuppression medications, and bed rest. Therefore, the philosophy about osteoporosis is prevention rather than catching up. When performed routinely, a bone density scan can monitor the rate of bone loss or improvement after a therapy is prescribed. The procedure itself is an hour-long painless x-ray. The image is shot from under the patient, measuring the bone mineral content and bone area. The result is a value called the *T-score*, which is the patient's bone density compared with a bone mass value usually reached at age 30 years. A T-score of $2\frac{1}{2}$ or more standard deviations below the normal peak bone mass is considered osteoporosis. The DEXA scan is completed yearly and is most reliable when performed on the same scanner. Preventive treatment may consist of the addition of multivitamins, calcium, and vitamin D daily. Treatment for osteoporosis may include all of those *plus* estrogen/progesterone replacement and/or Fosamax.

9. What is the average waiting time to transplant?

Transplant timing varies with blood type (O, A, B, and AB) and height of the candidate. It is very important for the lung transplant candidate and family to understand that waiting time, or seniority on the list, remains the primary means in determining which candidate is offered the donor organ(s). In other words, no matter how ill a candidate may become while waiting for a lung transplant, when a donor becomes available, the most suitable candidate with **the most waiting time**

accumulated on the UNOS list is transplanted. This method accounts for the unfortunate statistic that estimates 15–20% of patients do not survive the waiting time to lung transplantation. Waiting time for a donor varies in length because the donor pool is so unpredictable. The fragility of lungs, especially in a critically ill, ventilated donor, limits their functional use to about 15 of every 100 donors. Thus waiting time can vary from a few months to years depending on donor availability.

10. What is the success rate for lung transplantation?

Patients receiving lung transplants are living longer and returning to productive lives. According to the Scientific Registry of Transplant Recipients, single-lung recipients have a 1-year survival rate of 73.8%, and double-lung survival at 1 year is 77.3%. Nationally, 3-year survival rates are 54.2% for single-lung recipients and 57.4% for double-lung recipients. Individual transplant centers provide survival statistics for their programs that may compare favorably with the national data presented.

11. Describe routine posttransplant care.

Following transplant, the lung transplant team, composed of the physicians, surgeons, nurses, and ancillary professionals of the cardiothoracic surgical and pulmonary staff, cares for patients. Patients participate in an exercise regimen or rehabilitation program. They also are given home-care instructions surrounding surveillance testing and procedures. In addition, patient and family education is initiated regarding immunosuppression, medications, routine laboratory testing, and logging of home spirometry. Transplant physicians generally agree that direct microscopic examination of tissue is the most helpful in assessing for organ rejection, particularly in the early postoperative period. Therefore, surveillance bronchoscopy is completed 1–2 weeks after the transplantation or sooner, if necessary. During this procedure the physicians examine the bronchial anastomoses, complete a bronchoalveolar lavage (BAL), obtain bronchial washings for cultures, and perform a transbronchial biopsy .

12. What are the early complications associated with lung transplantation?

Ginns summarized the complications of lung transplantation into 3 major classifications:
• Complications due to the operation itself
• Complications due to the immunosuppressive agents including infection and their side effects
• Complications due to the immunologic complications (rejection)

In the first 2 weeks posttransplant, although rare, the greatest cause of death is related to the operation itself. Such complications include ischemic reperfusion injury or reimplantation response, airway anastomotic complications, and surgical complications such as pain, phrenic nerve dysfunction, atelectasis/retained bronchial secretions, pneumonia, hemorrhage, pneumothoraces, respiratory failure, and cardiac and hemodynamic complications.

13. Describe infectious complications associated with lung transplantation.

Infection is the most common cause of mortality and morbidity within 90 days posttransplantation. Common infections seen in lung transplant recipients include bacterial pneumonia, *Clostridium difficile* with diarrhea and colitis, fungal sinus or pulmonary infections, viral infection, and especially cytomegalovirus (CMV). Early bacterial pneumonia has decreased from an incidence of 43% before 1990 to 1.5% in 1994. The decrease resulted from the prophylaxis with antibiotics for 3–5 days posttransplantation. Late bacterial pneumonias (3 months to 3 years) are caused by various organisms, but the most troublesome is pneumococcus. The patient's pneumococcal history should be documented and medical personal should boost the initial vaccine every 2–3 years posttransplantation. In addition *Staphylococcus aureus* and gram-negative rods (i.e., *Klebsiella, Citrobacter, Serratia,* and *Xanthomonas*) are seen, but the most prevalent bacterial pathogen is *Pseudomonas aeruginosa*. Infection is a special problem in patients with chronic rejection because of its persistence in abnormal airways. The antibiotic treatment of these pneumonias should be monitored according to the results of the sputum culture and antibiotic sensitivity. The incidence of *Clostridium difficile* is high because of heavy antibiotic and steroid use.

Empiric treatment consists of oral metronidazole (Flagyl) for 10 days or vancomycin for more symptomatic cases.

Colonization with fungal organisms, especially *Aspergillus* species, is not unusual in recipients. Early treatment is used for patients with such risk factors as recent transplantation, recent rejection treatment, or more than 2 positive cultures. When invasive fungus is suspected, an aggressive work-up of the head, sinuses, and the chest is indicated, and treatment with itraconazole in combination with inhaled or, in more symptomatic cases, intravenous amphotericin B is given. Finally, parasitic infections such as *Pneumocystis carinii* pneumonia (PCP) have been virtually eliminated through prophylaxis with Bactrim 80 mg/400 mg every 2–3 days or, if the patient is allergic to sulfa, Dapsone (diaminodiphenylsulfone) 100 mg/week.

This narrows down the infectious field to investigations that currently center on viral infections. Transplant patients are susceptible to viruses transmitted with donor-recipient mismatches.

14. What viral infections are most commonly seen in lung transplant recipients?

Common viral infections infections include herpes simplex virus (HSV), Epstein-Barr virus (EBV), and, the most worrisome, cytomegalovirus (CMV). Currently there are two approaches to therapy: (1) prophylactic treatment for everyone, (2) preemptive treatment following a positive antigenemia (PP165, checked every week posttransplantation for the first 3 months, then monthly). The current medication regimen includes intravenous ganciclovir, although other antiviral medications, such as valacyclovir, are quickly proving their worth . Mismatches between donors and recipients can be a cause of viral infections posttransplantation. The table describes the relative risk associated with viral mismatches.

Viral Mismatches and Associated Risks for the Infection in the Recipient

High risk	Donor positive (+)	Recipient negative (−)
Moderate risk	Donor +	Recipient +
Low risk	Donor −	Recipient −

HSV mismatch: Although not usually fatal, reactivation can occur in patients not prophylaxed for CMV and intubated patients in the intensive care unit (ICU) multiply treated for longstanding rejection.

EBV mismatch is a high risk for symptomatic primary infection and post transplant lymphoproliferative disease (PTLD).

CMV mismatch: Before 1991, CMV infections were attributed to 5% of all perioperative deaths and another 5% of later deaths. Consequently, many centers still match on the CMV status of the recipient. However, CMV can be reactivated at any time, notably by augmented immunosuppression. Primary infection is strongly associated with tissue invasion, dissemination, relapse, and high mortality, if untreated. CMV cases that do recur bear strong ties to multiple episodes of rejection treatment. It should be emphasized that patients who receive long or multiple courses of ganciclovir should be monitored closely for neutropenia, which can become profound if not detected early. One must remember that intravenous ganciclovir is 90% bioavailable, oral ganciclovir is less than 8%, and the dosage must be adjusted according to renal function or dysfunction.

15. Describe the types of rejection associated with lung transplantation.

Histologically, lung rejection is classified in two forms: acute cellular rejection and chronic rejection. **Acute rejection** occurs at least once in all lung transplant recipients, usually in the first 3 months posttransplantation, although it can occur later. Acute rejection usually presents symptomatically with cough, dyspnea, and fatigue. Other symptoms include hypoxemia, pulmonary infiltrates, pleural effusions, and fever. A drop in the home microspirometry readings and a decrease in pulmonary function test results may accompany this rejection. Management of acute rejection consists of administration of high-dose corticosteroids, optimization of maintenance immunosuppression, and use of additional therapies when necessary. Acute rejection should be treated aggressively because it is a precursor of chronic rejection.

Chronic rejection usually occurs 1 year after transplantation. It is defined histologically as inflammation and fibrosis of the small airways (respiratory bronchioles) or obliterative bronchiolitis (OB). It is usually associated with an irreversible 20% decrease in the forced expiratory volume in 1 second (FEV_1) from a previously established posttransplant baseline. Management of OB is individualized, depending on the current immunosuppressive regimen, previous treatment, and other organ issues. The mortality rate at 3 years after diagnosis is 40% or higher.

16. What are the usual immunosuppressive medications used in lung transplantation?

The drugs used to control rejection are varied and are used by each center in a plethora of combinations. However, the regimens used for lung transplantation have evolved through research in the renal and heart transplant arena. Most patients are maintained for the remainder of their lives on a 3-drug regimen. The primary drug of immunosuppression is either cyclosporine or tacrolimus. Cyclosporine is the drug that revolutionized solid organ transplantation. It acts by inhibiting cell wall synthesis through interference with the transcription of several T-cell cytokines. Inhibition of the cytokines results in specific and reversible inhibition of the immunocompetent T-cell activation. Toxic effects include nephrotoxicity, hypertension, neurotoxicity, hirsutism, gingival hyperplasia, and hepatotoxicity. Tacrolimus is pharmacologically related to cyclosporine A. It also inhibits the cell-mediated immune response by inhibiting T-cell activation. It binds to a different immunophilin than cyclosporine. The complex FK-binding protein then inhibits the release of interleukin-2 and other cytokines. Toxic effects include toxicities similar to those for cyclosporine: nephrotoxicity, hypertension, and possible diabetes mellitus. In addition, most lung transplant programs use steroids as part of the regimen along with azathioprine or mycophenolate mofetil. Chapter 7 presents a comprehensive overview of immunosuppressive medications.

17. What is the potential of discontinuing immunosuppressive medications in lung transplantation?

In 1992, Starzl and colleagues demonstrated the presence of donor cells in tissue and blood of long-term organ recipients. In 1993, based on this research, Pham and associates initiated a trial combining the infusion of the same donor bone marrow (BM) when available from the donor with simultaneous thoracic organ transplantation. Between September 1993 and September 1996, 44 patients received either heart (n = 24) or lung (n = 20) allografts. In addition, they received an infusion of unmodified donor BM (3.0×108 cells/kg) and then were maintained on routine immunosuppression with tacrolimus and steroids. This group was compared with a similar group of 26 recipients (16 hearts, 10 lungs) who were controls. There were no events or side effects associated with the bone marrow infusion, and all but one recipient is alive with good graft function. In addition, there was no difference in survival between the two groups. The average number of rejection episodes (grade > 3A) was significantly decreased during the first 100 postoperative days in the BM patients as compared with the group without BM. When tested by mixed lymphocyte reaction, none of the patients had evidence of donor-specific immunomodulation. The conclusion of the investigators was that infusion of donor bone marrow was safe in the heart or lung transplant recipient and associated with an augmentation of donor cell chimerism, but the impact of this immunomodulation was yet to be determined. In 1999, McCurry and colleagues reevaluated this research in the survivors. There was no difference in the rate of acute cellular rejection (ACR) in lung recipients with and without bone marrow. However, only 1 out of 26 (3.8%) of the lung recipients who received BM developed obliterative bronchiolitis (OB), which was significantly decreased from that seen in the lung recipients without BM (4 out of 13 or 31% developed OB). In addition, 42% of the BM recipients demonstrated donor hyporeactivity as compared with only 28% of the lung controls. Although the numbers are small, this study suggests that lung transplantation combined with unmodified donor bone marrow results in less rejection.

18. What other method of controlling rejection is being researched in lung transplantation?

In 1993, a protocol was undertaken that targeted cyclosporine into the new lung by an aerosol inhalation. Researchers thought that **aerosolized cyclosporine** would deliver a higher concentration than that obtained by systemic routes alone and that the result would be a better method of controlling rejection. Eighteen consecutive recipients with persistent acute rejection were treated with aerosolized cyclosporine in addition to their routine immunosuppression. It was administered by a jet nebulizer (Aero Tech II, CisUs, Bedford, Mass.) driven by compressed air (50 psi) at a flow rate of 10 L/min.[4] Three hundred milligrams of cyclosporine (Novartis, Basel, Switzerland) was dissolved in 4.8 ml propylene glycol. Inhalation was done through a mouthpiece during spontaneous respiration. A fiberoptic bronchoscopy with transbronchial biopsy was done at approximately 4 weeks after the initiation of therapy and then at 2–3-month intervals. Samples were obtained from the same segments where acute rejection was first detected. Two patients were unable to tolerate the aerosol treatments because of "intractable cough and airways irritation" and were withdrawn from the study. In 14 (88%) of the remaining 16 subjects, the previous grade-two or higher rejection before treatment was significantly diminished to minimal levels (A1) or disappeared (A0). Because of the impressive results of this study, research regarding aerosolized cyclosporine was initiated in new transplant recipients besides their regular immunosuppressive protocol and continues. The aim of this NIH-funded study is to determine the efficacy of aerosolized cyclosporine in addition to routine immunosuppression on acute and chronic rejection in the early post-lung transplantation.

19. What is the best method to detect rejection in the new lung?

Although each transplant center has its own protocol for surveillance, a chest x-ray, pulmonary function tests, bronchoscopic examination, and the recipient's clinical course form the cornerstone of this evaluation. Most physicians agree that direct microscopic examination of lung tissue is the best assessment tool for organ rejection and infection, especially in the first year following transplantation. The bronchoscopic examination of the airway includes a bronchoalveolar lavage, which is generally performed from either the right middle lobe (in right lung recipients) or in the lingula (in left lung recipients) in the area of radiographic infiltrates, if present, and examined for neutrophilia. The lavage fluid is sent for culture and antibiotic sensitivities.

20. Are the surgical outcomes better with single- or double-lung transplantation?

Basically the procedure has not changed in the last 10 years. However, questions remain regarding the best operation for candidates with either primary pulmonary/secondary pulmonary hypertension and alpha$_1$-antitrypsin deficiency. A retrospective review of lung transplants found no significant differences posttransplant in single versus double lung transplantation in the following: median duration of intubation, ICU length of stay, and hospital stay in primary and secondary pulmonary hypertension. In addition, survival was similar at 1 month (81% single and 84% double), 1 year (both 67%), and 4 years (57%). Finally, late functional status was not statistically different for the groups. The authors concluded that the outcomes for patients with pulmonary hypertension were similar regardless of whether they received a single- or double-lung transplant. By contrast, the report of the International Registry states that the survival curves appear to be diverging after 3 years posttransplant with double-lung recipients having a survival advantage over single-lung and heart-lung recipients (p = 0.003).

21. What causes a poor outcome in lung transplantation?

Independent predictors of adverse outcome at 1 year include preoperative ventilator support, retransplantation, lung diagnosis other than emphysema, and age. In addition, female recipients have higher mortality than male recipients (p = 0.001), and female donors to female recipients have poorer outcomes than other gender combinations (p = 0.03). Comorbid conditions in the first 4 years posttransplantation include hypertension, renal dysfunction, hyperlipidemia, diabetes, and malignancy. The 8-year actuarial survival was 50% at 5 years for all lung recipients (single or double) and 40% at 5 years for heart-lung recipients. The two most common causes of death in both the adult and pediatric populations over the first 5 years posttransplantation include infection (especially in the first and second year) and obliterative bronchiolitis (OB) in years 3–5. Other causes of mortality include CMV, lymphoma, acute rejection. and malignancy.

22. What factors affect the recipient's quality of life?

In a recent study, the quality of life of candidates for lung transplant was compared with that of 59 lung transplant recipients. Results indicated that the quality-of-life visual analogue scale score was significantly higher posttransplantation than pretransplantation ($p < 0.001$), as were coping skills/COPE, level of optimism/LOT, and levels of depression ($p < 0.001$), anxiety ($p < 0.001$), and global severity index per the SCL-90R ($p < 0.001$). Furthermore, functional measurements (i.e., PFTs) demonstrated significant improvement posttransplantation ($p < 0.05$). The investigators of the study concluded that pulmonary functions of lung transplant recipients posttransplantation improved, coping abilities were maintained, optimism increased, and symptoms of psychological distress decreased, resulting in a significant improvement in recipients' overall quality of life.

SUMMARY

Many advances have occurred that allow patients with end-stage lung disease to have a second chance at life. In comparison with other solid organ transplants, lung transplantation is relatively young and donor organs are scarce. Nonetheless, recipients and transplant programs are growing exponentially. Despite all of the potential problems, lung transplant recipients are living longer (5–18 years) and returning to productive lives. It is hoped that through rigorous research endeavors, advances in organ transplantation such as these will continue to evolve and that control of rejection and infection will be a problem of the past.

BIBLIOGRAPHY

1. American Thoracic Society International Consensus Statement: Idiopathic pulmonary fibrosis: Diagnosis and treatment. Am J Respir Crit Care Med 161:646–664, 2000.
2. Annual Report of the Scientific Registry of Transplant Recipients. Available at: www.ustransplant.org. Accessed August 24, 2002.
3. Gammie JS, Keenan RJ, Pham SM, et al: Single versus double lung transplantation for pulmonary hypertension. J Thorac Cardiovasc Surgery 115(2):397–402, 1998.
4. Ginns LC, Cosimi AB, Morris PF: Transplantation. Malden, MA, Blackwell Science, 1999, pp 438–473.
5. Hertz MI: Manual of Lung Transplant Medical Care. Minneapolis, MN, Fairview Publications, 2001.
6. Hosenspud JD, Bennett LE, Keck BM, et al: The Registry of the International Society of Heart and Lung Transplantation: Seventeenth Official Report—2000. J Heart Lung Transplant 18:611–626, 2000.
7. International Guidelines for the Selection of Lung Transplant Candidates. Am J Respir Crit Care Med 158(1):335–339, 1998.
8. Keenan, RJ, Iacono A, Dauber JH, et al: Treatment of refractory acute allograft rejection with aerosolized cyclosporine in lung transplant recipients. J Thorac Cardiovasc Surg 113(2):335–341, 1997.
9. Keenan R, Duncan A, Zenati M: Improved immunosuppression with aerosolized cyclosporine in experimental pulmonary transplantation. Transplantation 53:20–25, 1992.
10. Manzetti JD, Vensak JL, Aquilino TM, et al: A comparison of quality of life from pre to post lung transplant: A pilot study [abstract]. J Heart Lung Transplant 19:59, 2000.
11. Mauer JR, Frost AD, Estenne M, et al: International guidelines for the selection of lung transplant candidates. J Heart Lung Transplant 17(7):703–709, 1998.
12. McCurry KR, Pham SI, Zeevi A, et al: Immunomodulatory effects of donor bone marrow infusion in heart or lung transplantation: Five year experience. J Heart Lung Transplant 18(1):72, 1999.
13. Nunley DR, Dauber JH: Lung transplantation: Implications for the general internist. Adv Intern Med 41:497–528, 1996.
14. Pham SM, Zeevi A, Rao A, et al: Three year experience of combined donor bone marrow infusion and thoracic organ transplantation [abstract]. J Heart Lung Transplant 16:114, 1997.
15. Williams P: Infections in lung transplant patients. Personal communication, 1997.
16. Zeevi A, Pham SM, Pavlick M, et al: Donor specific bone marrow infusion in lung transplant recipients: The impact on immune modulation and delayed graft rejection [abstract]. J Heart Lung Transplant 16:115, 1997.

9. HEART TRANSPLANTATION

Sandra A. Cupples, DNSc, RN

1. Is heart transplantation an experimental procedure?

No, the first human-to-human heart transplantation procedure was performed by Barnard in 1967 in South Africa. Three days later, the first heart transplantation was performed in the United States. These recipients lived for 18 days and 6.5 hours, respectively. Approximately 100 heart transplantations were performed during the following year, but most heart transplant centers closed because of dismal survival rates.

The development of the endomyocardial biopsy forceps, the categorization of a histologic grading system for rejection, and the discovery of the immunosuppressant cyclosporine A were three landmark events that significantly improved survival rates and propelled heart transplantation into the modern era. Heart transplantation is no longer considered experimental and has become an acceptable treatment modality for end-stage heart disease.

2 Approximately how many heart transplant procedures are done each year in the United States? What are the current survival rates?

Approximately 2500 heart transplant procedures are performed each year. The most recent International Society for Heart and Lung Transplantation data indicate that one- and three-year survival rates are 85.6 and 79.5 percent, respectively.

3. Approximately how many candidates are on the heart transplant waiting list? What is the average waiting time for a donor heart?

As of February 2002, there were 4163 patients on the national heart transplant waiting list. Each month, many more patients are added to the waiting list than there are available donor organs. The current average waiting time for a donor heart exceeds 300 days. The amount of time that heart transplant candidates may have to wait on the list depends on their blood type, height and weight, and severity of illness.

4. What types of patients are referred for heart transplantation?

Approximately 45% of adult patients referred for heart transplant evaluation have ischemic cardiomyopathy. Another 44% have nonischemic cardiomyopathy that may be classified as peripartum, inflammatory, familial, infiltrative, or idiopathic. The remaining 11% have congenital anomalies, refractory ventricular dysrhythmias, or valvular disease, or are undergoing retransplantation.[10]

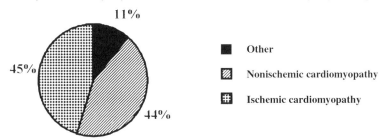

5. Before the formal transplant evaluation process begins, what must the transplant team first determine?

Before the formal evaluation process begins, the transplant team must first determine whether the patient has any other medical or surgical options that offer better long-term survival.

Patients with ischemic cardiomyopathy undergo tests to determine if they have any reversible ischemia that may be treated with either surgical or catheter intervention. The tests that may be done to detect reversible ischemia and viable or hibernating myocardium include the following:
- Radionuclide studies:
  - Planar rest and redistribution[201] thallium imaging
  - [99m]Technetium-labeled tetrofosmin
  - [99m]Technetium-labeled sestamibi imaging
- Positron emission tomography.
- Dobutamine echocardiography

Individuals with nonischemic cardiomyopathy are given a trial of maximal medical therapy that may include the following:
- Angiotensin-converting enzyme inhibitors
- Angiotensin receptor blockers
- Beta blockers
- Diuretics
- Digoxin
- Vasodilators
- Aldactone
- Inotropic agents

6. What is the purpose of the heart transplant evaluation process?
The purpose of the heart transplant evaluation is to:
- Determine the statistical likelihood that the patient will have improved life expectancy posttransplant.
- Ascertain the likelihood that the patient will be able to resume an active and relatively normal lifestyle posttransplant
- Assess the patient's potential to comply with a strict posttransplant medical regimen that involves lifelong daily medications and frequent follow-up visits.
- Reconfirm that there are no viable medical or surgical alternatives to transplantation.

The evaluation process involves a review of both physiologic and psychosocial criteria.

7. What is the first step of the evaluation process?
The first step is to establish the severity of the patient's functional impairment and prognosis. This is done by determining the patient's New York Heart Association classification, hemodynamic status, and maximal oxygen consumption if the metabolic exercise test can be tolerated by the patient.

8. How is the patient's maximal oxygen consumption determined?
The patient's maximal oxygen consumption is determined by a metabolic exercise test. This test is the gold standard by which patients are stratified; it is the most accurate predictor of survival. The metabolic exercise test, also known as a VO_{2max}, is typically performed after the ambulatory patient has achieved stability on a 2-week or longer course of optimal medical therapy.

9. What are the accepted, probable, and inadequate indications for heart transplantation?
According to guidelines formulated by the 24th Bethesda Conference on Cardiac Transplantation, the accepted, probable, and inadequate indications for heart transplantation are as follows:

PARAMETER	ACCEPTED INDICATIONS	PROBABLE INDICATIONS	INADEQUATE INDICATIONS
Maximal oxygen consumption	Maximal oxygen consumption < 10 ml/kg/min with achievement of anaerobic metabolism	Maximal oxygen consumption < 14 ml/kg/min with achievement of anaerobic metabolism and major limitations in activities of daily living	Maximal oxygen consumption > 15 ml/kg/min without other indications

(Cont'd. on next page.)

PARAMETER	ACCEPTED INDICATIONS	PROBABLE INDICATIONS	INADEQUATE INDICATIONS
Ischemia	Severe, limiting ischemia not amenable to surgical or catheter intervention	Recurrent, unstable ischemia not amenable to surgical or catheter intervention	
Other	Recurrent, symptomatic, refractory ventricular dysrhythmias	Instability of fluid balance and renal function not associated with patient noncompliance	Ejection fraction < 20% History of functional class 3 or 4 symptoms of heart failure Previous ventricular dysrhythmias

From Mudge GH, Goldstein S, Addonizio LJ, et al: 24th Bethesda Conference on Cardiac Transplantation: Task force 3—Recipient guidelines. J Am Coll Cardiol 22:21–30, 1993.

10. What tests are typically done during the evaluation process?

On completion of a thorough history and physical examination, patients typically undergo rigorous physiologic testing. In addition to the following tests, a number of consultations may be obtained as indicated, including consultations with a dentist/oral surgeon, endocrinologist, gynecologist, nutritionist, neuropsychologist, ophthalmologist, oncologist, or psychiatrist.

SYSTEM	TEST OR PROCEDURE
Cardiovascular	Electrocardiogram (ECG) Right heart catheterization Left heart catheterization Metabolic exercise test Echocardiogram (M-mode and 2-dimensional; Doppler) 24-hour Holter monitoring* Endomyocardial biopsy* Radionuclide ventriculography* Multigated blood panel imaging scan* Carotid and peripheral Doppler flow studies*
Pulmonary	Chest radiograph Pulmonary function tests Tuberculin purified protein derivative Skin test anergy battery Lung ventilation-perfusion scanning*
Renal	Urinalysis 24-hour urine for creatinine clearance and protein excretion
Gastrointestinal	Stool guaiac (three tests) Abdominal ultrasound Colonoscopy* Sigmoidoscopy*
Immunologic	Blood type and antibody screen Panel reactive antibody Human leukocyte antigen typing
General laboratory studies	Blood chemistries Renal and liver function panels Lipid profile Complete blood count with differential leukocytic count Prothrombin time, partial thromboplastin time, fibrinogen International normalized ratio

(Cont'd. on next page.)

SYSTEM	TEST OR PROCEDURE
General laboratory studies (cont'd.)	Carcinoembryonic antigen Glycosylated hemoglobin* Hemoglobin A_{1c}* Toxicology screen*
Infectious disease, general	History (travel, exposure, risk factors) Vaccinations Tuberculin skin test; anergy panel Stool culture Stool for ova and parasites
Infectious disease, serologies	Human immunodeficiency virus Hepatitis profile Herpes group virus Cytomegalovirus IgG and IgM antibodies Epstein-Barr IgG and IgM antibodies Rapid plasma reagin test Varicella titers Toxoplasma gondii IgG and IgM antibodies Fungal antibody screen Lyme titers*
Gender-specific tests	Mammography Papanicolaou test Prostate specific antigen Digital rectal examination Beta human chorionic gonadotropin*

* As indicated.
Adapted from Cupples SA, Boyce SW, Stamou SC: Heart transplantation. In Cupples SA, Ohler L (eds): Solid Organ Transplantation: A Handbook for Primary Health Care Providers. New York: Springer, 2002, pp 146–188, with permission.

11. What are the major physiologic contraindications to heart transplantation?
At this time, there are no universally accepted contraindications to heart transplantation. Each transplant center has its own policies regarding contraindications. However, some generally accepted physiologic contraindications are listed below:

SYSTEM	CONTRAINDICATIONS
General	Advanced age (typically > 60–65 years) Morbid obesity (≥ 30% of predicted ideal body weight) Severe cachexia Recent or active neoplasm
Pulmonary	Irreversible pulmonary hypertension (> 4–8 Wood units) Irreversible pulmonary parenchymal disease Recent unresolved pulmonary infarction Severe chronic bronchitis Severe obstructive/restrictive pulmonary disease (forced expiratory volume in 1 sec < 50% of predicted or ratio of forced expiratory volume in 1 sec to forced vital capacity < 40–50% of predicted)
Renal	Irreversible renal disease with serum creatinine > 2.0–2.5 mg/dl or creatinine clearance < 50 ml/min)
Hepatic	Irreversible hepatic disease (total bilirubin > 2.5 mg/dl)

(Cont'd. on next page.)

SYSTEM	CONTRAINDICATIONS
Cardiovascular	Significant, uncorrectable peripheral vascular disease Cerebrovascular disease Myocardial infiltrative and inflammatory disease
Gastrointestinal	Active peptic ulcer disease Current or recent diverticulitis
Skeletal	Severe osteoporosis
Other	Active infection Acquired immunodeficiency disorder Systemic granulomatous diseases Coexisting systemic disease likely to limit survival and/or rehabilitation Insulin-dependent diabetes mellitus with end-organ damage

Adapted from Cupples SA, Boyce SW, Stamou SC: Heart transplantation. In Cupples SA, Ohler L (eds): Solid Organ Transplantation: A Handbook for Primary Health Care Providers. New York, Springer, 2002, pp 146–188, with permission..

12. Why is fixed pulmonary hypertension a contraindication to heart transplantation?

Over time, the transplant candidate's native right ventricle gradually adapts to and is able to pump against elevated pulmonary pressures that may develop with chronic congestive heart failure. The naïve donor right ventricle, however, has not been exposed to pulmonary hypertension and will fail in its attempt to pump against irreversibly high pulmonary pressures. Therefore, patients with fixed pulmonary hypertension are generally not candidates for heart transplantation; however, they may be candidates for heart–lung transplantation.

13. What does the psychosocial evaluation generally involve?

At a minimum, the psychosocial evaluation for heart transplantation includes a consultation with a social worker for assessment of the patient's living environment, social support, emotional stability, neurocognitive status, compliance history, substance abuse history, insurance benefits, and commitment to the transplantation process. Depending on the patient's profile, the psychosocial evaluation may also include assessments by a psychologist, psychiatrist, neuropsychologist, or substance-abuse counselor.

14. List psychosocial contraindications to heart transplantation.

The major psychosocial contraindications to heart transplantation include the following:
- Current substance abuse
- Psychosocial instability
- Behavior patterns that are likely to preclude compliance
- Unmanaged mental illness
- Dementia
- Severe mental retardation
- Suicidal behavior or ideation

Patients who are currently using tobacco, alcohol, or illicit drugs are typically advised to enroll in a formal substance-abuse cessation program and to demonstrate abstinence for a given time period before listing.

15. Which strategies can help noncompliant patients to improve their adherence to medical therapy so that they can be placed on the transplant list at some time in the future?

Some transplant programs offer patients with a history of marginal compliance an opportunity to enroll in end-stage heart disease research protocols. Other programs conduct monthly support group meetings or develop behavioral contracts mutually with their noncompliant patients. Such strategies enable the transplant team to assess a patient's motivation and compliance over time and offer him or her a "second chance" at improving adherence.

16. What are the United Network for Organ Sharing categories for adult heart transplantation patients?

Adult patients who are accepted as candidates for heart transplantation are listed in one of the following United Network for Organ Sharing (UNOS) categories. However, because of the dynamic nature of congestive heart failure, certain patients may move back and forth among these categories while they are on the waiting list.

STATUS		REQUIREMENTS
1A	(a)	Mechanical circulatory support for acute hemodynamic decompensation that includes at least one of the following: • Left and/or right ventricular assist device implanted for ≤ 30 days • Total artificial heart • Intra-aortic balloon pump, and/or • Extracorporeal membrane oxygenator
	(b)	Mechanical circulatory support for > 30 days with objective medical evidence of the following significant device-related complications: • Thromboembolism • Device infection (ventricular assist device [VAD], pocket, or driveline) • Device malfunction • Life-threatening ventricular dysrhythmias
	(c)	Mechanical ventilation
	(d)	Continuous infusion of a single high-dose intravenous inotrope (e.g., dobutamine ≥ 7.5 µg/kg/min, or milrinone ≥ 0.5 µg/kg/min), or multiple intravenous inotropes in addition to continuous hemodynamic monitoring of left ventricular filling pressures
	(e)	The patient does not meet any of the criteria specified above, but is an inpatient at the listing transplant center hospital and has a life expectancy without a heart transplant of < 7 days.
1B		Left and/or right ventricular assist device implanted for > 30 days and/or continuous infusion of intravenous inotropes (hospitalized or at home)
2		Patient is waiting at home on oral medications

17. What are the key aspects of care for the outpatient transplant candidate?

Owing to the shortage of donor organs, transplant candidates may be on the waiting list for a prolonged period of time. Depending on their blood type, body size, and UNOS status, some patients may wait several years for a donor heart. Routine care of such patients may include the following:

• Periodic echocardiograms to evaluate current ejection fraction
• Periodic metabolic exercise tests to evaluate continued need for transplantation (Occasionally left ventricular function improves, thereby obviating the need for transplantation.)
• Routine cancer screening according to American Cancer Society guidelines
• Monitoring for infection, allergic reactions, weight changes (Significant increases or decreases in the candidate's weight may have ramifications in terms of acceptable donor weight and should be reported to UNOS.)
• If blood transfusions are required, administration of leukocyte-depleted blood or use of a leukocyte-removing filter
• Administration of cytomegalovirus (CMV)-negative blood for candidates who are CMV-seronegative (Administration of blood products at an institution other than the transplant center should be reported to the transplant team so that panel reactive antibody levels can be re-checked.)
• Administration of immunizations per established guidelines
• Frequent monitoring of serum electrolytes and renal and hepatic function; prothrombin time (PT) and international normalized ratio (INR) levels if on anticoagulation therapy

18. Why might a transplant candidate's prothrombin time and international normalized ratio levels be erratic and difficult to stabilize?

Heart transplant candidates often take warfarin sodium (Coumadin). As the patient's congestive heart failure becomes more pronounced, blood flow to the gut and liver becomes more compromised. If less of the anticoagulant is absorbed, the patient's prothrombin time (PT) and international normalized ratio (INR) levels may decrease. Compromised blood flow to the liver can exacerbate hepatic dysfunction, which in turn can potentiate the response to warfarin through impaired synthesis of clotting factors and decreased metabolism of warfarin. PT and INR levels may also be erratic because of drug interactions between warfarin sodium and other medications such as amiodarone.

19. What are panel-reactive antibodies?

Some transplant candidates have preformed human leukocyte antigen (HLA) antibodies that are reactive to the sera from a random group of individuals. Such antibodies are referred to as panel-reactive antibodies (PRAs). A high level of these antibodies increases the risk of posttransplant rejection, morbidity, and mortality. Some transplant centers periodically perform screening tests to determine the level of each transplant candidate's PRAs. Multiparous women and individuals who have previously received blood transfusions may be more likely to have elevated PRA levels.

20. What happens if a candidate's PRA level is elevated?

Candidates who have a high PRA level (typically > 8–10% reactivity) require a prospective lymphocytotoxic crossmatch with each potential donor. If the crossmatch with a given donor is negative, the transplantation procedure may be performed. This requirement for a negative prospective crossmatch may extend the length of time that the candidate has to wait for a suitable organ. Before transplantation, some transplant centers use plasmapheresis or prescribe an immunosuppressive agent to decrease a candidate's PRAs.

21. What is a left ventricular assist device?

A left ventricular assist device (LVAD) is an implantable pump that is used as a bridge to transplantation for patients with life-threatening heart failure. It is used to support the left ventricle. LVADs confer physiologic benefits by decreasing the workload of the heart and augmenting systemic circulation. Workload is reduced by decreasing preload and myocardial oxygen consumption. Systemic circulation is enhanced through the maintenance of an adequate and consistent cardiac output, which results in improved perfusion to all tissues and helps to prevent organ failure. (See chapter 10.)

22. Name the two major factors that determine whether a donor organ is suitable for a given candidate.

The two major factors that determine whether a donor organ is suitable for a particular candidate are blood type compatibility and height and weight ratio. In most cases, HLA matching is done retrospectively. However, patients with PRA levels above 10% require a prospective crossmatch.

23. What criteria are used to determine whether a donor organ is acceptable?

A donor heart is typically considered to be acceptable if the donor's age is less than 45–50 years and the donor has an arterial oxygen saturation > 80% on ventilatory support. In addition, seven "Ns" are required by most heart transplant programs:
- Negative serologies (e.g., human immunodeficiency virus, hepatitis B surface antigen, hepatitis C)
- No active systemic infection
- No significant ventricular dysrhythmias
- No extracranial malignancies

- No significant cardiac disease or trauma (e.g., myocardial infarction, coronary artery disease, cardiopulmonary resuscitation, or cardiac contusion)
- No cardiac abnormalities (e.g., global hypokinesis, valvular abnormalities, left ventricular hypertrophy)
- No history of intravenous drug use

Most transplant centers typically require coronary angiography for male and female donors over the age of 45 and 50 years, respectively, and any donor with risk factors for coronary artery disease. Some transplant centers have an alternative donor program in which allografts from older donors are used for older candidates (with the candidate's informed consent).

24. What does the immediate preoperative care of the transplant candidate involve?

The immediate preoperative care is similar to that of any patient undergoing open heart surgery. In addition to discontinuing and reversing any anticoagulation, transplant candidates require the following:

- Assessment for any signs or symptoms of infection
- Administration of immunosuppressants and prophylactic antibiotics
- Placement of a pulmonary artery catheter
- Reduction of any pulmonary vascular resistance with sodium nitroprusside, nitroglycerine, or prostaglandin E_1
- Review of the patient's current medical therapy for any medications that might affect the postoperative course (e.g., amiodarone [Cordarone] may increase chronotropic requirements and the risk of pulmonary complications).

25. Discuss the two types of heart transplantation procedures.

The two types of heart transplantation procedures are orthotopic and heterotopic transplantations. With orthotopic transplantation, the recipient's native heart is excised and replaced with a donor heart. Most heart transplantation procedures today involve the orthotopic technique. Heterotopic transplantation involves the placement of a donor heart into the recipient's right chest cavity. In this "piggyback" procedure, the recipient and donor aortae, superior vena cavae, and pulmonary arteries are connected by an end-to-side anastomosis. The heterotopic technique is rarely performed. It is typically reserved for situations in which a normal donor heart alone could not maintain adequate right ventricular function (e.g., in the presence of irreversibly elevated pulmonary pressures or if the donor heart is too small relative to the size of the recipient). Heterotopic transplantation has several disadvantages. It involves the risk of thromboembolism from the native heart; therefore, recipients must remain on anticoagulant therapy. In addition, recipients with ischemic cardiomyopathy may continue to have angina.

26. Describe potential problems that might arise in the immediate postoperative period.

Heart transplant recipients may experience many of the same postoperative complications as other types of open heart surgery patients. However, the transplant recipient is also at risk for unique problems related to the denervation of the transplanted heart and the global ischemia associated with explantation, transplantation, and implantation, particularly decreased diastolic compliance, impaired contractility, and depressed systolic function.

POTENTIAL PROBLEM	PRECIPITATING FACTORS	POTENTIAL TREATMENT OPTIONS
Compromised fluid status		
Hemorrhage	Preoperative anticoagulants	Blood products (whole blood,
	Previous cardiac surgery	packed red blood cells,
	Coagulopathy	fresh frozen plasma, platelets)
	Prolonged cardiopulmonary	Protamine sulfate or Aprotinin
	bypass (CPB) time	Surgical re-exploration
	Enlarged pericardial space	

(Cont'd. on next page.)

POTENTIAL PROBLEM	PRECIPITATING FACTORS	POTENTIAL TREATMENT OPTIONS
Compromised fluid status (*cont'd.*)		
Hypovolemia	Third spacing of fluids ↑ in intravascular space during rewarming Failure to maintain adequate preload	Optimize preload fluid volume Maintain higher filling pressures
Hypervolemia	Preoperative heart failure Cardiopulmonary bypass High-dose steroids Preoperative renal dysfunction Nephrotoxic immuno-suppressants	Diuretics Renal-dose dopamine
Myocardial dysfunction		
Right ventricular failure	Pulmonary hypertension Undersized allograft Prolonged ischemia (> 5 hours) Reactive pulmonary vasoconstriction due to cardiopulmonary bypass and/or protamine administration	Vasodilators Pulmonary vasodilators (isoproterenol, prostaglandin E_1, prostacyclin, nitroglycerin, nitric oxide, sodium nitroprusside, amrinone) Minimal use of vasopressors Mechanical right ventricular support
Left ventricular failure	Prolonged ischemia	Inotropic agents (dopamine, dobutamine, epinephrine, ephedrine) Intra-aortic balloon pump Extracorporeal membrane oxygenation Left ventricular assist device Retransplantation
Dysrhythmias (junctional rhythms, atrioventricular blocks, bradydysrhythmias)	Inadequate myocardial preservation Prolonged ischemia Sinus node dysfunction secondary to surgical trauma Pulmonary hypertension Cardiac edema Rejection Pretransplant amiodarone	Atrial ventricular pacing Isoproterenol Terbutaline Theophylline
Hypertension	Cyclosporine and steroid therapy	Antihypertensive agents (diltiazem, nifedipine, enalapril)

Adapted from Cupples SA, Boyce SW, Stamou SC: Heart transplantation. In Cupples SA, Ohler L (eds): Solid Organ Transplantation: A Handbook for Primary Health Care Providers. New York, Springer Publishing, pp 146–188, 2002, with permission.

27. Name three major types of immunosuppressive therapy.

Although immunosuppression protocols vary widely among transplant centers, immunosuppressants generally may be categorized according to the time they are administered and the purposes for which they are given. (See chapter 7.)

CATEGORY	TIME FRAME
Early prophylaxis	Immediately preoperatively, intraoperatively, and during the first several weeks after transplantation
Induction therapy	Induction therapy consists of intravenous agents that are given 7–14 days postoperatively to reduce the risk of rejection
Maintenance prophylaxis	For the remainder of the patient's life.
Rejection therapy	Immediately upon diagnosis of rejection

28. For heart transplant recipients, how is rejection defined?

Rejection is the process by which the immune system attempts to destroy the allograft. The Bethesda Conference Task Force on Cardiac Transplantation has defined rejection as "any clinical event, usually, but not always, accompanied by abnormal endomyocardial biopsy findings, that is treated with significant augmentation of immunosuppression"[14] (p. 42).

29. What causes rejection?

Rejection can be mediated by either cellular or humoral factors. Cellular and humoral rejection differ with respect to incidence, mediating factors, and pathophysiology.[20,22]

CHARACTERISTIC	CELLULAR REJECTION	HUMORAL (VASCULAR) REJECTION
Incidence	Most common type of rejection	Relatively rare in setting of prospective crossmatch
Mediating factor	Mediated by T cells	Mediated by antibodies
Pathophysiology	Surface cell antigens of allograft are recognized as foreign. Antigens are processed by recipient's antigen processing cells and presented to helper T cells. This process stimulates the production of interleukins and T-cell proliferation. Interleukins then recruit inflammatory cells and activate cytotoxic cells. Cytotoxic cells invade and attempt to destroy the allograft.	Antibodies bind to target antigens on the endothelial surface. This is followed by complement fixation and activation, which in turn induce platelet aggregation. Platelet aggregation and degranulation lead to the release of potent mediators such as platelet aggregating factor and initiate a complex biochemical cascade. Endothelial cell damage and increased vascular permeability facilitate the leakage of proteins into the vessel wall. Activation of the clotting cascade precipitates fibrin deposition. Other biologic mediators precipitate vasospasm. Blood flow to the organ is significantly reduced, resulting in damage to the coronary arteries, hypotension, and cardiogenic shock.

30. What are the different types of rejection?

TYPE	OCCURRENCE	CHARACTERISTICS
Hyperacute	Rare In the operating room or immediately after transplantation (within first few hours)	Humoral rejection Mediated by preformed circulating antibodies (e.g., blood group incompatibility or antibodies against specific endothelial antigens or human leukocyte antigen [HLA])

(Cont'd. on next page.)

TYPE	OCCURRENCE	CHARACTERISTICS
Hyperacute (cont'd.)		Characterized by rapid tissue necrosis and allograft failure Usually fatal
Acute	During the first few months after transplantation; incidence decreases thereafter, but can occur anytime after the transplant procedure.	Cellular rejection Characterized by interstitial and perivascular mononuclear cell infiltrates.
Chronic	After 6 months	Characterized by intimal thickening and vascular fibrosis Associated with cell-mediated and humoral injury to the endothelium

31. How is rejection diagnosed?

Ever since the introduction of the bioptome, the endomyocardial biopsy has become the gold standard by which rejection is diagnosed. This brief procedure typically involves inserting the bioptome into the right internal jugular vein, into the right atrium, across the tricuspid valve, and into the right ventricle. If the amount of scar tissue in the right internal jugular vein is significant, a femoral approach may be used. Several specimens of endomyocardial tissue are obtained from the right septal wall.

32. Are there any signs and symptoms of rejection?

Rejection may be associated with vague clinical manifestations such as fatigue, lethargy, shortness of breath, low-grade fever, and mood changes. Often, there are no clinical manifestations unless the rejection is severe. The mnemonic **REJECTION EPISODE** may be useful in remembering the signs and symptoms that may be associated with rejection.

R Rub (pericardial friction)*
E Electrocardiogram voltage decreased*
J Jugular venous distention*
E Edema (new onset, peripheral)*
C Cardiac dysrhythmias (atrial dysrhythmias, bradydysrhythmias)*
T Tiredness, fatigue
I Intolerance of exercise*
O Onset of low-grade fever
N New S3 or S4*

E Enlarged cardiac silhouette*
P Pulmonary crackles*
I Increase in weight*
S Shortness of breath*
O Onset of hypotension*
D Disturbances in mood
E Echocardiogram findings: decreased systolic function, change in left ventricular mass and wall thickness, decrease in left ventricular chamber size, shortening of isovolumic relaxation time, or increase in early transmittal filling velocity *

* May indicate severe rejection.

33. How is rejection graded?

Biopsy specimens are graded according to the International Society for Heart and Lung Transplantation standardized endomyocardial biopsy grading system.

GRADE	INTERPRETATION
0	No rejection
1A	Focal (perivascular or interstitial) infiltrates without necrosis
1B	Diffuse but sparse infiltrate without necrosis
2	One focus only with aggressive infiltrate and/or myocyte damage
3A	Multifocal aggressive infiltrates and/or myocyte damage
3B	Diffuse inflammatory infiltrates with necrosis
4	Diffuse aggressive polymorphous infiltrate with necrosis; with or without edema, hemorrhage, vasculitis

Adapted from Billingham ME, Cary NR, Hammond ME, et al: A working formulation for the standardization of nomenclature in the diagnosis of heart and lung rejection: Heart rejection study group. J Heart Lung Transplant 9:587–593, 1990.

34. What does *Quilty effect* on a biopsy indicate?

The term *Quilty effect* refers to a type of lesion characterized by flat or bulging lymphocytic proliferations. "Quilty" is the name of the patient in whom this lesion was first observed.

There are two patterns of Quilty lesions:

Quilty A: The lesion is confined to the endocardial tissue.
Quilty B: The lesion extends into the myocardium and may be associated with myocyte damage.

The pathogenesis and clinical significance of Quilty lesions are unknown. Quilty B may be mistaken for moderate rejection. The Quilty effect is not associated with decreased survival.

35. List the complications associated with endomyocardial biopsies.

The endomyocardial biopsy is a relatively safe procedure that is associated with low morbidity. However, the following complications can occur:

- Pneumothorax
- Hematoma
- Atrial or ventricular dysrhythmias
- Vasovagal reaction
- Perforation of carotid artery or myocardium
- Hemothorax
- Bleeding
- Damage to tricuspid valve
- Calcification of tissue on the septal wall

36. How frequently are endomyocardial biopsies done?

The frequency with which endomyocardial biopsies are performed varies from center to center. Generally, biopsies are performed more frequently during the first 6–12 months posttransplantation. Some centers discontinue biopsies after a given time period and resume them only if the recipient is symptomatic. If all biopsy results are relatively normal, a typical biopsy schedule might resemble the following:

INTERVAL POSTTRANSPLANT	FREQUENCY
Weeks 1–6	Weekly
Weeks 7–16	Bimonthly
Months 5–6	Monthly
Months 7–12	Every six weeks
Months 12–24	Every 3 months
Months 25–60	Every 6 months
After month 60	Only if symptomatic

37. What does routine, long-term follow-up of a heart transplant recipient involve?

Long-term follow-up varies among transplant programs. A typical follow-up protocol is depicted below.

TEST OR PROCEDURE	FREQUENCY
Complete blood cell count Basic metabolic panel Magnesium level Trough immunosuppression levels	With every endomyocardial biopsy or as indicated
Chest x-ray Lipid profile	Every 6–12 months or as indicated
Echocardiogram Electrocardiogram 24-hour urine for creatinine clearance, protein excretion Extensive screening for infection Cardiac catheterization (right and left* heart) or stress test (such as dobutamine echocardiogram)	Annually or as indicated

* Depending on recipient's current renal function.

38. Why are vomiting and diarrhea of concern after heart transplantation?

Vomiting and diarrhea may interfere with absorption of medications. Recipients who are not adequately absorbing their immunosuppression medications may be at increased risk for rejection. Often, transplant recipients must be readmitted to the hospital so that immunosuppressive agents may be administered intravenously.

39. What are the major causes of death after heart transplantation?

The causes of death vary with the interval posttransplant.[11]

First postoperative month	Perioperative complications of acute rejection, nonspecific graft failure, multisystem organ failure
Months 2–12	Infectious complications
After first year and thereafter	Coronary artery vasculopathy Malignancy

40. What are the major problems that confront heart transplant recipients?

The major posttransplant complications are infection, vasculopathy, hypertension, metabolic disorders (hyperlipidemia, obesity, osteoporosis, diabetes mellitus), renal insufficiency, gastrointestinal disorders, malignancy, and reduced exercise tolerance. (See chapters 20 and 21.)

41. What is the primary cause of posttransplant morbidity and mortality during the first year after transplantation?

Infection is the primary cause of morbidity and mortality during the first year after transplantation. Factors that increase the risk for infection include the following:
- Immunosuppression agents
- Surgical disruption of epithelial and endothelial barriers
- Exposure to nosocomial infections
- Deteriorated physical status before transplantation (See chapter 20)

42. What are some important points to remember about infection among heart transplant recipients?

Some important points about infection among heart transplant recipients follow:

Most common site of infection	Lung
Viral pathogens of major concern	Cytomegalovirus Epstein-Barr virus Herpes simplex 1 and 2 Varicella zoster virus
Single most common and most important pathogen	Cytomegalovirus
Most common site of cytomegalovirus (CMV) infection	Gastrointestinal tract
CMV infection with the highest morbidity and mortality	CMV pneumonitis
Bacterial pathogens of major concern	*Listeria monocytogenes*, *Nocardia asteroides*, *Legionella pneumophila*, and typical and atypical mycobacteria.

43. What is the major impediment to long-term survival following heart transplantation?

The major impediment to long-term survival is coronary artery vasculopathy (CAV). CAV is responsible for the majority of graft failures after the first posttransplant year and remains the most common reason for retransplantation. In 2000, the Registry of the International Society for Heart and Lung Transplantation listed the prevalence of CAV at 1 and 5 years after heart transplantation at 8% and 22%, respectively.

44. Does coronary artery vasculopathy differ from coronary artery disease?

Yes. CAV is an unusual form of coronary artery disease (CAD); it affects both epicardial and myocardial vessels. Other differences between CAD and CAV are summarized below:

CHARACTERISTIC	NATURAL CORONARY ARTERY DISEASE	TRANSPLANT CORONARY ARTERY VASCULOPATHY
Type of lesion	Asymmetric lesions	Concentric intimal lesions
Extent of lesion	Involves focal lesions	Diffuse process; affects entire length of vessel
Effect on small branches	Affects small branches	Typically does not affect small branches
Effect on internal elastic lamina	Internal elastic lamina disrupted	Internal elastic lamina intact
Effect on intramyocardial vessels	Does not affect intramyocardial vessels	Affects intramyocardial vessels
Calcification	Common	Rare
Course of development	Develops slowly over years	Develops rapidly (may develop over months)
Development of collateral vessels	Common	Rare
Development in children	Children typically not affected	Children affected

Adapted from Cupples SA, Boyce SW, Stamou SC: Heart transplantation. In Cupples SA, Ohler L (eds): Solid Organ Transplantation. A Handbook for Primary Health Care Providers. New York, Springer Publishing, pp 146–188, with permission.

45. Summarize the causes, clinical manifestations, diagnosis, and treatment of coronary artery vasculopathy.

The following table summarizes the causes, clinical manifestations, diagnosis, and treatment of CAV:

CAUSES		
IMMUNOLOGIC FACTORS	NONIMMUNOLOGIC RECIPIENT FACTORS	NONIMMUNOLOGIC DONOR FACTORS
Human leukocyte antigen (HLA) mismatching Acute rejection Chronic rejection Suboptimal immuno-suppression	Age Gender Obesity Hypertension Hyperlipidemia Diabetes mellitus Cytomegalovirus infection Smoking Oxidative injury	Age Gender Ischemic time Preexisting coronary artery disease (CAD)
CLINICAL MANIFESTATIONS	DIAGNOSIS	TREATMENT
Increasing fatigue Exertional dyspnea Elevated left ventricular filling pressures Signs and symptoms of graft failure: Congestive heart failure Dysrhythmias Sudden death Angina rare because allograft is denervated	Coronary angiography* Exercise electrocardiography* Myocardial nuclear imaging studies* IVUS more effective because it permits assessment of the actual lumen diameter	Percutaneous transluminal coronary angioplasty (PTCA)† Coronary artery bypass graft surgery (CABG)† Directional coronary atherectomy† Retransplantation: only definitive treatment‡

* Typically lack(s) sufficient sensitivity and underestimate(s) presence of coronary artery vasculopathy (CAV).
† Generally of limited use because of the diffuse, concentric nature of CAV.
‡ Not offered at all transplant centers because of the shortage of donor organs and the increased morbidity and mortality associated with retransplantation.

46. What are the prevalence, characteristics, and treatment options of common posttransplant complications among heart transplant recipients?

COMPLICATION	PREVALENCE	CHARACTERISTICS	TREATMENT OPTIONS
Hypertension	Most common complication during first year posttransplant; occurs in 61% of survivors[7] Prevalence increases over time; reported in 50 to 90% of all recipients.	More common in: Males Older recipients Recipients with pretransplant history of hypertension or ischemic cardiomyopathy Recipients with family history of hypertension, myocardial infarction or stroke Blood pressure may be higher in morning than in evening Etiologic factors include: Abnormal regulation of sodium balance secondary to cardiac denervation, cyclosporine, and renal impairment Structural changes in resistance arteries Immunosuppressive agents	Pharmacologic: Calcium antagonists ACE inhibitors Beta-blockers Nonpharmacologic: Reduction in salt intake Weight loss Exercise Smoking cessation

(Cont'd. on next page)

COMPLICATION	PREVALENCE	CHARACTERISTICS	TREATMENT OPTIONS
Hyperlipidemia	Occurs in 60–83% of recipients who are on triple-drug immunosuppressant therapy[12]	Increased cholesterol levels have been observed as early as 3 weeks after transplant; however, most elevations are observed within 6–18 months Total cholesterol levels typically increase 30–80 mg/dl over pre-transplant levels; higher levels have been observed in recipients who are not on lipid-lowering agents[11] Associated etiologic factors: History of pretransplant coronary artery disease (CAD) History of pretransplant hyper-lipidemia Obesity Male gender Diabetes Older age Renal dysfunction Thiazide diuretics Antihypertensive agents Immunosuppressive agents (cyclosporine, prednisone)[1,9]	Nonpharmacologic: Weight loss Exercise Smoking cessation National Cholesterol Education Program Step 2 diet Pharmacologic: Bile acid sequestrants Nicotinic acid Folic acid derivatives Hydroxy-methyl-glutaryl coenzyme A reductase inhibitors (especially for mixed hyperlipidemia)
Obesity	Similar to prevalence of hyperlipidemia	First transplant year: most recipients gain 5–10 kg Contributing factors: Immunosuppressive agents (especially cyclosporine and prednisone) Noncompliance with low-fat diet Lack of exercise	Low-fat diet Increased exercise
Osteoporosis	Rate of bone loss approaches 20% during first post-transplant year. Significant bone loss occurs in almost 100% of recipients.[7] Approximately 50% of recipients on long-term steroid therapy have osteoporosis.[25]	Etiologic factors: Immunosuppressive agents (especially calcineurin inhibitors and steroid therapy) Steroid therapy affects bone resorption and formation Contributing factors: Older age Renal failure Postmenopausal status Clinical manifestations include back pain, vertebral compression fractures, and avascular necrosis of weight-bearing joints.	Nonpharmacologic: Weight-bearing exercise Smoking cessation Pharmacologic: Antiresorptive agents Agents to increase bone formation Testosterone Supplements: calcium, vitamin D Substitute hydro-chlorothiazide for loop diuretics Decrease or dis-continue steroid therapy (if possible) *(Cont'd on next page.)*

COMPLICATION	PREVALENCE	CHARACTERISTICS	TREATMENT OPTIONS
Diabetes mellitus	Occurs in 20% and 16% of recipients at 1 and 5 years after transplant.[10]	Etiologic factors: Glucocorticoids: increase insulin resistance Cyclosporine: potentially toxic to beta cells; can decrease insulin production Tacrolimus: also diabetogenic Glucocorticoid-induced diabetes mellitus is dose dependent. Cyclosporine-induced diabetes mellitus is not dose dependent.	Diet therapy Exercise Oral hyperglycemic agents Insulin therapy (insulin-dependent recipients may require as much as a 3- to 4-fold increase in insulin)
Renal insufficiency	Occurs in approximately 12% of recipients at 1 and 5 years after transplant.[10]	Etiologic factors: Primary mechanism: cyclosporine- → renal vasoconstriction of afferent arterioles → increased renal vascular resistance → decreased renal plasma flow and glomerular filtration rate → chronic ischemia → renal fibrosis Secondary mechanism: direct tubular toxicity of cyclosporine A biphasic pattern of renal insufficiency may occur: There may be an initial, rapid decline in renal function during the first 6 months after transplant. As the cyclosporine dose is decreased over time, renal function often improves, and serum creatinine levels stabilize. After 7–8 years, there may be a more gradual but progressive decline in renal function. Clinical manifestations: Decreased creatinine clearance Disproportionate azotemia Hyperkalemia Increased serum uric acid levels Proteinuria Decreased sodium excretion Hypertension Fluid retention[11,21]	Keep cyclosporine or tacrolimus levels in therapeutic but not toxic range. Avoid or use with caution medications that increase calcineurin inhibitor levels or induce synergistic nephrotoxicity when used with calcineurin inhibitors (e.g., aminoglycosides, erythromycin, antifungal agents, nonsteroidal antiinflammatory agents). If these medications cannot be avoided, it is important to monitor calcineurin inhibitor levels and renal function before, during, and after these medications are given.
Gastrointestinal disorders	Gastrointestinal lesions (gastritis, esophagitis, duodenitis)	Contributing factor: glucocorticoid therapy	Antisecretory compounds H_2 histamine receptor antagonists
	Biliary tract disease[3]: most common problem. Incidence: 1–17%	Major predisposing factor: effect of cyclosporine on bile metabolism Other predisposing factors: Diabetes mellitus	Cholecystectomy

(Cont'd. on next page.)

COMPLICATION	PREVALENCE	CHARACTERISTICS	TREATMENT OPTIONS

Gastrointestinal disorders *(cont'd.)*	Biliary tract disease *(cont'd.)*	Other predisposing factors *(cont'd.)*
		  Female gender
		  Cholelithogenic antihyperlipidemic agents
		  Steroid-induced obesity
		  Perioperative ischemia
		  Vagotomy-induced gallbladder dysmotility[11,21]	

	Pancreatitis[25]:
	  2–8% of heart transplant recipients
		Contributing factors:
		  Perioperative hypoperfusion
		  Preexisting disease
		  Azathioprine
			Substitute mycophenolate mofetil for azathioprine

47. When is drug therapy for hyperlipidemia typically initiated?

The initiation of lipid-lowering therapy varies among transplant centers. Some programs start all recipients on statins, even those with normal cholesterol profiles. Other programs institute therapy if

- Total or low-density lipoprotein levels are elevated.
- A 3- to 6-month trial of nonpharmacologic interventions has been ineffective.
- Pretransplant compliance with the National Cholesterol Education Program Step 2 diet has been ineffective.
- Immunosuppression levels are at maintenance levels but lipid levels remain elevated.[12]

48. What are the goals of cholesterol therapy?

Typically, the goals for low-density and total cholesterol levels are < 100 mg/dl and < 200 mg/dl, respectively.

49. What precautions are associated with the use of various lipid-lowering agents?

A variety of lipid-lowering agents may be prescribed for heart transplant recipients. The precautions associated with the use of each type of medication are listed below.

MEDICATION	PRECAUTIONS

Bile acid sequestrants
  Cholestyramine
  Colestipol
	May interfere with the absorption of cyclosporine; cyclosporine and other medications should not be taken 1 hour before or 4–6 hours after bile acid sequestrants are taken.

Nicotinic acid Niacin	Concurrent cyclosporine use: may increase liver function tests and uric acid level; monitor recipient for hepatotoxicity and/or gout. Can cause hyperglycemia; not recommended for diabetic patients. Concurrent use of niacin with cyclosporine, lovastatin, and/or gemfibrozil may cause myositis and rhabdomyolysis; monitor liver function tests and creatine kinase. Concurrent prednisone use: may increase risk of peptic ulcer disease.

Folic acid derivatives
  Clofibrate
  Gemfibrozil
  Fenobibrate
	May cause gallstones (transplant recipients are already at increased risk for cholelithiasis)
	Concurrent use with lovastatin and cyclosporine can cause rhabdomyolysis.
	Gemfibrozil may potentiate the effects of warfarin.
	Use cautiously in diabetic patients: interacts with insulin and sulfonylureas.

(Cont'd. on next page.)

MEDICATION	PRECAUTIONS
Hydroxy-methylglutaryl coenzyme A reductase inhibitors	Can increase creatine kinase level and cause myositis and rhabdomyolysis, especially in patients taking other medications that are metabolized by the cytochrome P450 system.
Lovastatin Pravastatin	Monitor liver function tests, creatine kinase level, and recipient for musculoskeletal pain.
Simvastatin Fluvastatin	Cyclosporine inhibits the metabolism of lovastatin.

Adapted from Cupples SA, Boyce SW, Stamou SC: Heart transplantation. In Cupples SA, Ohler L (eds): Solid Organ Transplantation: A Handbook for Primary Health Care Providers. New York, Springer, 2002, pp 146–188, with permission.

50. What is the prevalence of malignancy among heart transplant recipients?

Prolonged administration of immunosuppression agents is associated with an increased risk of malignancy. Recent International Society for Heart and Lung Transplantation Registry data indicate that the incidence of malignancy among heart transplant recipients is approximately 4% and 10% at 1- and 5-year follow-up, respectively. The prevalence of skin cancer and lymphomas, the two most frequently occurring malignancies, is as follows:

	ONE-YEAR FOLLOW-UP	FIVE-YEAR FOLLOW-UP
Skin Cancer	35.1%	51.8%
Lymphoma	27.6%	15.2%

It is important to note that malignancies that are most common among the general population (e.g., tumors of the lung, breast, and colon) do not occur more frequently in heart transplant recipients.

51. What types of malignancies occur in heart transplant recipients?

Cincinnati Transplant Tumor Registry data indicate that the most frequently occurring types of malignancies in heart transplant recipients, in descending order, are the following:

1. Lymphomas
2. Skin and lip
3. Lung
4. Karposi's sarcoma
5. Head/neck
6. Colon/rectum
7. Kidney
8. Prostate
9. Hepatobiliary system

52. How do cutaneous neoplasms in heart transplant recipients differ from those in the general population?

The characteristics of cutaneous neoplasms in transplant recipients differ from those of the general population. These differences are summarized below. Because both basal and squamous cell carcinomas recur often, spread rapidly, and metastasize frequently, the approach to therapy and follow-up surveillance is aggressive.

HEART TRANSPLANT RECIPIENTS	GENERAL POPULATION
Squamous cell carcinomas outnumber basal cell carcinomas.	Basal cell carcinomas outnumber squamous cell carcinomas.
Occur at age 30–40 years.	Frequently occur at age 60–70 years.
Incidence of multiple skin carcinomas is high.	Incidence of multiple skin carcinomas is relatively low.
Squamous cell carcinomas are aggressive and metastatic; more deaths are due to squamous cell carcinomas than melanomas	Melanomas are aggressive and metastatic; most deaths are due to melanomas.

From Penn I: Tumors after renal and cardiac transplantation. Hematol/Oncol Clin North Am 7:431–445, 1993.

53. Why do some heart transplant recipients have reduced exercise tolerance?

Many heart transplant recipients can achieve high levels of exercise. Others, however, have impaired maximal exercise tolerance. This impairment is associated with several factors, including pretransplant deconditioning, chronotropic incompetence, diastolic dysfunction, glucocorticoid-induced myopathy, abnormalities in peripheral oxygen uptake and use, and arterial desaturation caused by elevated left heart filling pressures that interfere with ventilation.

54. What are the effects of cardiac denervation?

Donor cardiectomy results in both afferent and efferent cardiac denervation. The physiological effects and clinical implications of denervation are summarized below.

TYPE OF DENERVATION	EFFECT	CLINICAL IMPLICATION
Afferent	Impairment of renin-angiotensin aldosterone regulation	Hypertension
	Impairment of normal vasoregulatory response to changing cardiac filling pressures	Hypertension
	Elimination of subjective symptom of angina during ischemia	Recipient will have other symptoms of ischemia, such as shortness of breath, fatigue, decreased exercise tolerance.
Efferent	Parasympathetic: loss of vagally-mediated tone results in higher resting heart rate (approximately 100 beats per minute)	Resting tachycardia
	Sympathetic: blunting of usual rapid changes in heart rate and contractility normally observed during exercise, hypovolemia, or vasodilation	Enhancement of ventricular performance depends upon the stimulation of beta-adrenergic receptors by circulating catecholamines. Therefore, recipients require longer warm-up and cool-down periods before and after exercise.
		Administration of beta-blocking agents may be harmful, particularly during stress situations

55. What precautions should heart transplant recipients take when exercising?

Because of the effects of denervation, heart transplant recipients require longer (10–20 minutes) warm-up and cool-down periods. Weight-lifting may be limited to a certain number of pounds. Strenuous exercise should be temporarily suspended if glucocorticoids are used to treat rejection.

56. Why are cardiac rehabilitation programs helpful for heart transplant recipients?

By attending formal outpatient cardiac rehabilitation programs, heart transplant recipients achieve the following:

- Improved peripheral oxygen use
- Increased exercise tolerance
- Education about how to exercise safely
- Greater confidence in their ability to exercise

BIBLIOGRAPHY

1. Augustine SM, Baumgartner WA, Kasper EK: Obesity and hypercholesterolemia following heart transplantation. J Transplant Coord 8:164–169, 1998.
2. Augustine SM, Masiello-Miller MM: Heart transplantation. In Nolan MT, Augustine SM (eds): Transplantation Nursing: Acute and Long-term Management, Norwalk, CT, Appleton & Lange, 1995, pp 109–140.

3. Begos DG, Franco KL, Baldwin JC, et al: Optimal timing and indications for cholecystectomy in cardiac transplant patients. World J Surg 19:661–667, 1995.
4. Berry GJ, Billingham ME: Pathology of human cardiac transplantation. In Baumgartner WA, Reitz B, Kasper E, Theodore J (eds): Heart and Lung Transplantation, 2nd ed. Philadelphia, W.B. Saunders, 2002, pp 286–306.
5. Billingham ME, Cary NR, Hammond ME, et al: A working formulation for the standardization of nomenclature in the diagnosis of heart and lung rejection: Heart rejection study group. J Heart Lung Transplant 9:587–593, 1990.
6. Blum A, Aravot D: Heart transplantation: An update. Clin Cardiol 19:930–938, 1995.
7. Brann WM, Bennett LE, Keck BM, et al: Morbidity, functional status, and immunosuppressive therapy after heart transplantation: An analysis of the Joint International Society for Heart and Lung Transplantation/United Network for Organ Sharing Thoracic Registry. J Heart Lung Transplant 17:374–382, 1998.
8. Cupples SA, Boyce SW, Stamou SC: Heart transplantation. In Cupples SA, Ohler L, (eds): Solid Organ Transplantation: A Handbook for Primary Health Care Providers. New York, Springer Publishing, 2002, pp 146–188.
9. Cupples SA, Spruill LC: Evaluation criteria for the pretransplant patient. Crit Care Nurs Clin North Am 12:35–47. 2000.
10. Hosenpud JD, Bennett LE, Keck BM, et al: The registry of the International Society for Heart and Lung Transplantation: Seventeenth official report—2000. J Heart Lung Transplant 19:909–931. 2000.
11. Hunt S: Heart transplant recipient management. In Baumgartner WA, Reitz B, Kasper E, Theodore J (eds): Heart and Lung Transplantation, 2nd ed. Philadelphia, W.B. Saunders, 2002, pp 427–433.
12. Lake KL: Management of posttransplant obesity and hyperlipidemia. In Emery RW, Miller LW (eds): Handbook of Cardiac Transplantation. Philadelphia, Hanley & Belfus, 1996, pp 147–164.
13. Miller LW: Listing criteria for cardiac transplantation. Transplantation 66:947–951, 1998.
14. Miller LW, Schlant RC, Kobashigawa J, et al: 24th Bethesda conference on cardiac transplantation: Task force 5—complications. J Am Coll Cardiol 22:41–54, 1993.
15. Mudge GH, Goldstein S, Addonizio LJ, et al: 24th Bethesda conference on cardiac transplantation: Task force 3—recipient guidelines. J Am Coll Cardiol 22:21–30, 1993.
16. Ohler L, Morris KH, McCauley MF, et al: Cardiac transplantation: A review for critical care nurses. J Intensive Care Med 9:211–226, 1994.
17. Olbrisch ME, Levenson JL: Psychosocial evaluation of heart transplant candidates: An international survey of process, criteria and outcomes. J Heart Lung Transplant 10:948–955, 1991.
18. Penn I: Incidence and treatment of neoplasia after transplantation. J Heart Lung Transplant 12:S328–S336, 1993.
19. Penn I: Tumors after renal and cardiac transplantation. Hematol/Oncol Clin North Am 7(2):431–445, 1993.
20. Petrovic LM, Demetris AJ, Banner B, et al: Rejection of solid organ allografts: An overview of mechanisms and morphology. In Makowka L, Sher L (eds): Handbook of Organ Transplantation. Landes, TX, Ortho Biotech, 1995, pp 397–443.
21. Rickenbacher PR, Hunt SA: Long-term complications of transplantation. In Emery RW, Miller LW (eds): Handbook of Cardiac Transplantation. Philadelphia, Hanley & Belfus, 1996, pp 201–216.
22. Rohrer KS: Transplantation immunology. In Nolan MT, Augustine SM (eds.): Transplantation Nursing: Acute and Long-term Management, Norwalk, CT, Appleton & Lange, 1995, pp 1–15.
23. Rourke TK, Droogan MT, Ohler L: Heart transplantation: State of the art. AACN Clin Issues 10:185–201, 1996.
24. Tolman DE, Taylor DO, Olsen, SL, et al: Heart transplantation. In Makowa L, Sher L (eds): Handbook of Organ Transplantation. Austin, TX, Landes, 1995, pp 107–131.
25. Wagoner LE: Management of the cardiac transplant recipient: Roles of the transplant cardiologist and primary care physician. Am J Med Sci 314:173–184, 1997.
26. Weis M., von Scheidt W: Cardiac allograft vasculopathy: A review. Circulation 96: 2069–2077, 1997.

10. VENTRICULAR ASSIST DEVICES AS A BRIDGE TO CARDIAC TRANSPLANTATION:
A Comprehensive Overview of Device and Patient Management

Leslie C. Sweet, RN, BSN, and Lori Coleman, RN, CPTC

1. What is a ventricular assist device?

A ventricular assist device (VAD) is a surgically implanted mechanical circulatory support device (MCSD) that assists the native heart in sustaining adequate systemic circulation. The VAD may simply augment the native heart function or completely replace it. In the latter setting, the heart serves to funnel blood directly into the mechanical pump. The VAD is implanted in an effort to unload the failing heart until it can recover its native function or until a more definitive therapy can be provided (e.g., implantation of a suitable donor organ for cardiac transplant candidates).

2. How does a ventricular assist device differ from a totally artificial heart?

A VAD is connected to the native heart to augment the heart's intrinsic function. Should malfunction or failure of the VAD occur, the native heart remains intact and continues to function within its capabilities. The totally artificial heart (TAH), another type of MCSD, involves removal of the native heart at the time of implantation of the device, similar to removal of the native heart for transplantation. Because the TAH physically replaces the native heart, it is the only available mechanism to circulate the blood. Two TAH devices are currently involved in clinical trials in the United States under separate Investigational Device Exemptions (IDE) with the U.S. Food and Drug Administration (FDA). The CardioWest TAH (CardioWest Technologies, Inc., Tucson, AZ) is being implanted as a bridge to transplant in patients requiring biventricular support. The Abiocor TAH (ABIOMED, Inc., Danvers, MA) is available as an alternative to medical therapy in terminally ill patients with end-stage heart failure (ESHF) who are also deemed ineligible for cardiac transplantation. This indication constitutes end-destination therapy.

3. Why are ventricular assist devices necessary?

Over 4.5 million Americans have been diagnosed with congestive heart failure (CHF), with over 550,000 new cases diagnosed annually.[1] Although there are approximately 4000 ESHF heart transplant candidates on the waiting list at any given time, fewer than 2500 suitable donor hearts are available each year. With the epidemic levels of CHF and the disproportionate number of available donor organs for patients with medically refractory heart failure, VADs can provide an alternative therapeutic option as either short- or long-term therapy for maintaining the viability of these patients until a donor organ becomes available. In patients with VAD support for more than 30 days preceding cardiac transplantation, mortality rates at 1- and 5-years posttransplantation are 86% and 72% respectively.[2]

4. How many heart transplant candidates require ventricular assist device support as a bridge to transplant?

The first VAD implantation as a bridge to transplantation was performed in 1978. Since that time, the National Heart, Lung, and Blood Institute (NHLBI) estimates that over 4000 VADs have been implanted as a bridge to cardiac transplantation. In the United States, approximately 300 to 400 heart transplant candidates are bridged to transplantation each year.[10]

5. Is there more than one type of ventricular assist device?

Several different types of VADs are currently approved by the FDA as a bridge to cardiac transplantation. These VADs may be classified in the following ways:

- Duration of support (short-term versus long-term)
- Technical attributes of the pump (pulsatile flow versus continuous flow)
- Anatomic positioning of the pump (corporeal or internal versus paracorporeal or external).

For clarification, devices that support the left side of the heart are referred to as left ventricular assist devices (LVADs); devices that support the right side of the heart are right ventricular assist devices (RVADs); and devices that support both ventricles are biventricular assist devices (BVADs or BiVADs). The table below (columns continued on facing page) summarizes and differentiates several characteristics of the more commonly used FDA-approved VADs.

Characteristics of Several Ventricular Assist Devices

DEVICE	INDICATIONS FOR USE RELATED TO HEART FAILURE	DURATION OF SUPPORT	TYPE OF SUPPORT	PUMP FLOW DESIGN	VAD PUMP FLOWS (Range in lpm)
Bio-pump (Medtronic, Inc., Minneapolis, MN)	Bridge to myocardial recovery (postcardiotomy shock), bridge to long-term VAD support or cardiac transplant, temporary RVAD support post-LVAD implant	Short-term (usually 7–10 days)	LVAD, RVAD, or BVAD	Continuous flow	Up to 7
Abiomed BVS 5000/5000i (ABIOMED, Inc., Danvers, MA)	Bridge to myocardial recovery (viral myocarditis, postcardiotomy shock) or bridge to long-term VAD support, failed cardiac transplant, RVAD support post-LVAD implant	Short-term (usually 1–2 weeks)	LVAD, RVAD, or BVAD	Pulsatile	5000: up to 5 5000i: up to 6
HeartMate IP LVAS (Thoratec Corporation, Pleasanton, CA)	Bridge to cardiac transplantation	Long-term (months, up to several years)	LVAD only	Pulsatile	Up to 10
HeartMate XVE LVAS (Thoratec Corporation, Pleasanton, CA)	Bridge to cardiac transplantation (end-destination therapy for ESHF patients ineligible for cardiac transplant, pending final FDA approval)	Long-term (months, up to several years)	LVAD only	Pulsatile	Up to 10
Novacor LVAS (World Heart Inc., Audubon, PA)	Bridge to cardiac transplantation	Long-term (months, up to several years)	LVAD only	Pulsatile	Up to 12
Thoratec VAD (Thoratec Corporation, Pleasanton, CA)	Bridge to cardiac transplantation, bridge to myocardial recovery (postcardiotomy shock)	Short-term or long-term (weeks to several years)	LVAD, RVAD, or BVAD	Pulsatile	1.2–7.2

(Columns cont'd on facing page.)

BVAD = biventricular assist device, BSA = body surface area, BVS = biventricular support, ESHF = end-stage heart failure, FDA = U.S. Food and Drug Administration, IP = implantable pneumatic, LA = left atrium, lpm = liters per minute, LV = left ventricular, LVAD = left ventricular assist device, LVAS = left ventricular assist system, m² = meters squared, RA = right atrium, RV = right ventricle, RVAD = right ventricular assist device, VAD = ventricular assist device, XVE = extended lead vented electric.

6. How does the left ventricular assist device help the failing heart?

The physiologic benefits of an LVAD result from its ability to decrease the workload of the heart and augment the systemic circulation. An LVAD decreases myocardial workload by reducing preload and myocardial oxygen consumption. An LVAD augments systemic circulation by maintaining an adequate and consistent cardiac output, thereby improving organ perfusion. LVAD blood flow is dependent on intravascular volume and right ventricular function.

(Questions cont'd. on next page.)

Characteristics of Several Ventricular Assist Devices (Columns Continued)

PUMP PLACE-MENT	BSA REQUIRE-MENTS (m²)	INFLOW CANNULA-TION	OUTFLOW CANNULA-TION	INFLOW AND OUTFLOW VALVES	ANTI-THROMBO-EMBOLIC THERAPY	POWER SOURCE	DISCHARGE OPTIONS
Paracor-poreal	Unde-fined	RVAD: RA or RV LVAD: LA	RVAD: pulmonary artery LVAD: aorta	Valveless	Anticoagulation therapy	Electrical	Hospital use only
Paracor-poreal	> 1.3	RVAD: RA or RV LVAD: LA or LV apex	RVAD: pulmonary artery LVAD: ascending aorta	Angioflex mechanical	Anticoagulation therapy	Electrical	Hospital use only
Corporeal	> 1.5	LV apex	Ascending aorta	Porcine biopros-thetic	Antiplatelet therapy	Electrical	Hospital use only
Corporeal	> 1.5	LV apex	Ascending aorta	Porcine biopros-thetic	Antiplatelet therapy	Electrical, portable batteries	Hospital or outpatient use
Corporeal	> 1.5	LV apex	Ascending aorta	Porcine biopros-thetic	Anticoagulation and antiplatelet therapy	Electrical, portable batteries	Hospital or outpatient use
Paracor-poreal	Unde-fined	RVAD: RA or RV LVAD: LA or LV apex	RVAD: pulmonary artery LVAD: ascending aorta	Bjork-Shiley mechanical	Anticoagulation therapy ± antiplatelet therapy	Electrical, portable driver	Hospital or medical facility (home use pending FDA approval)

BVAD = biventricular assist device, BSA = body surface area, BVS = biventricular support, ESHF = end-stage heart failure, FDA = U.S. Food and Drug Administration, IP = implantable pneumatic, LA = left atrium, lpm = liters per minute, LV = left ventricular, LVAD = left ventricular assist device, LVAS = left ventricular assist system, m² = meters squared, RA = right atrium, RV = right ventricle, RVAD = right ventricular assist device, VAD = ventricular assist device, XVE = extended lead vented electric.

7. How does the right ventricular assist device help the failing heart?

As the LVAD supports the left ventricle (LV), the RVAD supports the right ventricle (RV). By unloading the RV and augmenting pulmonary circulation, RVAD placement provides the RV an opportunity for myocardial recovery without compromising right-sided cardiac output. RV failure, which occurs less frequently than LV failure, may be precipitated by several pathophysiologic mechanisms, including myocardial infarctions of the RV, pulmonary hypertension, and viral myocarditis. RV failure may also be precipitated by implantation of an LVAD, secondary to the physiologic changes associated with unloading the LV.

8. What are the clinical applications of ventricular assist devices?

The following table summarizes the current clinical uses of VADs (LVADs and/or RVADs):

CLINICAL APPLICATION	DEVICE FUNCTION
Bridge to cardiac transplantation	Provides circulatory support until a suitable donor organ becomes available.
Bridge to myocardial recovery	Provides circulatory support until the myocardium recovers adequate native function.
Bridge to a bridge	Provides short-term circulatory support until a long-term VAD can be implanted as a bridge to transplant.
Destination therapy	Provides permanent circulatory support as an alternative to maximal medical therapy in ESHF patients deemed ineligible for cardiac transplantation. (Only the HeartMate XVE LVAS has FDA panel recommendation for approval for this indication at this time.)

ESHF = end-stage heart failure, FDA = U.S. Food and Drug Administration, LVAS = left ventricular assist system, VAD = ventricular assist device, VE = extended lead vented electric.

9. When should congestive heart failure patients be considered for ventricular assist device implantation?

Consideration of eligibility for VAD implantation involves evaluation of clinical parameters, including cardiac hemodynamics as indicators of myocardial function and multisystem organ function. This evaluation is balanced with individual institutional parameters, such as the availability of donor organs and mean waiting times in the local area. Historically, patients were considered for VAD implantation in emergent situations when survival of the patient to transplant appeared unlikely. The current trend is to consider a more elective implantation to minimize the morbidity and mortality associated with the clinical deterioration of the emergent patient. Given the magnitude of this surgical procedure, the decision regarding the timing of VAD implantation must take into consideration the patient's current clinical status (i.e., whether the patient has adequate multisystem organ function to survive the complex surgery and postoperative course) and rate of deterioration (i.e., whether the patient can survive until a suitable donor heart becomes available).

Patients undergoing initial evaluation for cardiac transplantation may benefit from preliminary screening for VAD eligibility to identify treatment options should medically refractory heart failure develop before a suitable donor organ becomes available. The screening is specifically applicable to patients with common blood types (e.g., blood type O) in regions with few donor organs. An initial awareness of potential advantages or limitations of device use in a particular patient may influence the consideration of VAD implant, particularly with respect to timing of the implantation and device selection.

Emergent evaluation for VAD placement should be initiated when pharmacologic interventions become less effective and the heart failure becomes medically refractory. This may occur not only in eligible transplant candidates, but also in patients not previously requiring transplant evaluation, such as those experiencing acute postcardiotomy shock or those who present in the emergency department in acute cardiogenic shock, as is seen in viral myocarditis or postpartum cardiomyopathy. In the latter settings, a temporary VAD may be implanted, allowing stabilization of the patient until heart transplant eligibility is confirmed. A permanent VAD may be implanted later if the patient's heart failure remains refractory and requires long-term bridge support.

Elective implantation of a VAD allows time for maximizing the patient's clinical status before the major implant surgery. Whether elective or emergent, VAD implantation before the onset of irreversible end-organ failure secondary to prolonged hypoperfusion is preferable. Patients with irreversible end-organ failure glean little benefit from a well-functioning VAD because ultimately they likely will succumb to the other comorbidities such as multisystem organ failure (MSOF) or sepsis. Preoperative evaluation of systemic organ function and the identification of any preoperative infections are pivotal considerations before VAD implantation.

Earlier clinical trials with VAD implantation had strict hemodynamic selection criteria. Today, with hemodynamic criteria used as general guidelines, VAD implantation is considered in the following settings:

- Cardiac transplant candidate
- Decompensated cardiomyopathy (ischemic, idiopathic, viral myocarditis, postpartum) refractory to maximal medical therapy, including inotropic agents, with or without intraaortic balloon pump (IABP) support with consideration of the following specific clinical indicators:[11]
    - $CI < 2$ L/min/m^2
    - Systolic blood pressure < 80 mmHg (mean arterial pressure < 65 mmHg)
    - Pulmonary capillary wedge > 20 mmHg
    - Systemic vascular resistance > 2100 dynes/s/cm^5
    - Urine output < 20 ml/hr despite diuretic therapy
- Acute myocardial infarction with cardiogenic shock
- Inability to wean from cardiopulmonary bypass
- Refractory ventricular arrhythmias.

LVAD patients with severe right ventricular failure may also need to be evaluated for placement of an RVAD. The LVAD performance will be severely compromised if the RV is unable to adequately eject blood through the pulmonary vascular bed to the left atrium (LA) and ventricle. It is possible that a patient undergoing LVAD implant only may subsequently and unexpectedly require RVAD support because of the physiologic effects on the RV secondary to unloading the LV. Depending on the myocardial reserve of the RV, the RVAD support may be either short- or long-term. Additionally, RV failure may be present independent of LV failure. In either scenario, the RV is evaluated for myocardial recovery after 1–2 weeks of RVAD support, at which time the RVAD is weaned and explanted, or, if necessary, converted to a more long-term VAD, providing BVAD support in the patient with irreversible biventricular failure.

Long-term BVAD support occurs infrequently because the incidence of irreversible biventricular failure is relatively low. However, the occasional patient with concomitant LV failure and refractory ventricular tachyarrhythmia may also ultimately require BVAD support if the arrhythmic RV is unable to adequately fill and subsequently eject blood to the LV. In such cases, patients with BVAD support may remain in sustained ventricular tachycardia or fibrillation without significant hemodynamic or clinical decompensation.

10. What are the contraindications to left ventricular assist device placement in a transplant candidate?

Contraindications to LVAD placement typically include the following:

CONTRAINDICATION	RATIONALE
Inadequate body surface area	Results in inability to implant corporeal VADs because of the size constraints of the pumps (usually if BSA is < 1.5 m^2).
Aortic valve incompetence	Results in a "continuous loop" of blood circulation between the pump, the aorta, and the regurgitant blood flow back to the left ventricle, with compromised forward blood flow.

(Cont'd. on next page.)

CONTRAINDICATION	RATIONALE
Mechanical valves	Result in increased risk of thromboembolic events post-LVAD implantation.
Active sepsis	Results in increased surgical risk or risk of seeding the VAD, with increased morbidity and mortality rates.

BSA = body surface area, LVAD = left ventricular assist device, VAD = ventricular assist device.

Important considerations, but not absolute contraindications, for LVAD implantation may include the following:

RELATIVE CONTRAINDICATION	RATIONALE
Right heart failure	LVAD flows may be compromised due to inadequate RV ejection; concurrent short- or long-term RVAD support may be required if inotropic therapy is insufficient.
Patent foramen ovale	Hypoxia may result from right to left shunting following LV unloading with LVAD implant; should be closed surgically at the time of device implant.
Ischemia	Anginal symptoms or ischemic arrhythmias may persist post-LVAD implant; concurrent CABG may be performed with LVAD implant.
Arrhythmias	May result in inadequate RV ejection and subsequent inadequate LVAD flows; refractory arrhythmias may warrant BVAD implant.

BVAD = biventricular assist device, CABG = coronary artery bypass grafting, LVAD = left ventricular assist device, RV = right ventricle, RVAD = right ventricular assist device

11. What is the average duration of the ventricular assist device implantation surgery?
The duration of the VAD implantation surgery averages from 4–8 hours. Factors influencing the operative time may include:
- Type of VAD implanted (LVAD versus BVAD, corporeal versus paracorporeal)
- History of prior sternotomy and/or CABG
- Preexisting comorbidities (e.g., coagulopathy)

It is helpful for the patient's families and friends to be aware of the potential length of the procedure as they await the arrival of the patient in the intensive care unit (ICU).

12. What are the intraoperative strategies for minimizing infection in patients undergoing ventricular assist device implantation?
With implantation of an artificial device, it is imperative to minimize the potential for infection. To this end, various policies have been developed and adopted by implantation centers, which may include the following:
- Strictly enforced limited access of staff to the operating room suite in which the implant is occurring
- Use of special head-to-toe sterile suits by the implant team
- Use of strict sterile techniques while priming the pump, especially the corporeal pumps.

13. After pump implantation, what are the expected left ventricular assist device flow rates?
VAD flow ranges vary according to the device implanted, but they all provide maximum flows of 5–10 liters per minute (lpm). Typically, relatively stable intraoperative VAD flows fluctuate in the immediate postoperative period as the extravascular and intravascular volumes begin to equilibrate. Barring any concurrent medical issues, VAD flows should stabilize by the second postoperative day. Excessively high LVAD flows do not necessarily indicate improved VAD performance, but rather systemic vasodilatation associated with active sepsis.

Recognizing that LVAD flows are dependent on a patient's body surface area and the device being used, the following chart provides a reference for the expected flow rates with the HeartMate LVAS.[3]

TIME	EXPECTED FLOW RATE
Operating room	3–5 liters per minute
First 6 postoperative hours	2.5–3.5 liters per minute
Second postoperative day and thereafter	3.5–5 liters per minute

14. What postoperative complications are associated with ventricular assist device implantation?

Recognizing device-specific influences, the table below summarizes the complications typically associated with LVAD implantation. The most common complications are infection and bleeding.

EARLY POSTOPERATIVE COMPLICATIONS		LATE POSTOPERATIVE COMPLICATIONS	
• Bleeding	• Arrhythmias	• Infection/sepsis	• Psychosocial
• Hypovolemia	• Thromboembolism	• Thromboembolism	maladaptation
• Tamponade	• Neurologic events	• Neurological events	• Device-related
• Right heart failure	• Reoperation	• Hypovolemia	malfunction/failures
• Pulmonary hypertension		• Arrhythmias	

15. Of the more common types of complications experienced by ventricular assist device patients, what are the possible causes, manifestations, and interventions?

Management of complications in the postoperative VAD patient involves consideration of strategies for both standard post–open heart care as well as post-VAD implant issues. The following table is a review of patient management issues more specifically related to VAD implantation. VAD-related considerations and interventions vary depending on the type of VAD implanted.

Infection

CAUSE		MANIFESTATIONS		CONSIDERATIONS/INTERVENTIONS	
Patient-Related	VAD-Related*	Patient-Related	VAD-Related*	Patient-Related	VAD-Related*
Bacterial or fungal organisms in blood, sputum, urine, stool		Hyperthermia Sinus tachycardia Hypotension ↓ SVR Elevated WBC	Excessively high VAD flows Decreased pneumatic VAD pressure requirements	Prophylactic antimicrobial therapy, initiated intraoperatively through 48–72 hours postoperatively Administer organism-specific antibiotics Consider infectious disease consultation	
Invasive lines Surgical incisions Prolonged immobilization and hospitalization Prolonged intubation Reoperation Poor nutritional status	Transcutaneous cannula or driveline exit sites Corporeal pump pocket site Inflow/outflow valves			Frequent and thorough handwashing Remove all invasive lines and catheters as soon as possible Aggressive pulmonary toilet; extubate as soon as possible Monitor CBC and differential Monitor wound site(s) for signs of infection (redness, swelling, exudate) Monitor temperature; pan culture if > 38.3°C or 101°F	Strict sterile dressing changes using antiseptic solution (not creams) and occlusive dressing at least daily Increased frequency of dressing changes per signs of infection Consider antibiotic irrigation of exit site, including driveline tunnel where applicable

* Device-specific.

(Cont'd. on next page.)

Infection (Continued)

CAUSE		MANIFESTATIONS		CONSIDERATIONS/INTERVENTIONS	
Patient-Related	VAD-Related*	Patient-Related	VAD-Related*	Patient-Related	VAD-Related*
				Administer pharma-cologic agents to ↑ SVR and BP	
				Consider fluid resuscitation	
				Maximize nutritional status; consider small bowel feeding tube	
				Mobilize patient as soon as possible	

Bleeding

CAUSE		MANIFESTATIONS		CONSIDERATIONS/INTERVENTIONS	
Patient-Related	VAD-Related*	Patient-Related	VAD-Related*	Patient-Related	VAD-Related*
Coagulopathy related to liver dysfunction or preoperative anticoagulation	Cannulation site (inflow or outflow) Fibrinolysis related to pump	Chest tube drainage > 100 ml/hr within first 12 hours post-op	↓ VAD flows Incomplete VAD filling or or ↓ VAD SV	Monitor CBC and coagulation profiles	Use aprotinin during implant
Platelet dysfunction related to prolonged CPB time or preoperative antiplatelet therapy		Hypotension Sinus tachy-cardia ↓ CVP/LAP ↓ Hgb/Hct		Correct coagulation profiles with leuko-cyte-depleted, CMV-negative blood products (*Note:* administration of blood products may precipitate RHF, or ↑ the patient's PRA level)	
Postoperative hemolysis				Correct acidosis	
Clotting factor deficiency				Maintain slightly ele-vated filling pressures	
Hypothermia				Volume resuscitation	
History of cardiac surgery				Consider inotropic therapy	
				Administer pharmaco-logic agents as needed (e.g., protamine)	
				Consider delaying post-operative anticoagu-lation therapy	
				Increase PEEP	
				Warming blanket for hypothermia	

Tamponade

		Patient-Related	VAD-Related*	Patient-Related	
		Sudden drop in CT drainage ↑ RAP and CVP Hypotension, narrow pulse pressure Sinus tachycardia ↓ SaO$_2$ Diminished or absent periph-eral pulses Cyanosis	↓ VAD flows Incomplete VAD filling or ↓ VAD stroke volume	Reoperation to identify and stabilize bleeding site, evacuate hematomas (Note: Prophylactic antibiotics should be administered to minimize high risk of infection associated with reoperation)	

* Device-specific.

(Cont'd. on next page.)

Bleeding *(Continued)*

Tamponade *(Cont'd.)*

Patient-Related	VAD-Related*
↓ Urine output TEE confirmation of tamponade ↑ cardiac silhouette on CXR	

Hemolysis

CAUSE		MANIFESTATIONS		CONSIDERATIONS/INTERVENTIONS	
Patient-Related	VAD-Related*	Patient-Related	VAD-Related*	Patient-Related	VAD-Related*
CPB machine Blood transfusions Hepatic failure Coagulation deficiencies	Movement of blood through mechanical device	↓ Hgb/Hct Hematuria ↑ Plasma-free Hgb	↓ VAD flows (outflow) ↓ VAD inflow or ↓ SV, incomplete filling of pump	Monitor CBC, coagulation profile, plasma-free Hgb Monitor vital signs Administer blood products judiciously	Monitor VAD function, including TEE to evaluate cannulae position and VAD valve integrity Maximize filling of pump to minimize trauma to blood cells

Thromboembolism

CAUSE		MANIFESTATIONS		CONSIDERATIONS/INTERVENTIONS	
Patient-Related	VAD-Related*	Patient-Related	VAD-Related*	Patient-Related	VAD-Related*
Inadequate anticoagulation	Incomplete VAD ejection Kinking or obstruction of cannulae Low VAD flows Low VAD SV	Signs and symptoms of other organ or peripheral arterial occlusion Signs and symptoms of TIA/CVA (e.g., mental status changes, seizures, etc.) Abnormal computed tomography scan, EEG, ultrasound	Obstruction of inflow or outflow valves → decreased filling or emptying of VAD	Monitor coagulation profile Maintain adequate anticoagulation per device-specific protocols Antihypertensives Consider TEE to evaluate native heart or VAD thrombus	Prevent kinking of cannulae or pneumatic cables to optimize flow through the pump Confirm and maintain adequate VAD ejection and flows

Right Heart Failure

CAUSE		MANIFESTATIONS		CONSIDERATIONS/INTERVENTIONS	
Patient-Related	VAD-Related*	Patient-Related	VAD-Related*	Patient-Related	VAD-Related*
Preoperative risks for RHF include pulmonary edema,	Physiological implications associated with unloading the LV	↑ RAP ± ↓ LAP ↑ PVR ↓ SaO₂ Signs and symptoms of	Poor LVAD filling or ↓ SV of LVAD ↓ LVAD outflow	Inotropic agents: milrinone, epinephrine Pulmonary vasodilatory agents	Implant RVAD Adjust VAD parameters, when possible, to maximize forward flow

* Device-specific.   *(Cont'd. on next page.)*

Right Heart Failure (Continued)

CAUSE		MANIFESTATIONS		CONSIDERATIONS/INTERVENTIONS	
Patient-Related	VAD-Related*	Patient-Related	VAD-Related*	Patient-Related	VAD-Related*
(cont'd.) ↑ temperature, ↑ inotropic therapy Bleeding Multiple blood transfusions → volume overload → ↑ PVR → RHF Pulmonary HTN Pulmonary infarct RV infarct or septal defects Dysrhythmias		*(cont'd.)* RHF: liver congestion, jaundice, peripheral edema Atrial arrhythmias Per TEE: dilated RV, acute TR, inadequate filling of LA/LV, leftward septal shift		*(cont'd.)* (including NO) Hyperventilation, especially patients with ↑ PVR Fluid management to avoid overloading the RV Judicious use of blood transfusions for bleeding and anemia issues	
				Consider TEE to evaluate native heart and VAD function	

Dysrhythmias

CAUSE		MANIFESTATIONS		CONSIDERATIONS/INTERVENTIONS	
Patient-Related	VAD-Related*	Patient-Related	VAD-Related*	Patient-Related	VAD-Related*
Myocardial ischemia or infarction Drug toxicity Hypoxia Electrolyte imbalance Invasive monitoring lines Response to a systemic problem	Manipulation or irritability of native ventricle related to device cannulation	Dysrhythmias Hypotension Shortness of breath Deterioration in mental status Thrombus formation in native heart Pulmonary edema	↓ VAD flows	Assess patient to evaluate clinical/hemodynamic significance of dysrhythmia Monitor and correct electrolyte balances Wean inotropic support as soon as possible Remove invasive cardiac monitoring lines Consider antiarrhythmic pharmacologic agents Electrical cardioversion Consider anticoagulation therapy for dysrhythmia	Assess VAD for compromised performance If patient is on LVAD and rhythm remains refractory, may need to implant RVAD Depending on the type of dysrhythmia and VAD support, may not need to cardiovert if VAD keeps patient hemodynamically stable

Device-Related Issues

	CAUSE		CONSIDERATIONS/INTERVENTIONS	
Condition	Patient-Related	VAD-Related*	Patient-Related	VAD-Related*
Incomplete filling Low SV	Bleeding Cardiac tamponade Hypovolemia RHF in LVAD implant	Cannulae position Inflow cannula obstruction or or kinking	Reposition patient Reoperation for bleeding or tamponade	Adjust device parameters to maximize filling (↓ rate, ↑ vacuum, ↓ EJD, ↓ % systole)

* Device-specific.

(Cont'd. on next page.)

Device-Related Issues *(Continued)*

	CAUSE		CONSIDERATIONS/INTERVENTIONS	
Condition	Patient-Related	VAD Related*	Patient-Related	VAD-Related*
	RV ischemia Dysrhythmia Myocardial recovery Pulmonary HTN	Inflow valve obstruction Incorrect adjustment of VAD parameters ($\uparrow$ rate, $\uparrow$ EJD, $\downarrow$ vacuum, $\uparrow$ % systole) Incorrect positioning of paracorporeal VADs	Volume resuscitation Inotropic agents Pulmonary vasodilators Antiarrhythmic agents Cardioversion Aggressive anticoagulation for persistent low flow states Monitor patient vital signs and urine output to confirm adequate perfusion Perform echocardiogram to evaluate native heart and VAD function	Verify cannulae are free of kinking; reposition paracorporeal pump as needed Verify pneumatic line is free of kinking, air leak, or condensation accumulation Verify vent line is free of kinking or obstruction Consider RVAD implantation in LVAD-supported patient Consider exchanging cables, controllers, consoles
Incomplete emptying Low flow (output)	Systemic HTN, specifically with low output	Cannulae position Outflow cannula obstruction or kinking Outflow valve obstruction Pneumatic cable disconnect, obstruction, or air leak ($\rightarrow \uparrow$ pump rate, $\downarrow$ SV, $\uparrow$ venting) Incorrect adjustment of VAD parameters ($\downarrow$ eject pressure, $\downarrow$ rate, $\downarrow$ EJD, $\downarrow$ % systole) Incorrect positioning of paracorporeal VADs	Antihypertensives	Adjust device parameters to maximize pump emptying ($\uparrow$ ejection pressures, $\uparrow$ pump rate, $\uparrow$ % systole, $\uparrow$ EJD) Be prepared to manually pump if needed
High flow (output)	Aortic regurgitation Sepsis	Inflow valve regurgitation or incompetence	Echocardiogram to evaluate integrity of both native and device valves Monitor temperature; pan culture if > 38.3°C or 101°F Treat infections with culture-sensitive antibiotics	Consider changing pump mode from automatic/adjustable to fixed at a lower, controlled rate with a lower output as tolerated

Device Malfunction

	CAUSE		MANIFESTATIONS		CONSIDERATIONS/INTERVENTIONS
Patient-Related	VAD-Related*	Patient-Related	VAD-Related*	Patient-Related	VAD-Related*
Patient mismanagement of the pump	Motor failure of corporeal VAD Kink or air leak of pneumatic cables Kink or obstruction of vent line	Decompensating hemodynamics and associated signs and symptoms (e.g. altered LOC, cool and clammy extremities, cyanosis)	Audible or visual alarm status Absence of visual or audible indicators of pump function Severely low to no VAD filling (SV) or emptying (flow or output)	Volume resuscitation Pharmacologic support, including inotropic and chronotropic therapy	Prepare to manually pump to avoid blood stasis and subsequent clotting Consider systemic anticoagulation Check all connections

* Device-specific.   *(Cont'd. on next page.)*

Device Malfunction (Continued)

CAUSE		MANIFESTATIONS		CONSIDERATIONS/INTERVENTIONS	
Patient-Related	VAD-Related*	Patient-Related	VAD-Related*	Patient-Related	VAD-Related*
	Fluid in vent port Fractured wires in driveline cables Console malfunction Power source malfunction				Correct pneumatic or vent line obstructions Replace consoles, controllers, and/or cables Replace power source Access back-up consoles, etc. Consider exchanging the pump, specifically paracorporeal (increased risk of mortality associated with exchanging corporeal pumps)

* Device-specific.
BP = blood pressure, CBC = complete blood count, CMV = cytomegalovirus, CPB = cardiopulmonary bypass, CT = chest tube(s), CVA = cerebrovascular accident, CVP = central venous pressure, CXR = chest x-ray, EEG = electroencephalogram, EJD = ejection duration, Hct = hematocrit, Hgb = hemoglobin, HTN = hypertension, LA = left atrium, LAP = left atrial pressure, LOC = level of consciousness, LV = left ventricle, LVAD = left ventricular assist device, ml/hr = milliliters per hour, NO = nitric oxide, PEEP = positive end-expiratory pressure, PRA = panel reactive antibody, PVR = pulmonary vascular resistance, RAP = right atrial pressure, RHF = right heart failure, RV = right ventricle, RVAD = right ventricular assist device, SaO$_2$ = oxygen saturation, SV = stroke volume, SVR = systemic vascular resistance, TEE = transesophageal echocardiogram, TIA = transient ischemic attack, TR = tricuspid regurgitation, VAD = ventricular assist device, WBC = white blood cell.

16. Can patients with left ventricular assist devices be defibrillated?

Yes, patients with LVADs can be defibrillated. Depending on the device, connections between the pump and controllers or consoles may require separation before cardioversion or countershock to protect the external electronic components. The connections must be reestablished as soon as possible to reinitiate pump function, thereby minimizing blood stasis and subsequent blood clot formation within the pump.

17. Can patients receive cardiopulmonary resuscitation?

Regardless of which device is implanted, pharmacologic and pacing interventions are acceptable. However, external compressions of the heart are typically undesirable because of potential pump or cannulae dislodgement and subsequent bleeding complications. Instead, manual pumping of the device is initiated to optimize cardiac output.

18. Can patients be weaned from a ventricular assist device?

The concept of weaning transplant candidates from VAD support is still evolving. The long-term benefits and successes have been inconsistent, probably because of multiple variables, including the initial ESHF pathology. Viral myocarditis patients may be most eligible for consideration because their pathology is typically acute and potentially reversible, as may acute myocardial infarction or postcardiotomy shock patients. These patients typically have a short-term VAD (e.g., Abiomed BVS 5000/5000*i* [ABIOMED, Inc., Danvers, MA] or the Bio-Pump [Medtronic, Inc., Minneapolis, MN]) implanted initially so that they may be more easily evaluated for myocardial recovery and potential weaning. With the long-term VADs, consideration for weaning is more complicated. Some implantation centers have developed weaning protocols, based on the results of echocardiograms or neurohormonal measurements, to evaluate the potential for permanent myocardial recovery that would warrant explantation of the device.

19. What are the goals of patient management?

The postoperative care of a patient with an LVAD involves a multidisciplinary approach. Specific postoperative goals for the patient with an LVAD include the following:

- Maintain adequate preload so as to maintain optimal VAD output.
- Wean intravenous pharmacologic support as tolerated.
- Extubate and remove invasive lines promptly.
- Avoid hypertension that may affect pump output; use pharmacological agents as necessary.
- Prevent infection, specifically related to the driveline or cannulae exit site(s).
- Optimize nutritional status to promote healing and prevent infection; monitor albumin and prealbumin levels.
- Maximize physical rehabilitation with the support of occupational and physical therapists.
- Maximize psychosocial support, which may include professional counseling.
- Educate the long-term VAD patient and significant others on VAD management and troubleshooting in anticipation of hospital discharge while on support.

20. Specifically, what is involved with ventricular assist device monitoring?

VAD performance, which is unique for each device, typically includes monitoring and documentation of the following:

- Patient's vital signs, hemodynamics, neurological status, blood work, and urine output
- VAD function
  - Pump operation mode (e.g., automatic vs fixed)
  - Pump rate
  - Pump stroke volume
  - Pump flows
- Manually adjusted pump parameters when applicable
- Assessment of the integrity of external components, including
  - Visualization of pump filling and emptying with paracorporeal pumps
  - Presence of blood clots in paracorporeal pumps
  - Kinks or obstructions of transcutaneous cannulae or pneumatic/vent lines
  - Security of external connections.

21. What is the most common type of assist device used to bridge patients to cardiac transplantation?

Because left heart failure occurs more frequently than right heart failure, LVADs are used more frequently. The HeartMate Left Ventricular Assist System (LVAS) [Thoratec, Inc., Pleasanton, CA], which has two different designs, is the more commonly used LVAD for bridge to heart transplantation. Both designs incorporate an implantable blood pump with a percutaneous driveline cable that exits the skin and connects to an external console or system controller and power source. The original clinical design is a pneumatically driven (air-driven) system that shunts trapped air between the pump and an external console, thereby causing the pump's internal diaphragm to move blood in and out of the pump. The HeartMate implantable pneumatic LVAS (IP LVAS) requires the patient to be hospitalized while on support because of the size of the external console and the limited 30-minute battery capability.

The HeartMate Vented Electric LVAS (VE LVAS) design received FDA approval subsequent to the IP LVAS, and it has become the more popular design because of its portability. Since that time, it has undergone several design improvements and is now known as the XVE (Extended Lead Vented Electric) LVAS. The XVE LVAS, as its predecessors, is a motor-driven, implantable pump that may be converted to an air-driven system with manual pumping capabilities should mechanical failure occur. With this device, patients may connect to electricity while sleeping, but may otherwise connect to portable batteries worn in a battery holster throughout the day. This portability allows patients to more fully rehabilitate and to return home on the device and possibly even to work or school while waiting for a suitable donor organ.

One limitation of this device is that it is capable of supporting the left ventricle only. For patients with irreversible biventricular failure, the Thoratec VAD [Thoratec, Inc., Pleasanton,

CA] may be preferable because it provides short- and long-term support of both ventricles. This pneumatically driven device consists of an external pump for each side of the heart, with transcutaneous inflow and outflow cannulae for connection of the pumps to the heart and greater vessels. An electrically powered, moderately sized, external console drives the pumps. A portable driver, currently approved for use in a medical facility, is now under clinical investigation through the FDA for home use. In the interim, however, patients must remain in a medical facility capable of managing patients on the device.

22. What are the components of the vented electric left ventricular assist system?
The XVE LVAS consists of an implantable, pulsatile pump with a transcutaneous driveline, an external system controller, and an external power source (electricity or battery). The device may also be manually driven by hand pumping in case of an emergency, such as loss of power (both electrical and battery) or mechanical failure.

The blood pump contains a flexible diaphragm, which separates the motor from the blood chamber. Porcine valves are located in the inflow and outflow cannulae to ensure unidirectional blood flow through the pump. The pump is implanted subdiaphragmatically, either in a pre-peritoneal pocket or intraabdominally. The percutaneous driveline, which is typically tunneled subcutaneously to exit the right upper quadrant of the abdomen, connects the blood pump to the system controller. The driveline contains both the electrical wires that transmit information between the pump and system controller, and a vent line that allows air displacement behind the diaphragm during the pump cycle. The displaced air moves in and out of the driveline via the vent module and filter, which are anchored over the airholes of the driveline.

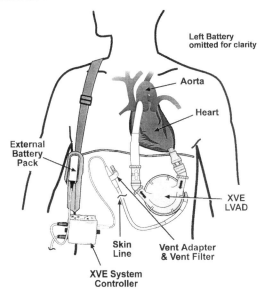

Implanted and worn components of the HeartMate XVE LVAS. (Reprinted with permission from Thoratec Corporation.)

23. What are the specific features of the blood pump for the vented electric left ventricular assist system?
The XVE LVAS weighs approximately $2\frac{1}{2}$ pounds. It consists of a titanium pump that is divided into two chambers by a flexible diaphragm. One chamber receives the oxygenated blood as it passes through the pump; the other chamber houses the pump motor. All blood-contacting surfaces of the pump are textured. The textured surfaces promote the development of a pseudointimal layering by the blood, which helps to minimize blood clot formation within the pump. The maximum

output of the device is 10 liters of blood per minute (lpm), with a stroke volume of 83 milliliters. Whereas a healthy heart ejects approximately 5 lpm, the XVE LVAS averages 5–7 lpm. The blood flow of the XVE LVAS is volume dependent, so the patient who was on fluid restrictions preimplant may be encouraged to increase fluid intake postimplant to maintain adequate pump flows.

24. How does the vented electric left ventricular assist system actually work?
The system controller is primarily responsible for pump function, as well as alarm activation when it detects problems. During normal pump function, the controller activates the motor, which rotates and displaces the diaphragm for emptying and filling of the pump. Displacement of the pump diaphragm results in pressure changes within the pump, which are similar to the internal pressure changes of the native heart during diastole and systole. These pressure changes effect the appropriate opening and closing of the unidirectional valves. The pressure changes are described as follows:
1. The blood within the left ventricle fills the pump through the inflow valve. Once the blood chamber is full, the pump motor rotates, causing vertical displacement of the flexible diaphragm.
2. The internal pump pressure exceeds the LV pressure, closing the inflow valve as "pump" systole begins.
3. There is isovolumetric pressurization as the pump pressure continues to increase but does not exceed aortic pressure. During this phase, both the inflow and outflow valves remain closed.
4. The increasing pump pressure quickly exceeds the aortic pressure, and the outflow valve opens, allowing for pump ejection (systole).
5. Pump ejection ends as the motor ceases displacing the diaphragm.
6. The diaphragm returns to its resting position. The blood pump fills as pump diastole begins, in preparation of another cycle.

25. What are the power source options for the vented electric left ventricular assist system?
Electricity or two portable batteries may power the XVE LVAS. The power base unit (PBU) is a bedside console, which connects to the system controller via a 20-foot cable. Connection of the system controller to the PBU provides electrical power to the XVE LVAS. The PBU contains an internal, back-up battery, which provides uninterrupted, interim power during power failures, allowing the patient continued pump function while safely changing to the portable batteries or the 24-hour emergency battery pack. Power failure also triggers an audible and visible alarm to alert the patient.
Connection to the PBU obviously limits the patient's mobility and, hence, is used primarily when the patient is sleeping. Otherwise, the patient may connect to two portable batteries, which are worn in a battery holster over the patient's shoulders. A pair of batteries provides 4–6 hours of power, depending on the pump rate and motor demands. When ambulating on batteries, patients are required to carry at least one extra set of back-up batteries. The system controller provides visual and audible indicators of relative battery power reserve.
The power source configurations for the Novacor LVAS [World Heart, Inc. Audubon, PA], the other long-term, implantable LVAD, are similar to those of the HeartMate XVE LVAS and include a bedside console and wearable battery packs. The Thoratec VAD, however, has a bedside console and a portable driver that resembles a large briefcase. The driver is transported using a lightweight luggage carrier. Although it is slightly more cumbersome than wearable batteries, most patients are capable of ambulating independently with the portable driver.

26. How long may a patient be supported with a vented electric left ventricular assist system?
Time to transplantation depends on the number of patients listed per blood type and donor organ availability in a particular region. However, the longest time a patient has been successfully supported on a VE LVAS is now in excess of 900 days. As with all of the currently available long-term VAD technology, factors influencing the length of support include not only donor availability, but also other patient comorbidities and management factors such as postoperative infection, coagulation issues, PRA levels (which may be elevated due to blood transfusions), and device durability.

27. Can a patient with a vented electric left ventricular assist system resume normal activities after implantation of the device?

As with all of the long-term corporeal VADs, the patient is expected to undergo significant physical rehabilitation postoperatively, depending on the extent of deconditioning before device implantation. The VAD patient should at least return to the preoperative level of activity because cardiac output and end-organ perfusion are usually significantly improved. Hence, it is imperative that occupational and physical therapy work closely with the VAD patient, beginning in the intensive care unit. It may even be possible for a patient to return to work or school after a sufficient period of recovery. Sexual activity can usually resume in 6–8 weeks or when approved by the physician.

28. What specific activities should a patient with the vented electric left ventricular assist system avoid?

Certain activities are excluded according to the type of VAD implanted. Even with the portable XVE LVAS, patients may not participate in contact sports nor in activities that involve submersion in water (e.g., bathing or swimming). In that displaced air is moving in and out of the vent filter, submersion of the vent filter in any fluid allows that liquid to be pulled into the motor chamber, potentially damaging the motor and causing pump failure. A specially designed shower kit, which protects the external components of the XVE LVAS, is available to allow patients to shower. (Patients on the external VADs, i.e., the Thoratec VAD, are usually restricted to sponge baths.) The following is a list of specific restricted activities for XVE LVAS patients:

- Participating in activities that involve submersion in water (e.g., bathing, swimming, etc.)
- Participating in sports that involve jumping, jogging, or physical contact (e.g., football)
- Sleeping on the stomach
- Touching television, computer screens, or other surfaces that can emit a potentially disruptive static charge to the system controller
- Becoming pregnant
- Driving or sitting in a passenger seat with an airbag
- Undergoing magnetic resonance imaging tests.

29. What medications may be required specifically for patients supported by the vented electric left ventricular assist system?

Medications frequently prescribed after XVE LVAS implantation are summarized in the following table:

MEDICATION	INDICATION	COMMENTS
Antiplatelet therapy (both aspirin and dipyridimole)	To minimize the potential for thromboembolic events	Warfarin is not required because of textured surfaces and tissue valves.
H_2 antagonist (e.g., ranitidine)	To prevent gastric reflux	Gastrointestinal distress, potentiated by the abdominal placement of the pump, can compromise nutritional status.
Metoclopramide	To promote upper gastric motility	Premature satiation, potentiated by abdominal placement of the pump, can compromise nutritional status.
Antihypertensive agents	To prevent hypertension	To maintain adequate XVE LVAS output, systolic blood pressure should not exceed 140 mmHg.
Diuretics	To prevent fluid overload	Third-spacing of fluid secondary to ESHF may require pharmacologic support initially as immediate postoperative extra- and intravascular volumes equilibrate.

(Cont'd. on next page.)

MEDICATION	INDICATION	COMMENTS
Antimicrobial therapy	To prevent or treat infection	Both the device and the patient are susceptible to infection. Infection may result in life-threatening sepsis.

ESHF = end-stage heart failure; XVE LVAS = extended lead vented electric left ventricular assist system.

30. If infection is one of the more common postoperative complications associated with the vented electric left ventricular assist system, what interventions can be instituted to prevent it?

INTERVENTIONS	RATIONALE
Transcutaneous tunneling of the velour-covered driveline	Maximizing the distance of the exit site to the pump pocket minimizes the potential for bacteria to seed the pocket; velour covering of driveline promotes tissue ingrowth and thereby provides a bacterial barrier.
Postoperative prophylactic systemic antibiotics for 48 hours	Prevention of iatrogenic infections in open heart surgical patient.
Prompt removal of invasive lines and drains	Prevention of iatrogenic infections in open heart surgical patient.
Daily, sterile driveline exit site dressings, including ½ strength chlorhexidine solution; surgical gowns, caps, and gloves; and occlusive dressings	Infection of the exit site may spread to the pump pocket or pump and become systemic; prophylactic topical agents should not be used because they may irritate the skin surrounding the exit site or potentiate the development of resistant organisms.
Immobilization of external driveline with modified abdominal binder	Maintains integrity of healing exit site.

31. What is involved in preparing the patient with a vented electric left ventricular assist system for discharge home?

Multidisciplinary Approach

Regardless of the implanted device, a multidisciplinary approach is crucial to a successful discharge program. The patient's physical condition, knowledge base, and support systems must be evaluated to determine eligibility for discharge. Ideally, preimplantation evaluations by the social worker, physical therapist, and psychiatrist are completed. Physical rehabilitation, with the assistance of the physical and occupational therapy teams, is initiated in the intensive care unit and continued until discharge. The ultimate goal is to return the patient to a New York Heart Association (NYHA) class of I–II prior to discharge to ensure optimal independence with daily activities, while minimizing burdens to the companion(s).

The social worker assesses both the patient and the significant others for emotional and physical needs and financial concerns. The VAD coordinator along with the social worker evaluates potential domestic structural needs. Domestic structural considerations include device technical support concerns, such as the availability of a three-prong plug (which is not controlled by a wall switch) for placement of the bedside console or, for patients dwelling in apartment complexes, the availability of an elevator versus stairs for ease of moving equipment in and out of the home. The psychiatrist or other professional counselor provides insight into strategies to optimize the patient's coping mechanisms and enhance knowledge retention regarding device and medication education.

VAD Education and Training

VAD-supported patients and their caregivers must become proficient in the daily management of the device, including troubleshooting strategies for all alarms and device failures. The necessary education is extensive and is most commonly initiated by the VAD coordinator once the patient has recovered sufficiently from surgery and can retain information. In that it is recommended that the patient have trained companions available, any interested family members, friends, or companions should be included in the training sessions. These persons may actually begin training before the postoperative patient, if so desired. Because of the emotional component associated with responsibility for device failure management, the age and maturity level of potential companions should be taken into consideration.

Maintenance of the integrity of the transcutaneous exit sites is crucial in minimizing potential exit-site infections that could ultimately progress to devastating sepsis. It is imperative, then, that patients and caregivers also be trained in the detailed dressing-change protocol. Following verbal instruction and direct observation of the dressing-change procedure, the patient and caregivers should perform this task with staff supervision before discharge.

The VAD patient and all trained companions must demonstrate competency in all areas of VAD management before discharge. Certification may include a written test and a skills' demonstration test, including not only daily management and preventive maintenance of the device, but also very specific interventions for each alarm scenario, such as back-up manual pumping of the VAD and accessing appropriate emergency response teams. In order to build the patient's confidence for handling device failures, some centers have the patient, and possibly trained companions, hand-pump the patient's VAD before discharge.

Depending on insurance constraints, many centers "wean" the VAD patient from the hospital setting by initially allowing him or her to leave the unit with a staff member, and then independently. Short day trips, followed by overnight trips away from the hospital, are recommended before hospital discharge—again, to build the confidence of both the patient and the trained companions.

32. What is involved in preparing the community for discharge of the patient with a vented electric left ventricular assist system ?

Community education is another essential component of a successful VAD patient discharge program. Decisions must be made about how to best support the discharged VAD patient with the local emergency response teams. Many centers train the patient's local emergency medical system (EMS), with the expectation that the local EMS team will be most accessible to the patient in the event of an emergency. One consideration with this plan is the feasibility of ensuring EMS VAD competency, because EMS involvement with the VAD patient is usually very infrequent.

Other centers with a hospital-based EMS or trauma response team, specifically with helicopter transport capabilities, train that team instead. The local EMS teams are notified of the presence of an LVAD patient in their region and of the 24-hour/day, 7-days/week availability of the hospital-based VAD-certified emergency response team. The expectation is that the local EMS or emergency department will stabilize the patient and the VAD-certified EMS team will arrange to transport the patient back to the implant center. Patients are advised to obtain a medical identification bracelet that identifies the type of VAD and the VAD-certified EMS dispatch contact, if applicable.

The role of the visiting nurse and the outpatient physical rehabilitation teams must also be considered before patient discharge. If these personnel are to be involved in the management of the VAD, programs must be developed to train, certify, and recertify them in order to establish and maintain their proficiency. As with the EMS programs, the fact that the patient and companions are trained on the VAD, together with the number of VAD patients in the community, may influence decisions regarding the extent of involvement of these important ancillary services. Regardless of the intricacies of VAD function, the visiting nurse may be most instrumental in supporting the patient in proper exit-site dressing care and management. Therefore, specific dressing care guidelines should be given to the visiting nurse before the patient's discharge.

The local power company is another community service organization that must be notified prior to hospital discharge of the VAD patient. The power company must be aware that a patient on a life-support system (i.e., the VAD) has been discharged to a home in their jurisdiction and that in the event of a power outage, restoration of electricity to that home is a high priority. This communication usually requires written documentation, either as a letter from the implanting surgeon or by completion of a power company form signed by the surgeon. The documentation may have to be renewed on an annual basis. Because this notification should be in place with the power company before patient discharge, the VAD coordinator needs to initiate the process, usually 2 weeks before discharge. Similarly, the patient's telephone company should be notified.

Finally, should the patient desire to return to work, training and certification of employers and/or fellow employees should ideally be completed before patient discharge and certainly before the first day of work. The extent of training should be similar to the patient's training, with the exception of issues that are specific to the home environment (e.g., driveline exit-site care). A sufficient number of people should be trained to maximize the patient's resources in the work environment. The same concepts also apply to VAD patients who desire to return to school.

33. Are there any other considerations involved in discharging the patient with a vented electric left ventricular assist system?

Before a patient is released for discharge, it may be helpful to create a checklist to ensure that all necessary procedures have been completed. The following list is not intended to be all-inclusive; each center may have individual variations.

- Has the patient and/or companion completed XVE LVAS training and certification, including exit-site care?
- Has a predischarge, two-dimensional echocardiogram been performed to evaluate native aortic valve opening with the XVE LVAS at a fixed rate of 50 beats per minute? This test may provide insight into native heart capabilities should device mechanical failure occur.
- If applicable, has the patient completed one or more day passes before discharge?
- Has a multidisciplinary group meeting occurred to ensure coverage of all aspects of the patient's discharge needs?
- Has all necessary equipment for home use of the XVE LVAS been ordered and supplied to the patient?
- Is there confirmation that the necessary domestic structural supports for the XVE LVAS (e.g., 3-prong power plug, bedside stand) have been obtained?
- Has the patient been provided with means to obtain exit-site dressing change supplies?
- Does the patient have access to a pager?
- Does the patient have emergency reference cards available with the necessary emergency contact numbers and guidelines about whom to call and when?
- If applicable, has the patient obtained a medical identification bracelet?
- Has the patient's local EMS been notified of the patient's discharge date? Has the responsible emergency response team been trained and certified on the device (either local or hospital-based)?
- Have the telephone and electrical power companies been notified of the patient's discharge date?
- Has the patient been provided with a follow-up appointment schedule?

34. What are the follow-up requirements for ventricular assist device patients who are discharged home?

Each institution establishes its individual follow-up plan for discharged VAD patients. Because these patients have VADs implanted as a bridge to cardiac transplantation, it may be helpful to establish a VAD follow-up regimen that mirrors the early posttransplant follow-up regimen, starting with weekly visits and extending to monthly visits. It is also important to instruct patients on clinical situations that warrant office visits separate from the scheduled times (e.g., signs of infection or altered integrity of the driveline exit site, significant or persistent device alarms or device failure). Patients are expected to arrive for the clinic visits with the required emergency back-up supplies, including the emergency hand pump, extra batteries, and a back-up system controller. Incorporated into the office visits are the following assessments:

- Clinical status of the patient, including blood pressure measurement
- Integrity and performance of the device (a hospital PBU should be available for documentation of the VAD performance and parameters)
- Integrity of the driveline exit site, including the healing process and signs of infection
- Assessment of emergency back-up supplies, including integrity of the hand pump and system controller
- Device supplies or inventory needs for the patient at home
- Patient's recall of device and alarm management issues
- Psychosocial needs of the patient and companions as they adapt to the discharge status.

35. What are the limitations of the currently available bridge-to-transplant ventricular assist devices?

The primary limitations of VADs are as follows:
- Minimum BSA requirements that may exclude some patients from long-term VAD support because of the size of the implanted pumps.
- Exit-site infections due to the size and/or rigidity of the percutaneous drivelines or cannulae
- Bleeding complications that may require reoperation or blood transfusions, which may subsequently increase panel-reactive antibody (PRA) levels
- Thromboembolic events that may result in contraindications to transplantation (e.g., a cerebral vascular accident with irreversible deficits)
- Device failures and/or durability issues that may limit the duration of support or require high-risk surgical replacement of the VAD.

It is hoped that future technological advancements, some of which are incorporated in devices presently used in European and U.S. investigational trials, will minimize the comorbidities and mortality rates associated with existing assist devices. In the interim, the current LVAD technology offers a viable option for the transplant candidate whose end-stage heart failure becomes refractory to maximal medical therapy.

BIBLIOGRAPHY

1. American Heart Association: Heart and Stroke Statistical Update. Dallas, TX, American Heart Association, 2002.
2. Cattaneo SM, Greene PS: Mechanical circulatory assistance before heart transplantation. In Baumgartner WA, Reitz B, Kasper E, Theodore J (eds): Heart and Lung Transplantation, 2nd ed. Philadelphia, Saunders, 2002, pp 120–132.
3. Duke T, Perna J: The ventricular assist device as a bridge to cardiac transplantation. AACN Clin Issues 10:217–228, 1999.
4. Frazier OH, Rose EA, Oz MC, et al: Multicenter clinical evaluation of the HeartMate vented electric left ventricular assist system in patients awaiting heart transplantation. J Thorac Cardiovasc Surg 122:1186-1195, 2001.
5. Holman WL, Ormaza S, Seemuth K, et al: How to run an outpatient VAD program: Overview. Am Soc Artif Intern Organs J 47:588–589, 2001.
6. Jessup M: Mechanical cardiac-support devices-dreams and devilish details. N Engl J Med 345:1490–1492, 2001.
7. Myers TJ, Catanese KA, Vargo RL, Dresslers DK: Extended cardiac support with a portable left ventricular assist system in the home. Am Soc Artif Intern Organs J 42:M576–M579, 1996.
8. Richenbacher WE, Seemuth SC: Hospital discharge for the ventricular assist device patient: Historical perspective and description of a successful program. Am Soc Artif Intern Organs J 47:590–595, 2001.
9. Seemuth SC, Richenbacher WE: Education of the ventricular assist device patient's community services. Am Soc Artif Intern Organs J 47:596–601, 2001.
10. Stevenson LW, Kormos RL, Bourge RC, et al: Mechanical cardiac support 2000: Current applications and future trial design. J Am Coll Cardiol 37:340–370, 2001.
11. Williams MR, Oz MC: Indications and patient selection for mechanical ventricular assistance. Ann Thorac Surg 71:S86–S91, 2001.

11. KIDNEY TRANSPLANTATION

Mary Jo Holechek, MS, CRNP, CNN, and Melinda M. Paredes, RN, MS

1. Name the most common causes of end-stage renal disease in the United States.

Diabetes, hypertension, and glomerulonephritis are the three most common causes of end-stage renal disease (ESRD). Diabetes mellitus is now the number one cause of ESRD, accounting for 43% of patients who started dialysis in 1998. Hypertension was responsible for 23% of patients who began dialysis that year and glomerulonephritis for 12%.[20] Recent studies have shown that genetic predisposition, age, elevated blood pressure, gender, hyperglycemia, smoking, and ethnicity can contribute to the development and progression of nephropathy. Some factors are amenable to intervention. Patients must be taught about the variables that they can control to some extent, including high blood pressure and elevated blood glucose levels.

2. What are the median waiting times by blood group for potential kidney transplant candidates?

The median waiting time is the amount of time it takes for 50% of the individuals registered on the cadaveric transplant list for a kidney in a specific blood group to actually be transplanted. Waiting times vary from blood group to blood group. Median waiting times by blood group give patients a gross estimate of how long the wait might be to receive a cadaveric organ.

BLOOD TYPE	MEDIAN WAITING TIME (DAYS)
O	1213
A	862
B	1426
AB	479

From United Network for Organ Sharing: 2000 Annual Data Report: The US Scientific Registry of Transplant Recipients and the Organ Transplantation Network: Transplant Data 1990–1999. Rockville, MD, United Network for Organ Sharing, 2000.

Patients with blood types B and O wait the longest for a cadaveric transplant.

3. Why are the waiting times for cadaveric renal transplants so long?

The waiting times are prolonged because the number of candidates awaiting transplantation far exceeds the number of available donors. At the end of 1999, approximately 46,000 candidates were waiting for a cadaveric renal transplant. During that year about 8000 cadaveric transplants and 4500 living-donor transplants were done. Only about 27% of patients awaiting transplantation were actually transplanted. Unless new strategies are developed to increase both the cadaveric- and living-donor pools, there will always be great disparity between the number of patients awaiting transplantation and the number of patients actually transplanted. Because of long waiting times, many patients die before receiving a transplant. In 1999, 3073 candidates died while waiting for a transplant.[20]

4. What can be done to decrease the prolonged waiting times for cadaveric renal transplants?

Transplant centers must be vigilant in identifying and scientifically testing alternative cadaveric-donor sources. The use of non–heart-beating donors is one strategy. A non–heart-beating donor (NHBD) does not meet strict brain death criteria but has sustained an injury from which there is no hope of recovery. The individual is allowed to die naturally after the family has decided to withdraw life support. When the donor is pronounced dead, 4–10 minutes are allowed to elapse before the procurement procedure can proceed. Unlike standard cadaveric donation, NHBD donation requires a period before procurement when the organs are not perfused, which can result in significant acute tubular necrosis (ATN) and delayed function. Nevertheless, several studies have found that graft survival rates for standard cadaveric-donor recipients and NHBD recipients are similar, but recipients of NHBD organs require dialysis more frequently in the immediate postoperative period and have longer hospital stays.

Another strategy to increase the cadaveric organ donor pool is to use marginal donors whose problems might normally preclude the use of their organs—problems such as a history of hypertension, diabetes, substance abuse, or hepatitis C; age outside the normal limits for transplantation; procurement injuries; and prolonged cold (ischemic) times.

For donors with a history of diabetes and hypertension, the donor kidneys can be biopsied, and if they are found to have no or limited damage (i.e., < 20% sclerotic glomeruli) related to the chronic disease, the organs can be offered for transplantation. Organs from donors with a history of substance abuse can be used if current serologies are negative for diseases such as HIV, hepatitis B, and hepatitis C and if potential recipients are informed about the slight risk that potential donors' serologies have not yet converted to positive.

If a donor has hepatitis C, a kidney can be offered to a potential recipient with a history of hepatitis C. The recipient must be informed of the chance that a different strain of hepatitis C might be contracted, but that these kidneys usually function well and present no long-term problems. Patients willing to accept a hepatitis C kidney often have much shorter waiting times.

Generally, cadaveric kidney donors should be at least 2 years old and less than 65 years old; but in certain circumstances, organs from younger and older donors can be used. If kidneys are used from donors less than 2 years old, both kidneys should be transplanted into the same recipient. A skilled surgeon is essential for this complex surgery, and heparinization is required postoperatively to prevent thrombosis of the small pediatric vessels. A capsulotomy is also done on the kidneys to ensure that they will not be compressed by the capsule as they increase in size rapidly. Because the capsule facilitates post-biopsy hemostasis, the absence of the capsule puts the patient at greater risk for bleeding if a biopsy is needed. To minimize the risk of rejection and the need for biopsy, the recipients of pediatric kidneys are usually given daclizumab or another drug for induction. Pediatric kidneys take weeks to months to achieve the nephron mass necessary to support adult renal function, so dialysis is usually required for a period after surgery.

Kidneys from older donors have decreased nephron mass and should be biopsied and pumped before being used for renal transplantation. If the nephron mass in one of the kidneys is inadequate but the two kidneys collectively have adequate nephron mass, the kidneys can be offered together to one recipient. This type of transplant is called a two-for-one because both kidneys are used.

Organs that sustain injury at the time of procurement are often discarded, but a skilled surgeon should examine them before this occurs. Sometimes vessel lacerations and ureteral damage can be repaired, and the organs can then be used as transplants. The potential recipient must be informed of any risks associated with the repairs that were done.

Traditionally, it is preferred that kidneys be transplanted within 24–36 hours after they are procured, but with the complex system involved in organ distribution this is not always possible. Kidneys that are beyond the usual time limits can be biopsied and pumped to assess their function. If they do well, then the ischemic time should not be a limiting factor. The greater the ischemic time, the more likely that there will be ATN initially. The ATN can last weeks to a month or more. Kidneys with ischemic times of 40 hours or more are being transplanted successfully, but dialysis is often required for several weeks.

Marginal donors can provide excellent organs, but great care must be taken to examine each donor and recipient carefully. The surgeon must ensure that the benefits outweigh the risks and that the recipient is fully informed.

5. What is being done to increase living kidney donation?
Increasing the number of living donors has the potential to decrease the number of patients on the cadaveric waiting list. Living unrelated-donor and altruistic-donor programs are being

used to encourage more living donation. Initially, only blood relatives were considered as donors for family members. Blood relatives were thought to provide the best matched kidneys and were likely to donate freely without coercion or concerns about ethical issues. However, many patients do not have close family members or their family members are unable to donate for various reasons. This has led to the initiation of living unrelated-donor programs through which unrelated individuals can donate to potential transplant recipients. The donors are usually spouses, friends, neighbors, or church members, but they can be strangers (altruistic donors). As with any transplant, the donor must receive medical and psychosocial clearance for the transplantation to proceed. The tissue match is not critical. The short cold time afforded by these elective transplantations is what makes them so successful.

For many potential donors, concerns about postoperative pain, time lost from work and child- or elder-care, physical disability, financial disincentives, and cosmetic concerns have impeded them from offering to be a donor for a family member, friend, or unknown recipient. With these factors in mind, Kavoussi and Ratner, building on the work of Clayman and Gill, developed the first human laparoscopic donor nephrectomy procedure. The donor kidney can be removed using minimally invasive laparoscopic surgical procedures. The laparoscopic donor procedure is associated with less pain than the conventional nephrectomy procedure and requires a shorter hospital stay. Donors are able to resume activities of daily living and return to work sooner. There are only four small incisions made during this surgery. As a result of this procedure, many individuals who never would have agreed to be organ donors have donated. In some centers this procedure had increased living organ donation rates by 100%.

6. How is a laparoscopic donor nephrectomy done?

In 95% of cases the left kidney is removed because it is technically easier. The donor is placed on the right side in the lateral decubitus position with the hips rolled slightly to the posterior. Three ports are inserted through which the camera and laparoscopic equipment are introduced into the abdominal cavity. The three 5–10 mm port incisions are made at the following locations: (1) lateral to the rectus muscle, halfway between the umbilicus and iliac crest; (2) at the umbilicus (primary camera port); and (3) halfway between the umbilicus and the xiphoid process.

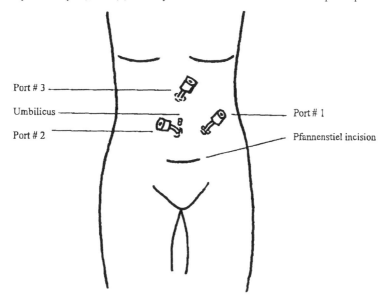

Positioning of 3 ports for the laparoscopic donor nephrectomy procedure: Port #2 is the primary camera port. The remaining ports are for the introduction of instruments. The Pfannenstiel incision is below Port #2 and the umbilicus.

After the ports are sutured in place, the actual procedure can begin. With the use of a Veress needle, CO_2 is instilled to float the abdominal organs, allowing for maximal visualization and preventing organ perforation. Using the camera via the umbilical port and forceps and scissors through the other ports, the surgeon releases the kidney from surrounding structures including the spleen, colon, and Gerota's fascia. The renal vein and artery are identified and separated from surrounding structures. The ureter is located and released from adjacent structures. Double clips are applied to the ureter; then the ureter is ligated between the two clips. When the kidney is completely free except for its vascular attachments, a 5-cm Pfannenstiel ("bikini" cut) incision is made below the umbilicus through which the donor kidney will be removed. Double staples are placed first on the artery, and the vessel is ligated between the staples. The same procedure is followed for the vein. The kidney is now free and ready for removal. A mesh endocatch bag is inserted through the incision, and then using the equipment through the ports, the surgeon, giving special attention to the ureter, places the kidney completely in the bag. The bag is gently pulled back through the Pfannenstiel incision. The donor kidney is given to the recipient transplant team while the donor transplant team completes the donor surgery. The 5-cm incision is closed, and the surgeon then observes through the camera port for any bleeding from the sites of ligation and cautery. Once it is certain there is no bleeding, the ports are removed and the port incisions are sutured and clipped.

7. How does the laparoscopic donor nephrectomy (LDN) procedure compare with the conventional nephrectomy procedure?

Comparison of Conventional and Laparoscopic Nephrectomies

	CONVENTIONAL	LAPAROSCOPIC
Operative time	3 hr, 15 min	~ 4 hr
Cost	=	=
Length of stay	4–7 days	2–4 days
Graft/patient survival	=	=
Pain	>	<
Degree of disability	>	<
Financial losses	>	<
Time lost from work, child- or elder-care	3–9 wk	1–5 wk
Estimated blood loss	150–700 ml	~ 200 ml
Complications	=	=
Cosmetic changes	>	<

=, equivalent; >, greater than; <, less than.

The LDN procedure takes longer than the conventional nephrectomy procedure because it is done indirectly with a laparoscopic camera that directs the equipment required to remove the kidney. This technique increases operating room costs as does the need for about $1000–$2000 of disposable equipment used for each surgery. Nevertheless, the cost of the two procedures breaks even because the length of stay for LDN patients is shorter. There is no difference in patient or graft survival or in complication rates between the two procedures. LDN patients recover more quickly and are able to return to their regular activities sooner. LDN patients are usually off pain medication in 7-10 days, while conventional patients may require pain medicine for as long as a month. The much larger incision is responsible for the increased level of pain. With LDN patients the estimated blood loss is also less and cosmetic changes are fewer. These features are what have made the LDN procedure more attractive to people who may not have otherwise donated an organ.

8. What is an altruistic donor?

An altruistic donor is a person who has agreed to donate an organ to someone who is a stranger. The altruistic donor simply wants to do good for another person. The donor does not have any input into who receives the organ. There are altruistic-donor programs in individual hospitals as well as programs that represent entire cities. Trained health care professionals screen altruistic donors who call and offer a kidney for transplantation. These transplant professionals then determine which patient would be the best recipient for the altruistic donation. For programs that represent an entire city or region, the patient at the top of the cadaveric list is often selected. Other programs may give priority to children. If the donor is cleared from medical and psychosocial standpoints and a suitable candidate is found, the transplantation can proceed. There will likely be greater regulation of altruistic programs in the future.

9. Is a patient with a malignancy automatically excluded from transplantation?

Patients with cancer are not automatically excluded from consideration for a transplant, but they must be cancer free for a specified period to ensure that the immunosuppressants would be less likely to cause a recurrence. Dr. Israel Penn, who developed the Transplant Tumor Registry, recommended a waiting period of 2–5 years after surgical removal or medical treatment of the malignancy, depending on the type of tumor.[14] Patients should be made aware that the cumulative effect or long-term use of immunosuppressants could cause recurrence of the original disease or development of de novo malignancies. The transplant team with input from the patient must determine whether the benefits of transplantation under these circumstances outweigh the potential risks.

10. Where is the transplanted kidney surgically placed in the recipient?

It is preferred to place the kidney extraperitoneally in the iliac fossa when possible. The right side is preferred for a first renal transplant. This placement facilitates anastomoses and allows easy access if a biopsy is required. Placing the kidney in the right iliac fossa decreases the incidence of ileus because the left colon is not manipulated. The left side may be utilized if the patient has had a previous transplant on the right or if a pancreas transplant is planned in the future. It is generally preferred to place the pancreas on the right to avoid kinking of the blood vessels that could lead to thrombosis.

11. Describe the usual immunosuppression protocol used for kidney transplant recipients postoperatively.

Most patients are on triple therapy that includes a corticosteroid, a calcineurin inhibitor, and mycophenolate mofetil. Methylprednisolone remains the cornerstone of most immunosuppression protocols. A common dosing regimen is 6 intravenous doses of 125 mg of methylprednisolone after the surgery. The patient is then converted to oral prednisone at a dose of about 30 mg daily, which can be tapered to 20 mg when the level of the calcineurin inhibitor is therapeutic.

Tacrolimus or cyclosporine is the preferred calcineurin inhibitor. In cases in which there is concern about the length of the cold ischemia time or a history of calcineurin inhibitor toxicity or graft thrombosis, the calcineurin inhibitor is held for a period of about 3–5 days, and the patient receives induction therapy. Polyclonal antibodies (Thymoglobulin) and monoclonal antibodies (e.g., muromonab-CD3) can be used for induction. Humanized antibodies such as daclizumab (Zenapax) and basiliximab (Simulect) have been used as well. Once there is evidence of improved kidney function, such as increased urinary output and decreased serum creatinine, the calcineurin inhibitor is slowly titrated up to a therapeutic level.

Mycophenolate mofetil (CellCept) is given at a dose of 1–1.5 gm twice a day. African Americans are given the higher dose because of their greater incidence of rejection. The dose is adjusted for those who develop significant gastrointestinal symptoms, including diarrhea, nausea, and vomiting. The dose can be adjusted to 4 times/day (e.g., 500 mg 4 times/day) or decreased if necessary.

12. Why is ketoconazole sometimes used in patients who have difficulty achieving a thera-peutic calcineurin inhibitor (tacrolimus [Prograf], cyclosporine [Neoral]) level despite high dosages?

The inability to reach a therapeutic calcineurin inhibitor level can occur for no apparent reason or can be related to another medication that increases the metabolism and excretion of cal-cineurin inhibitors such as phenytoin (Dilantin) or rifampin. A patient may take tacrolimus doses of 8–10 mg twice a day or cyclosporine doses of 300 mg twice a day or higher and still not reach a therapeutic level, which poses two problems:

• Failure to achieve a therapeutic level puts the patient at risk for rejection.
• Large doses of calcineurin inhibitors are expensive.

Both ketoconazole and calcineurin inhibitors are excreted via the P450 cytochrome pathway. If both are present in the blood, they compete for excretion, slowing the excretion of both drugs and increasing their serum concentrations. For example, it has been found that doses of tacrolimus can be decreased as much as 30–80% because of the slowed metabolism caused by ketoconazole. A daily dose of ketoconazole (200 mg) costs about $3. A 10-mg, twice-daily dose of tacrolimus costs approximately $64. Using ketoconazole to increase the tacrolimus levels and decrease the dose can save patients a significant amount of money. If a patient is taking a 10-mg dose of tacrolimus and it is decreased by 80% to 2 mg twice daily, the total cost of the tacrolimus ($12) and ketoconazole ($3) is about $15 a day. If the tacrolimus level remains subtherapeutic, the ketoconazole dose can be increased to twice daily, and this increase does not substantially in-crease the cost. Additionally, ketoconazole may be the only way to achieve a therapeutic level for a patient on phenytoin or any other drug that increases the metabolism of calcineurin inhibitors.

If ketoconazole is used for the purpose of elevating the calcineurin inhibitor level, frequent laboratory tests are essential for the first few weeks until the level stabilizes. If for any reason the ketoconazole is discontinued, the tacrolimus dose needs to be increased substantially. This regi-men is suitable only for compliant patients with consistent drug levels.

13. Describe the routine anti-infective agents that are administered postoperatively.

One of the most significant side effects of the immunosuppressant drugs is that they lower the patient's ability to fight infection, particularly in the first few months after transplantation. Most centers use prophylactic antibacterial, antiviral, and antifungal agents to prevent the most common infections. A cephalosporin is usually given for about 24 hours after surgery to provide broad-spectrum coverage.

Trimethoprim/sulfamethoxazole (TMP/SMZ, Bactrim SS) is given for 1 year to protect the patient from *Pneumocystis carinii* pneumonia (PCP), urinary tract infections (UTI), and possibly toxoplasmosis. If a patient has a sulfa allergy, thrombocytopenia, or drug-induced nephritis, then dapsone 100 mg daily or pentamidine 300 mg by inhalation can be substituted for the TMP/SMZ. These drugs provide only PCP coverage, and another antibiotic such as amoxicillin is needed for UTI coverage.

Acyclovir (Zovirax) is used for 3 months after transplantation to prevent herpes simplex in-fections. However, if a patient is CMV negative and received a kidney from a CMV-positive donor, valganciclovir is substituted to protect against active CMV disease as well. Oral ganciclovir (Cytovene) may also be used. Both valganciclovir and oral ganciclovir require renal dosing, and valganciclovir should not be used if the patient remains dialysis dependent.

Clotrimazole troches (Mycelex) 10 mg is given 4 times/day for 3 months to combat fungal infections. Nystatin swish and swallow 500,000 units can be substituted if the patient is intolerant of the clotrimazole troches.

14. What is acute tubular necrosis?

Acute tubular necrosis (ATN) is an ischemic injury sustained by the kidney during organ procurement and preservation. It is characterized by anuria or oliguria that can last for several days to weeks. ATN also can be caused by reperfusion when there is a sudden rush of oxygen free radicals into the tissues. Certain donor factors are known to contribute to ATN, including older age, cold ischemia time > 24 hours, hemodynamic instability before procurement, the type of solution used to perfuse the kidney (Collins vs. University of Wisconsin [UW]), and whether the kidney was pumped or not. Additionally, patients who have had a previous transplant or have high panel-reactive antibody (PRA) levels are more prone to ATN.

15. How is ATN managed?

There is no treatment for ATN except to maintain the patient on dialysis until the kidney functions. If ATN is expected to be a problem, induction therapy with a monoclonal or polyclonal antibody may be initiated intraoperatively and the calcineurin inhibitor held for several days to spare the kidney from the nephrotoxic effects.

It is important to rule out other causes of renal dysfunction because ATN is a diagnosis of exclusion if a biopsy has not been done. Ultrasonography should be done to ensure vessel patency. A nuclear scan can identify a urine leak. If ATN persists for a week after transplantation in the absence of any other problems, a biopsy should be done to confirm the diagnosis and ensure that there is not a component of rejection as well. If the patient still has ATN at the time of discharge, he or she is referred back to the home dialysis unit. Blood work needs to be done twice a week with weekly biopsies until the kidney functions.

16. What surgical complications can occur after renal transplantation?

During the first 24 hours after transplantation, **bleeding** may occur due to bleeding disorders, anticoagulation, or small vessels that were not ligated during the operative procedure. The patient experiences significant and increasing abdominal pain, and the hematocrit falls steadily. An ultrasound will show evidence of fluid collection around the kidney, as will a CT scan. If the hematocrit does not stabilize and a fluid collection is present, an emergency exploratory laparotomy (EL) is indicated.

Thrombosis can be either arterial or venous. It may be due to clots, technical problems, and, on rare occasions, the cytokine release that occurs with the administration of muromonab-CD3. If a patient has good renal function and one of the major vessels thromboses, there will be a sudden cessation in urinary output. Thrombosis is more difficult to diagnose if there is minimal urinary output. Other symptoms include graft tenderness, elevated creatinine, and hematuria (with venous thrombosis). If thrombosis is suspected, the patient should return to the operating room immediately for an EL. If the kidney is thrombosed and without viable tissue, which is usually the case, a transplant nephrectomy must be done.

Wound infections may occur due to immunosuppressant drugs that increase susceptibility to infection and delay wound healing. Patients with diabetes are at even higher risk because diabetes slows wound healing as well. A cephalosporin is given for the first 24 hours after surgery to prevent infection.

Lymphoceles can develop if all the lymphatic vessels were not properly tied off intraoperatively. As a result, the lymph fluid accumulates around the transplanted kidney. Lymphoceles can grow so large that they compress the kidney, impairing function. They can put pressure on the bladder, causing frequent urination, pain, and incontinence. They can also obstruct the iliac vein, causing edema in the affected extremity. Lymphoceles can be identified using ultrasound. Small lymphoceles can be drained but often recur. Recurrent or large lymphoceles need surgical drainage and repair to prevent chronic problems.

Urine leaks usually occur where the ureter is anastomosed to the bladder and can be mistaken for rejection because both conditions cause the creatinine to rise and the urine output to decrease. If a patient has good urine output, there may be an increase in yellow serous drainage from the wound. The wound drainage should be sent for creatinine measurement. If the creatinine in the fluid from the wound is several times higher than the serum creatinine, a leak is likely. If the patient has minimal output or confirmation of a leak is needed, a renal scan can be done. If the leak is small, decompression of the bladder with a catheter helps to seal it. A percutaneous nephrostomy tube with a stent may also be placed to divert the urine while the leak heals. If the leak persists or is large, surgical repair is required.

Renal artery stenosis is a late surgical complication that occurs several months to a year after transplantation and is often related to technical complications at the anastomosis. The patient presents with uncontrolled hypertension and worsening renal function. A bruit can usually be heard over the stenotic artery. An arteriogram is needed to confirm the diagnosis; however, it should be done with minimal dye to prevent further injury to the kidney. The stenosis can be treated with angioplasty, but surgical intervention is required for recurrent stenosis.

17. What is the Banff 97 grading system for acute rejection on a renal biopsy?

The Banff 97 grading system rates the severity of an acute rejection episode based on microscopic evaluation of biopsy samples. Each biopsy is given a grade from 1–3 that indicates the severity of the rejection based on the presence or absence of tubulitis, intimal arteritis, transmural inflammation, and fibrinoid necrosis.

The grade also provides an indication of whether the rejection episode can be reversed. The lower the grade, the less severe the rejection, and the more likely that it can be reversed. Some patients are considered to have borderline rejection when the changes are very mild. The grade also guides treatment selection:

• Borderline to grade 2A–2B: high-dose intravenous methylprednisolone (SoluMedrol)

• Grade 2B–3B: monoclonal antibodies (muromonab-CD3 [OKT3]), polyclonal antibodies (antilymphocyte globulin, antithymocyte globulin)

Banff Grading System for Renal Rejection

GRADE OF REJECTION	TUBULITIS	ARTERITIS	EXPECTED OUTCOME OF REJECTION
Borderline	Interstitial inflammation; mild tubulitis; 1–4 cells/cross section	None	Clinical significance and need to treat unclear
Grade 1A	Mononuclear inflammatory cell infiltrates in greater than 25% of interstitium of cortical tissue present; 5–10 cells/cross section	None	Usually easily reversed
Grade 1B	As with Grade 1, but > 10 cells/cross section	None	Usually easily reversed
Grade 2A	+/– tubulitis	Occlusion of < 25% of the lumen of the most involved artery by inflammatory cells and edema	More difficult to reverse
Grade 2B	+/– tubulitis	As with 2A, but > 25% of lumen occluded	More difficult to reverse than 2A
Grade 3	+/– tubulitis	Transmural inflammation or fibrinoid necrosis in one or more arteries	Often irreversible

18. What is seen on biopsy if a patient has tacrolimus or cyclosporine toxicity?

The Banff system provides criteria to describe tacrolimus or cyclosporine toxicity. Drug toxicity would show the following:

• Isometric vacuolization of the proximal tubular epithelium

• Thrombotic microangiopathy

If these problems are seen on biopsy, the tacrolimus or cyclosporine dose should be lowered accordingly.

19. If a transplant recipient's white blood cell count drops precipitously, what should be the first concern?

Viral infections can cause a rapid fall in the white blood cell (WBC) count. One of the most common viral infections in transplant recipients is cytomegalovirus (CMV). If the WBC falls and the patient complains of fatigue and fever, CMV should be suspected. The patient should have a CMV antigenemia drawn. A positive CMV antigenemia is indicative of active disease, and the result is generally available in 24 hours. CMV cultures can take weeks for a result. There are many other possible causes of a low WBC count, including medications such as mycophenolate mofetil, acyclovir, ganciclovir, and fluconazole, and systemic illnesses, but CMV should be high on the list of likely diagnoses in a transplant recipient.

20. What are the graft and patient survival rates for cadaveric- and living-donor renal transplants?

Graft and Patient Survival Rates for Cadaveric and Living Donors

	ONE YEAR	THREE YEARS	FIVE YEARS
Cadaveric graft survival	89.4%	76.3%	64.7%
Live-donor graft survival	94.5%	87%	78.4%
Cadaveric donor patient survival	94.8%	88.9%	81.8%
Live-donor patient survival	97.6%	94.6%	91%

From United Network for Organ Sharing: 2000 Annual Data Report: The US Scientific Registry of Transplant Recipients and the Organ Transplantation Network: Transplant Data 1990–1999. Rockville, MD, United Network for Organ Sharing, 2000.

21. What are the different types of kidney transplant rejection?

Despite great progress in tissue typing and various new potent and efficacious immunosuppressive drugs, rejection remains the number one cause of graft loss. Hyperacute, accelerated, acute, and chronic rejection are the recognized forms of rejection.

Hyperacute rejection generally occurs within minutes of releasing the cross-clamps. It is caused by the presence of preformed cytotoxic antibodies to the donor and is almost always irreversible. The kidney becomes edematous and deeply cyanotic with marked interstitial hemorrhage. This type of rejection is rarely seen as the final preoperative crossmatch usually identifies the presence of preformed antibodies.

Accelerated rejection is antibody-mediated like hyperacute rejection, but it occurs more slowly possibly because the number of preformed antibodies present at the time of transplant is inadequate to cause rejection. Over the course of several days the antibodies multiply rapidly, and the rejection episode becomes evident. Fever, oliguria, and tenderness over the graft are common complaints. Accelerated rejection is diagnosed by a positive repeat crossmatch, rising antibody titers, and the presence of complement degradation products (C4D) on biopsy. It is treated with plasmapheresis, which removes the antibodies to the donor kidney. Plasmapheresis is followed by an infusion of intravenous immunoglobulin that decreases the production of the antibody and decreases the response of the immune system to the antigen. The exact mechanism of these immunomodulatory effects of the immunoglobulin are unclear.

Acute cellular rejection can occur days to months after transplant. It is the most common type of rejection and is responsive to treatment. Acute cellular rejection is diagnosed by an ultrasound-guided biopsy. Histologically, it is characterized by interstitial edema, tubulitis, and mononuclear infiltration, and it may have components of arteritis and fibrinoid necrosis. High-dose methylprednisolone is usually an effective treatment, but monoclonal or polyclonal antibodies may be required if severe arteritis or fibrinoid necrosis are present.

Chronic rejection occurs insidiously over months to years after transplant. The cause of chronic rejection is not well defined. Both immune and nonimmune mechanisms are implicated. Chronic changes are seen in the arteries, tubules, interstitium, and glomeruli. On biopsy, there is tubular atrophy, glomerulosclerosis, and interstitial fibrosis. There is no treatment for chronic rejection. Some patients experience improved function when the calcineurin inhibitors (tacrolimus, cyclosporine) are discontinued, because they are nephrotoxic. The patient then begins a regimen of mycophenolate mofetil with prednisone. Sirolimus (Rapamune) has also been used. These medications do not reverse the rejection but may slow the progression to ESRD in some circumstances.

22. When is acute rejection most likely to occur after a renal transplantation?
Acute rejection usually occurs during the first 3 months after transplant. It is one reason that most centers draw laboratory work 1–2 times a week during this time period. Acute rejection must be identified and treated early because each rejection episode shortens the life of the kidney. About 90% of rejection episodes are cell-mediated; the remaining 10% are antibody-mediated (humoral).

23. Describe the standard treatment regimen for mild-to-moderate acute cellular rejection.
Intravenous methylprednisolone followed by high-dose oral prednisone is usually the treatment of choice. Initially methylprednisolone is given at a dose of 500 mg for 3 consecutive days. It is then tapered daily for 3 more days at doses of 250 mg, 125 mg, and 75 mg. When this 6-day course is complete, prednisone is started on the following schedule: 60 mg/day for 2 days, 40 mg/day for 2 days, and 30 mg/day. The prednisone is tapered further over time based on laboratory results and the clinical status of the patient. Glucose levels must be monitored carefully because of the diabetogenic effect of high-dose steroids.

24. Describe the standard treatment regimen for moderate-to-severe acute cellular rejection.
Polyclonal antibodies (e.g,. Atgam, Thymoglobulin) or monoclonal antibodies (muromonab-CD3) are preferred. Atgam is produced by the immunization of horses with human thymus lymphocytes. Thymoglobulin is produced by the immunization of rabbits with human thymocytes. Muromonab-CD3 is formed by the hybridization of B-lymphocytes with a myeloma cell line.

The polyclonal antibodies deplete circulating lymphocytes, particularly the T cells that are responsible for cellular rejection. Thymoglobulin is the polyclonal antibody of choice because it has been found to be more efficacious, more likely to reverse rejection, and more cost effective than Atgam. Thymoglobulin is given at a dose of 1.5 mg/kg, whereas the dose for Atgam is 10–15 mg/kg. Muromonab-CD3 blocks the ability of the T cell to recognize the antigen. The usual dose is a 5-mg intravenous push, but the dose can be increased to 10 mg if the patient fails to respond. The course of treatment with antibodies is usually 7–14 days, depending on the patient's response.

25. What causes the moderate-to-severe flulike symptoms seen with monclonal and polyclonal antibody treatments?
When monoclonal antibodies are given, the T-cell count falls rapidly, releasing cytokines into the circulation. Most of the significant symptoms seen with muromonab-CD3 are attributed to a cytokine-release syndrome. Complement activation has also been implicated. The symptoms include fevers, chills, rigors, and complaints of muscle and joint pain. On rare occasions, symptoms can progress to shock.

Symptoms seen with polyclonal antibodies are similar but are attributed to the introduction of a foreign animal protein into the circulation. The polyclonal antibodies usually produce less severe symptoms, but anaphylaxis can occur.

For minimization of these symptoms, patients are usually premedicated before the first 3 doses. The premedications include the following:
- Methylprednisolone, 500 mg intravenously about 1–4 hours before administration of the antibody
- Diphenhydramine, 50 mg orally about a half hour before dose
- Acetaminophen, 650 mg orally about a half hour before dose

The medications suppress the fever and other inflammatory symptoms arising from the cytokine release and response to the foreign protein. By the third day, the number of T cells is drastically reduced and symptoms are usually significantly improved or absent at this point.

26. How can the success of the monoclonal and polyclonal antibody therapies be monitored?

Both monoclonal and polyclonal therapies rapidly deplete T cells in a matter of hours to days. Transplant practitioners usually follow the CD3 T-cell subset, although some centers may monitor other subsets. A normal range for the percentage of CD3 cells is about 51–91%. The percentage should be about 5% or less to ensure adequate treatment. Some centers follow the absolute CD3 T-cell count. The actual number of CD3 cells is counted with this method. It is preferred that the absolute count be 50 or less.

If the CD3 count does not fall quickly, the dose may need to be increased, or it is possible that the patient has antibodies to the antibody preparation. For muromonab-CD3, an antibody titer can be drawn. If the level of antibody is greater than 1:1000, it is unlikely that the patient will respond to therapy. Generally, only patients who have received muromonab-CD3 before have developed antibodies. It is important to check for antibodies before a patient is given a second course of muromonab-CD3.

27. Can polyclonal antibodies be given via a peripheral line?

Thymoglobulin or Atgam should be given through a large high-flow central vessel because it can cause thrombophlebitis and thrombosis. If central access is not available, the addition of 20 mg of hydrocortisone and 1000 u heparin to the infusion solution can prevent these problems.

28. Are maintenance immunosuppressants removed by dialysis?

The following immunosuppressants are **not** removed by dialysis:
- Cyclosporine
- Sirolimus
- Mycophenolate mofetil
- Tacrolimus
- Prednisone

Because many transplant recipients require dialysis for varying periods after transplantation, the nurse should be aware if any of the medications being administered are removed by dialysis. Any medications that are removed by dialysis should be held until after the treatment is completed.

29. Name the symptoms that the transplant recipient should be taught to observe and report.
- General infection: fever, chills, and muscle/joint aches or pain
- Wound infection: fever; redness, warmth, or purulent drainage at surgical wound or any other site
- Respiratory infection: fever, persistent cough, pleuritic chest pain, and shortness of breath
- Wound dehiscence: increased pain and increased drainage
- Urine leak: increased yellow drainage from wound and decreased urine output
- Gastrointestinal problems: nausea, vomiting, dysphagia, abdominal cramps, and diarrhea
- Urinary tract infection: pain on urination, frequency, urgency, and hematuria
- Renal dysfunction: decreased urinary output; swelling of hands, eyelids, or lower extremities; weight gain of 1–2 kg/24 hours; tenderness over graft

30. What restrictions are placed on a renal transplant patient postoperatively?
- No driving for 4 weeks after surgery
- No strenuous exercise or heavy lifting for 3-4 months to prevent the development of incisional hernia and promote wound healing
- No contact sports to avoid damage to the superficially placed transplant kidney
- Avoidance of undue stress to knees and hips to prevent the avascular necrosis associated with steroids
- Avoidance of crowded areas with poor air circulation (e.g., movie theaters, planes)
- No cleaning of cat litter boxes and birdcages to avoid contracting toxoplasmosis and psittacosis, respectively
- Following a low-sodium, low-fat, low-cholesterol diet to facilitate blood pressure control and prevention of cardiovascular disease.

31. What precautions do transplant recipients need to take regarding live vaccines?

A transplant recipient should never receive any live vaccines or be exposed to the body fluids of a person who has recently received a live vaccine. Because transplant recipients are immunocompromised, use of a live vaccine or exposure to a virus shed in the body fluids of other individuals can cause active disease. The following vaccines are live:

- Measles, mumps, and rubella (MMR)
- Oral polio vaccine (OPV)
- Varicella/chicken pox vaccine
- Typhoid, TY21a
- Yellow fever
- Bacille Calmette-Guérin (BCG)
- Smallpox (Vaccinia)

Transplant recipients who are in close proximity to anyone who has received a live vaccine should be advised not to handle the body fluids (urine, stool, vomitus) of the individual for 1 month after the vaccination to prevent exposure to the shed virus in the fluids.

32. Should kidney transplant recipients receive the influenza vaccine?

All transplant patients should receive the influenza vaccine unless they have an allergy to eggs. Influenza can be a life-threatening illness in the immunocompromised transplant recipient. The influenza vaccine is inactive and should be administered in mid-October each year. The vaccine is composed of both influenza A and influenza B types that are expected to be most common during the current flu season. The influenza season is most active from December through February, and receiving the vaccine in October allows the patient to mount an appropriate immune response before the season begins. If a patient is transplanted in October, the influenza vaccine can be deferred until mid-December. If the vaccine is given in the immediate postoperative period when the immunosuppression is at its highest level, the immune system may not be able to mount a normal response that would confer immunity. It is important to educate patients about the influenza vaccine because many refuse the vaccine fearing that it can cause influenza.

33. Should kidney transplant recipients receive the pneumonia vaccine?

All transplant recipients should receive the pneumonia vaccine to protect them from *Streptococcal pneumoniae*. They are at risk for this type of pneumonia because of their immunocompromised state. It is preferable to receive this vaccine before transplantation so that a normal immune response can be mounted. Once a patient is transplanted, the vaccine should be readministered every 5–6 years. There is some argument that more frequent immunization is needed, but there are no data to support this practice at this time.

34. Describe the appropriate dental prophylaxis for a transplant recipient.

All transplant recipients should receive antibiotic prophylaxis before any dental work, including teeth cleaning for 6 months after transplant to decrease the risk of oral pathogens causing a systemic infection. After 6 months only high-risk patients require dental prophylaxis. High-risk patients include anyone with any of the following: acute or chronic rejection with increased immunosuppression, neutropenia, active CMV disease, severe gingivitis, dental abscesses, or cardiac abnormalities The American Heart Association Guidelines for endocarditis are followed:

- For patients with no allergies: Amoxicillin, 2 gm orally, 1 hour before procedure
- For patients with a penicillin allergy: Clindamycin, 600 mg orally, 1 hour before procedure

35. What causes hypophosphatemia in kidney transplant recipients?

The causes of hypophosphatemia are multifactorial:

1. An **elevated parathyroid hormone (PTH) level:** High levels of PTH increase the urinary excretion of phosphate. Although PTH levels fall dramatically after transplant in many patients, others have persistently high levels.

2. **Low levels of activated vitamin D:** Low levels result in impaired absorption of phosphate from the intestines. Levels can remain low in some patients despite transplantation.

3. **Corticosteroids:** Steroids reduce the tubular reabsorption of phosphate in the proximal tubule.

4. **Immunosuppressants:** Immunosuppressants such as cyclosporine have effects on the renal tubules and are thought to play a role in increased excretion of phosphate, but the exact mechanism is unknown.

Some of these causes present short-term problems, but others will be present throughout the life of the transplant.

36. What is the best treatment regimen for hypophosphatemia?

The first step is to make sure that the patient is no longer on a phosphate binder. Vitamin D supplements can be given in the form of calcitriol (Rocaltrol). Numerous phosphate supplements can also be given. The supplement that provides the largest dose of phosphate with the least potassium in the most palatable form is K-Phos Neutral. This preparation contains 250 mg of phosphate in a pill form but contains only 1.1 mEq of potassium. K-Phos Neutral, 250–500 mg, can be given 3 or more times a day depending on the degree of hypophosphatemia.

Another phosphate preparation is Neutraphos, which contains 250 mg of phosphate but has 7.13 mEq of potassium. Hyperkalemia can occur easily in patients on multiple doses of this formulation. This preparation comes in a powder that must be mixed with a liquid, and many patients find it unpalatable. There are phosphate supplements with as much as 14 mEq of potassium, so great caution must be taken to ensure that the correct supplement is ordered and administered.

Correction of hypophosphatemia is essential because phosphate plays an important role in calcium regulation, bone formation, acid–base maintenance, carbohydrate and lipid metabolism, and energy production. A level of 3–4.5 mg/dl is desired. Phosphate supplements can cause diarrhea.

37. What causes hypomagnesemia after renal transplant? How can it be treated?

Both tacrolimus and cyclosporine cause increased secretion of magnesium in the urine. As neither of these drugs can be eliminated from the immunosuppression regimen, magnesium supplementation is the best treatment. The preparation that contains the largest dose of elemental magnesium is Mg-Ox 400, which is a 400-mg tablet that contains 241.3 mg of elemental magnesium. Doses of 400–800 mg may be given 3–4 times a day depending on the degree of the hypomagnesemia. The nurse should keep in mind that any magnesium-containing product can cause diarrhea, and patients should be advised to report this symptom. Decreasing the dose can improve the diarrhea.

Magnesium supplementation is important because it is involved in many metabolic and enzymatic processes and neuromuscular functions. It is also known to increase HDL cholesterol and has a possible link to better blood pressure control. A level of about 1.3–2.0 mg/dl is desired.

38. What is the most common cause of death after transplantation?

The most common cause of death after a renal transplant is a cardiovascular event (e.g., myocardial infarction, congestive heart failure, stroke). Cardiac events are more common than cerebrovascular events. Transplant patients are at risk for these complications for several reasons, including comorbid conditions (e.g., diabetes, hypertension), older age, and the effects of immunosuppressants on the progression or development of atherosclerosis and lipid disorders. A history of smoking, hypercoagulability, transplant rejection, obesity, erythrocytosis, and infections; elevated homocysteine levels; or a family history of early cardiac death are other risk factors for cardiovascular events.

39. What can be done to reduce the risk of a cardiovascular event occurring after renal transplantation?

- Aggressive preoperative evaluation for cardiovascular problems that may be worsened by anesthesia, surgery and immunosuppression. Diagnostic testing may include echocardiogram, stress test, cardiac catheterization, and carotid Doppler studies.

- Preoperative cardiac bypass surgery or carotid endarterectomy for patients with critical lesions
- Tight blood glucose control
- Good blood pressure control
- Control of hyperlipidemia:
    - Nutrition therapy: Lipid and caloric restrictions.
    - Exercise
    - Drug therapy: (Single or multiple drug regimens may be required.)
      HMG-CoA reductase inhibitors (e.g., atorvastatin)
      Nicotinic acids (e.g., niacin)
      Bile acid sequestrants (e.g., cholestyramine)
      Fibric acid analogues (e.g., gemfibrozil)
    - Lower doses of cyclosporine, steroids, and tacrolimus, if possible. If the patient is taking cyclosporine, consider switching to tacrolimus because it causes less increase in the lipid levels.
- Smoking cessation
- Regular exercise
- Aspirin therapy to prevent the development of a hypercoagulable state
- Folic acid therapy to lower homocysteine levels
- Weight reduction

40. What recommendations should be made to transplant recipients regarding sexual activity and pregnancy?

After a successful transplant, libido often returns along with fertility. Sexual activity can resume several weeks after the transplant when it is physically comfortable for the patient and his or her partner. Women of childbearing age should be counseled to postpone pregnancy for at least 18 months after transplantation. Pregnancy should only be attempted in patients with normal renal function after careful consultation with the transplant surgeon, nephrologist, and high-risk obstetrician. Drugs such as prednisone and calcineurin inhibitors are believed to be relatively safe in pregnancy, but the safety of azathioprine and mycophenolate mofetil is not fully understood. Consultation regarding necessary medication adjustments is critical to ensuring the safety of the fetus and mother.

Birth control is essential not only to prevent pregnancy but also to avoid contracting sexually transmitted diseases. Protected sex through the use of condoms, spermicides, and other devices is necessary for both male and female transplant recipients.

41. What is a positive crossmatch transplant?

A positive crossmatch transplant is done when a transplant candidate has a healthy, willing donor but the candidate has antibodies to one of the donor's HLA antigens. In the past, a positive crossmatch before transplantation led to the cancellation of the proposed transplantation because hyperacute humoral rejection (antibody-mediated rejection) was guaranteed to occur, which would result in the loss of the transplant. Now, due to technological advances (plasmapheresis) and new medications (tacrolimus, mycophenolate mofetil, intravenous immunoglobulin [IVIG], and daclizumab), living-donor positive crossmatch transplants are possible and successful.

The key to this procedure is to remove as much of the antibody to the donor (donor-specific antibody) as possible from the recipient through plasmapheresis. Plasmapheresis involves removing the entire plasma volume via a dual lumen venous catheter, separating the plasma from the blood components, discarding the plasma, returning the whole blood components to the patient, and replacing the plasma with an equal volume of albumin or donor plasma. The plasma is removed because most of the antibodies in the body are found in it. Each plasmapheresis treatment is followed by the infusion of IVIG, which contains "good" antibodies to bacteria, viruses, and fungi. IVIG replaces these beneficial antibodies, but more importantly, it exerts an immunomodulatory effect.

Over time, by a mechanism that is unclear the IVIG modulates the immune system so that the production of the donor-specific antibody is reduced or eliminated. Depending on how high the transplant candidate's donor-specific antibody titer is, 1–6 plasmapheresis treatments may be ordered every other day preoperatively. It is desired to bring the titer level, which is reported as a ratio, down to about 1:16 or less.

To ensure that the immune system is well suppressed, both tacrolimus and mycophenolate mofetil are started on the first day of plasmapheresis. On the day of transplantation, daclizumab is given intraoperatively to further suppress the immune system, and 4 additional doses are given every other week postoperatively. Intensive immunosuppression to prevent a rebound of the donor-specific antibody is a crucial component of this protocol.

Usually two plasmapheresis treatments are given every other day after surgery, but more may be required if the donor-specific antibody titer rises. Positive crossmatch transplants are being done at several centers across the United States. Graft survival rates are similar to living-donor transplants with a negative crossmatch. In this era of severe organ shortages, this is yet another way to increase the living kidney-donor pool.

42. What is an ABO-incompatible transplant?

An ABO-incompatible transplant is done when a transplant candidate has a healthy, willing donor but the candidate's and donor's blood groups are incompatible. In the past, as with positive crossmatch transplants, ABO incompatibility precluded transplantation. Hyperacute rejection would occur immediately after transplantation due to the presence of antibodies to the incompatible blood group. With the availability of plasmapheresis and potent immunosuppressants and immunoglobulins, ABO-incompatible transplants have become a reality.

The most experience with this procedure is in Japan where cadaveric donors are virtually nonexistent, forcing the physicians to find novel methods of transplantation from living donors. Plasmapheresis is used to remove the antibodies to the incompatible blood group. Usually no less than 6 treatments are required to remove 99% of the IgG antibodies to the incompatible blood type (see question 41 for a description of plasmapheresis). The last three treatments before surgery are usually done on 3 consecutive days to avoid antibody rebound.

After each plasmapheresis, IVIG is given to replenish the "good" antibodies to bacteria, viruses, and fungi. IVIG also exerts an immunomodulatory effect that by a unknown mechanism reduces the production of the donor-specific antibody somewhat. Even more important, it seems to dampen the immune response to the antibodies if the antibody titer rises postoperatively.

Tacrolimus and mycophenolate mofetil are started at the time of the first plasmapheresis. The patient also receives daclizumab intraoperatively and then every other week for four more doses. Significant immunosuppression is a key factor for the success of this protocol.

At the time of transplantation, a laparoscopic splenectomy is done. The spleen is removed because it is one of the largest repositories of antibodies in the body. ABO-incompatible transplants that have been done without splenectomy have had a much lower success rate. Because of the splenectomy, the ABO-incompatible recipient should be vaccinated for pneumococcal pneumonia, meningitis, and tetanus several months before the transplant. The recipient also needs penicillin postoperatively to provide additional protection from pneumonia.

After surgery the recipient receives at least two more plasmapheresis treatments and possibly more if there is any indication of rejection. A low platelet count is one of the first signs of rejection. Although antibody titers are followed postoperatively, they are not a good indicator of function because the immune system has accommodated to the presence of the incompatible blood group antigens.

Surprisingly, the graft survival rates are close to those for living-donor transplants with compatible blood typing. Patients who agree to this type of transplant should be aware that the success rate is not as good and that the most significant problems arise shortly after transplantation. About 4–5 years after transplantation, there is no difference in the rate of chronic rejection between ABO-compatible and ABO-incompatible recipients.

43. Describe some challenges facing transplant centers in the future?
- Finding alternative donor sources because of the short supply of cadaveric donors
- Determining whether xenotransplantation is a realistic option considering the risks of cross-species transmission of pathogens and hyperacute rejection
- Developing strategies to keep the aging transplant population healthy, especially considering the increasing number of comorbid conditions
- Finding immunosuppressants with more specificity and less toxicity
- Creating new procedures and techniques to reduce some of the problems associated with living-donor organ donation
- Determining whether chimerism or induced tolerance can be consistently reproduced in humans so that transplantation can be done without immunosuppression
- Developing presumed consent laws by which anyone who dies suddenly is presumed to be a donor unless specified otherwise premortem
- Finding methods to grow kidneys from individual cells
- Ensuring that all transplant distribution methods and transplant protocols are ethical

BIBLIOGRAPHY

1. Avery R: Immunizations in adult immunocompromised patients. Cleve Clin J Med 68:337–347, 2001.
2. Bakris G, Williams M, Dworkin L, et al: Preserving renal function in adults with hypertension and diabetes: A consensus approach. Am J Kidney Dis 36:646–661 2001.
3. Bleyer AJ, Chen R, D'Agostino RB, Appel RG: Clinical correlates of hypertensive end-stage renal disease. Am J Kidney Dis 1:28–34, 1998.
4. Danovitch G: Handbook of Kidney Transplantation, 3rd ed. Philadelphia, Lippincott Williams & Wilkins, 2001.
5. Davidson I: Handbook of Kidney and Pancreas Transplantation. Austin, Landes Bioscience, 1998.
6. Ginns L, Cosimi A, Morris P: Transplantation. Malden, MA, Blackwell Science, 1999.
7. Greenberg A: Primer on Kidney Diseases, 2nd ed. San Diego, Academic Press, 1998.
8. Kasiske B, Vasquez M, Hatmon W: Recommendations for the outpatient surveillance of renal transplant recipients. J Am Soc Nephrol 11:S1–S86, 2000.
9. Lancaster L (ed): Core Curriculum for Nephrology Nursing, 4th ed. Pitman, NJ, Anthony J. Janetti, 2001.
10. Levi M: Post-transplant hypophosphatemia. Kidney Int 59:2377–2387, 2001.
11. Lewis D, Valerius W: Organs from non-heart beating donors: An answer to the organ shortage. Crit Care Nurs 19:70–74, 1999.
12. Owen W, Pereira B, Sayegh M: Dialysis and Transplantation. Philadelphia,W.B. Saunders, 2000.
13. Parker J (ed): Contemporary Nephrology Nursing. Pitman, NJ, Anthony J. Janetti, 1998.
14. Penn I: De novo cancers in organ allograft recipients. Curr Opin Organ Transplant 3:188–196, 1998.
15. Racusen L, Solez K, Colvin R: The Banff 97 working classification of renal allograft pathology. Kidney Int 55:713–723, 1999.
16. Racusen L, Solez K, Burdick J: Kidney Transplant Rejection, 3rd ed. New York, Marcel Dekker, 1998.
17. Ratner L, Montgomery R, Kavoussi L: Laparoscopic live-donor nephrectomy: The four year Johns Hopkins University experience. Nephrol Dial Transplant 14:2090–2093, 1999.
18. Ritz E, Tarng DC: Renal disease in type 2 diabetes. Nephrol Dial Transplant. 16:11–18, 2001.
19. Shapiro R, Simmons R, Starzl T: Renal Transplantation. Stamford, CT, Appleton & Lange, 1997.
20. United Network for Organ Sharing: 2000 Annual Data Report: The US Scientific Registry of Transplant Recipients and the Organ Transplantation Network: Transplant Data 1990–1999. Rockville, MD, United Network for Organ Sharing, 2000.

12. PANCREAS AND SIMULTANEOUS PANCREAS-KIDNEY TRANSPLANTATION

Janet B. Mize, RN, BSN, CCTC, CCM

1. What is the rationale for pancreas transplantation?

The primary reason for pancreas transplantation is to replace insulin therapy. In addition, the potential to maintain normal blood glucose levels may have a profound affect on preventing the secondary complications of diabetes, including diabetic neuropathy, gastroparesis, retinopathy, nephropathy, and accelerated cardiovascular disease.

2. What has prompted the need to perform pancreas transplantation?

As the incidence of diabetes increases and affects every age group and culture, the need to find a cure for the disease and the ability to better control the long-term complications have become the focus in diabetes medicine today. Kidney failure secondary to diabetes is one of the leading causes of end-stage renal disease. Kidney transplantation has long been an approved treatment modality for end-stage kidney disease. Transplanting a kidney in a patient with diabetes may cure renal failure; it may also stabilize and, in some cases, slow the complications of diabetes, such as neuropathy, diabetic gastroparesis, and retinopathy. However, it is not the answer to controlling blood glucose levels or preventing long-term progression of disease.

Pancreas transplantation has the potential to arrest the progression of diabetes complications and can have a profound effect on an individual's lifestyle. The first pancreas transplant was performed in 1966. Over the next 2 decades, variable success was reported with pancreas transplants. With improved surgical techniques and newer immunosuppression, the outcomes of pancreas transplantation improved in the early 1980s. The number of pancreas transplants increased from 72 in 1991 to 418 in 2000. Approximately 80% of pancreas recipients have been reported to achieve insulin independence for 1 year. Controlling the effects of diabetes could lead to reduction of renal insufficiency, thereby reducing the need for renal transplantation.

3. What is the incidence of diabetes in the end-stage renal disease population?

Statistics have shown that diabetes is second only to glomerular disease as an indication for kidney transplant and is the cause for approximately 20% of all transplants each year. About 45% of the end-stage renal disease (ESRD) population have diabetes; 15% of the cases are classified as having type I diabetes, and approximately 30% have poorly controlled type II diabetes.

4. Who are potential candidates for pancreas transplant ?

Pancreas transplantation is reserved for patients with type I diabetes and, on rare occasions, for prevention of diabetes in the patient requiring a total pancreatectomy. This specific group of patients does not have the means of producing insulin because of dysfunctioning islet cells. Islet cells, for reasons of trauma or disease caused by an immune-mediated response, make little or no insulin to allow blood glucose regulation. Patients with type II diabetes are not usually considered as candidates for pancreatic transplantation.

5. Why are patients with type II diabetes not candidates for pancreas transplantation?

Unlike type I diabetes, type II disease is caused by underutilization of the insulin produced by islet cells within the pancreas. Islet cells within the pancreas of a patient with type II diabetes continue to produce insulin, often at a normal or accelerated rate; however, the insulin is not able to actively reduce glucose levels. Transplantation of a pancreas into a patient with type II diabetes would not yield an insulin-free result.

6. How is pancreas transplantation justified medically and economically?

Opinions differ on pancreas transplantation in contrast to other organ transplantations. The pancreas is not a life-sustaining organ, so its value must be evaluated in relation to the alternative therapy. Insulin therapy is both inexpensive and effective, especially with some of the modern developments such as insulin pump therapy. However, providing a means of improving quality of life and reducing the complications of long-term insulin use in the diabetic patient must be viewed with an open mind. According to The Diabetes Control and Complications Research Group, diabetes is the most common endocrine disease in the world. The incidence of diabetes is estimated to be up to 16/100,000 in childhood, 260/100,000 by the age of 20 years, and 1050/100,000 for type I diabetes and 10,030/100,000 for type II diabetes by the age of 70 years. It is the fourth leading cause of death in Western countries and accounts for 15% of the hospitalizations per year. The reduction of long-term complications and improvement in quality-of-life issues point toward pancreas transplantation as a suitable and cost-effective means to control diabetes in the appropriate candidate.

7. What options are available for people who are considering pancreas transplantation?

There are three options for pancreas transplantation:
1. Transplantation of pancreas alone (PA)
2. Transplantation of pancreas simultaneously with kidney (SPK)
3. Transplantation of pancreas after kidney transplantation (PAK)

8. When is transplantation of pancreas alone the optimal choice?

Transplantation of pancreas alone is often considered a therapeutic alternative for patients with recurrent ketosis resulting in frequent admissions and aggressive management of "brittle" diabetes. In addition, it may be recommended for patients suffering from hypoglycemic unawareness that results in life-threatening complications. Such candidates must have substantial signs and symptoms of progressive disease, be pre-uremic, and have a normal serum creatinine and a normal 24-hour creatinine clearance/glomerular filtration rate.

9. What is the risk-to-benefit ratio for transplantation of pancreas alone?

Normal blood glucose levels as a result of pancreas transplantation decrease further progression of neuropathy, nephropathy, retinopathy, and vascular diseases associated with diabetes. However, returning glucose levels to normal does not resolve existing disease associated with long-term diabetes. There are some reports of symptoms improving following transplantation. However, one must consider the risks of major surgery and the long-term side effects of immunosuppression.

10. Can diabetic patients with a previous kidney transplant be considered for pancreas transplantation?

Yes. Many patients with successful kidney transplants continue to be burdened with the ill effects of diabetes. With PAK transplantation the risk of immunosuppression is not as significant because the patient has already taken immunosuppressive drugs for some time. The major risk in this scenario is the surgical procedure and the short-term boost in the immunosuppressive therapy postoperatively. However, long-term immunosuppression in such patients usually remains unchanged. The most that patients can look forward to with PAK transplantation is the possibility of becoming insulin-free and of reducing the risks of progressive diabetic disease.

11. Is there an advantage to simultaneous pancreas-kidney transplantation?

Simultaneous pancreas-kidney transplantation is the treatment of choice for diabetic patients with progressive kidney failure. Most transplant centers encourage dual-organ transplant for this group of patients. The clear advantage is that it involves one surgical procedure and uses a single donor, reducing the risk of antigens from multiple donors. SPK transplantation has been established as an effective means of treatment for patients with type I diabetes who have ESRD. Research has demonstrated that SPK transplantation improves patients' quality of life and reduces the side effects of progressive diabetes. The need for dialysis is eliminated. Transplantation is a more cost-effective therapy when compared with traditional treatments of long-term ESRD.

12. How are patients listed with the United Network for Organ Sharing ?

Appropriate candidates for SPK transplants are usually listed with the United Network for Organ Sharing (UNOS) for whole pancreas at the same time as being listed for a kidney. SPK candidates must meet the requirements for kidney transplant: a glomerular filtration rate of 20 ml/min or less or a serum creatinine level of 4–5 mg/dl. Single listing for whole pancreas does not have specific criteria for listing. As the waiting times for organs increase, patients listed for single organs may need to be listed for a second organ as medical conditions warrant. (See chapter 1 for more information about UNOS.)

13. Are there differences in patient and graft survival among the three options?

Yes. The table below describes patient and graft survival for PA, PAK and SPK transplants.*

TRANSPLANT TYPE	PATIENT SURVIVAL	1-YR GRAFT SURVIVAL	5-YR GRAFT SURVIVAL
Pancreas alone	95%	76.6%	63.9%
Pancreas after kidney	95%	71%	65.8%
Simultaneous pancreas and kidney	94%	Pancreas, 83% Kidney, 90%	Pancreas, 81.6% Kidney, 86.7%

* UNOS registry, 1999

Statistics have shown survival rates to be better in the patients receiving SPK transplants than in those receiving PA and PAK transplants. No scientific evidence has been published with regard to patient survival rates in each subgroup of pancreas transplantation. In recent years, this type of data has proved interesting. It is currently collected along with graft survival statistics by UNOS annually.

14. Do insulin requirements predict the need for pancreas transplantation?

No, with the refinement and variety of insulin therapies available today, many people with diabetes take less insulin than was taken years ago. Varieties of long- and short-acting combinations have reduced daily insulin requirements as well as reduced the large swings in blood glucose levels seen historically with the older types of therapy. In addition, if diabetic patients have significant nephropathy and require dialysis before transplantation, their insulin requirements are usually diminished to the point of controlling blood glucose levels with very small amounts of insulin or oral hyperglycemic medication.

15. Are there contraindications for PA, SPK, and PAK transplants?

Contraindications to pancreas transplants whether alone, at the time of kidney transplantation, or after kidney transplantation, do exist as with any other whole organ transplant. The absolute contraindications include overwhelming sepsis, metastatic disease, severe irreversible cardiovascular disease, and severe chronic obstructive pulmonary disease (COPD). In addition, a patient may not be an appropriate candidate for pancreas transplantation if there are considerable risk factors such as persistent incapacitating peripheral vascular- and neuropathy-related disease. Once again, potential candidates as well as the transplant team must recognize that the pancreas is not a life-sustaining organ. Therefore, a patient's condition should be thoroughly evaluated, with full weight given to the benefit-to-risk ratio of the procedure.

16. What are the preoperative challenges for patients in need of pancreas transplantation?

The major challenge in the evaluation of the diabetic patient for transplantation is ruling out the possibility of coronary artery disease. Approximately one-third of diabetic patients have some degree of coronary artery disease. Often these patients do not have signs or symptoms of disease. In addition, the potential pancreas recipient should be thoroughly screened for the extent of neuropathy, renal function, and retinopathy.[6] The presence of any of these symptoms should not eliminate a possible candidate, but the symptoms provide a baseline for future reference following pancreas transplantation.

17. What should be included in the evaluation?

In addition to the routine testing that transplant centers require for a potential organ transplant recipient, some tests require special attention in evaluations of candidates for a pancreas transplant. The cardiovascular assessment is usually the most important portion of the evaluation. Potential candidates require testing to detect cardiovascular abnormalities, a major concern in the diabetic candidate. Routinely, any candidate who is over 45 years old or who has had diabetes for more than 20 years requires not only a Doppler echocardiogram, but a stress test as well. Most often, the stress test requires the use of medication to stress the heart adequately. If any abnormalities are identified, a heart catheterization may be required to assess the extent of the coronary vessel disease. Additional interventions may be required to stabilize or improve cardiovascular disease before considering pancreas transplantation. Carotid arteries should also be examined for stenosis influencing hemodynamic flow.

Nerve conduction studies are needed to provide valuable information about baseline neuropathy, and an extensive ophthalmologic examination is required to evaluate retinopathy and visual acuity. Keep in mind, visual acuity can change rapidly in these patients as a result of fluctuating blood glucose levels. Metabolic studies such as C-peptide level, pro-insulin level, and hemoglobin A1-C should be a part of the laboratory values checked before transplantation.

18. How often should testing be repeated while patients wait for pancreas transplantation?

Cardiac reevaluation should be done every 6 months to monitor for possible progression of cardiovascular disease. Eye examinations should be included in the annual reevaluation testing required by transplant centers. Hemoglobin A1-C should be tested at least every 3 months to ensure adequate blood glucose control.

19. Where is the pancreas placed during transplantation?

The pancreas is normally placed intraperitoneally because of the rich vascular field within the peritoneum and the ability to absorb pancreatic "sweat." The transplanted graft is most often placed in the right iliac fossa for PA and SPK transplantations. The left iliac fossa is reserved for the transplanted kidney in the case of SPK transplantation. In cases of PAK, the pancreas is transplanted on the opposite side of the previously transplanted kidney.

20. What happens to the native pancreas?

The native pancreas remains in place and is not altered during pancreas transplantation. No longer able to produce insulin, the native pancreas continues to supply enzymes and performs its exocrine functions. The new pancreas is transplanted only to supply the insulin required to correct blood glucose levels. The enzymes produced by the new pancreas are drained in two fashions: (1) enteric drainage or (2) bladder drainage, both of which are surgical technique options.

21. What is enteric drainage?

Enteric drainage involves the drainage of exocrine secretions into the bowel. The whole pancreas along with a segment of donor duodenum is transplanted onto the recipient small bowel. All enzymes are drained into the bowel and excreted with the stool.

22. How does urinary drainage differ?

With urinary drainage the enzymes are drained into the bladder and excreted with the urine.

23. Is there an advantage to the different surgical techniques used to drain enzyme secretions for the transplanted pancreas?

For years there has been a controversy over the better method of draining the newly transplanted pancreas. The major advantages of enteric drainage are fewer urinary tract infections, a lower incidence of pancreatitis because risks of reflux are reduced, and fewer metabolic complications. A lower surgical complication rate and the use of urinary amylase for rejection monitoring are some of the advantages to the urinary drainage surgical technique.

24. What are the disadvantages to each method of drainage?

The major reported problem with the enteric drainage technique is the risk of anastomotic leak. This type of leak can complicate the transplant process by causing pancreatitis and/or sepsis. For bladder-drained patients, urology complications are the biggest challenge. Approximately one-fourth of the patients with bladder drainage need to be converted to enteric drainage by 6 months following transplantation to minimize urinary symptoms.

25. What are the postoperative complications associated with pancreas transplantation?

The most frequent complications following pancreas transplantation are thrombosis, pancreatitis, anastomotic leaks, and sepsis.

26. How is vascular thrombosis recognized and treated?

Vascular thrombosis can be caused by either arterial or venous thrombosis; pancreatic vascular thrombosis presents with acute abdominal pain, consistently high blood glucose levels, and a rise in serum amylase levels. If vascular thrombosis is suspected, exploration may be necessary to confirm the diagnosis. More prevalent is venous thrombosis in which, upon reentry, the pancreas appears large, engorged, and dark-blue in color. When vascular thrombosis is present, the graft has to be removed to prevent serious infection.

27. How common is pancreatitis following pancreas transplantation?

The handling of the donor pancreas and preservation techniques may induce a mild elevation of amylase immediately after transplant, which may be of no significance in the majority of pancreas transplants. However, caution must be observed in these patients because pancreatitis can be a sign of acute rejection in all pancreas transplants. Any consistent rise in serum amylase, and/or abdominal tenderness over the graft site should be considered rejection until ruled out. Anastomotic strictures can also produce a pancreatitis in patients later after transplantation.

28. Are anastomotic leaks prevalent in pancreas transplantation?

Leaks within the first 3 months after transplantation are common and are the most frequent postoperative complication. Patients often present with severe abdominal pain and an elevation in serum amylase. Radiological testing can detect most leaks, and for the most part these leaks require reexploration with repair of the anastomosis. Some smaller anastomotic leaks can be treated successfully by stent placement.

29. Is sepsis more common in pancreas transplantation?

Sepsis is the most common cause of death following pancreas transplantation. It is more common in pancreas transplant than kidney transplant alone, and it occurs more frequently than in other organ transplants. Sepsis can be attributed to the acidity of the enzymes excreted by the pancreas to aid in digestion of food. Often, this acidic atmosphere can erode the anastomosis causing a septic peritonitis. The peritonitis can go undetected until the patient presents with fever, extended and/or tender abdomen, and rising blood glucose levels. As in most cases of sepsis, once it is diagnosed, hospitalization for aggressive intravenous antibiotics, medical management of fluid intake and output, and close monitoring of blood glucose levels are essential. All cases of sepsis in the post-pancreas transplant patient have serious consequences and often require urgent exploratory laparotomy. Percutaneous drains to exchange abdominal fluid with a continuous flush of antiseptic solutions may be required.

30. What immunosuppressive regimen is used for the pancreas transplant recipient?

All forms of pancreas transplant (PA, SPK and PAK) use the same immunosuppression combination as kidney transplant alone. Currently, a combination of tacrolimus (Prograf), mycophenolate

mofetil (Cellcept) with or without prednisone is used as maintenance in most pancreas transplants. A more aggressive therapy with antibody induction has proven to be successful short-term
in reducing the risk of early rejection.

31. When can rejection be recognized in the pancreas transplant recipient?

During the initial phases of rejection in the pancreas transplant recipient, the insulin-produc-
ing islet cells are spared and glucose levels remain normal. Unfortunately, if rejection is missed
in its early stages, it can cause inflammation resulting in fibrosis of the graft and certain destruction of the islet cells. It is only at this time of destruction that a rise in blood glucose levels will
occur. Once a recipient becomes hyperglycemic, the rejection has become irreversible. Biopsy of
the head of the pancreas is the definitive diagnosis; however, such biopsies can be complicated
and have risks. The difficulty in diagnosing and initiating treatment for rejection in these recipients probably accounts for the lower graft survival rates within these subgroups.

In SPK transplantation, the transplanted kidney usually is the first to become involved. The
typical signs and symptoms of kidney rejection that occur are a sharp rise in serum creatinine, pain
at the transplant site, and possibly fever. Ideally, all pancreas transplant recipients should be biopsied if rejection is a question. In the case of the SPK, a biopsy of the kidney should be done before
initiating treatment for rejection. There is a high probability the pathology will confirm the diagnosis of rejection, and it can be assumed to involve both grafts. Once again, in SPK transplantation blood glucose levels do not elevate until after damage is done to the pancreatic islet cells.

**32. When should treatment for rejection be initiated in the PA, PAK or SPK transplant
recipient?**

If there is a consistent rise in serum amylase and/or creatinine and if biopsy is not feasible,
as in the case of the PA and PAK transplants, symptoms should be treated as rejection with rejection protocols specific to the transplant center. If caught early enough, medication addition and/or
adjustments will provide the desired results.

33. How does pancreas transplantation affect long-term secondary diabetic complications?

Pancreas transplantation has been shown to improve quality of life beyond that of kidney
transplantation alone. It has rendered many recipients with type-I diabetes insulin-free. Much research has been done on normalizing blood glucose levels and improving carbohydrate metabolism in relation to the positive effect of reducing complications in diabetic patients. Long-term
complications of diabetes such as nephropathy, neuropathy, retinopathy have been reduced, and
in some cases progression has been arrested following pancreas transplantation. Studies have
suggested improvement in some of the debilitating side effects in pancreas transplant patients
who remain insulin-free. Further research into the long-term treatment of diabetes with pancreas
transplantation needs to be done to demonstrate its long-term effectiveness.

34. Is pancreas transplantation cost-effective?

SPK transplantation has proved to be successful and to improve quality of life for recipients.
The treatment is not only effective but also cost-efficient when compared with the costs of complications and lifetime dialysis in the diabetic renal failure patient. Cost analysis and research
continue to evaluate the cost-effectiveness of PA and PAK. However, the general consensus is
that the reduction in diabetic complications is money well spent.

35. What if there is a possibility of a live donor for a diabetic renal failure patient?

A live-donor kidney transplant is always the best choice, when available, for three reasons:
1. Shorter time on dialysis
2. An ideal HLA match (most living donors are not HLA-matched) and decreased ischemic
   time
3. Scheduled procedure optimizing health status

Once the kidney has been transplanted and immunosuppression has been stabilized, a PAK
transplant can be considered.

36. What are the UNOS waiting times for pancreas transplantation?

Candidates with type-I diabetes listed for SPK transplantation have a shorter wait time on the UNOS waiting list because of the combination of organs. The advantages to SPK transplantation give the edge to candidates waiting for dual organs. PA and PAK candidates can wait upwards of 2 years, depending on the demographic area, blood type, and HLA matching.

37. Are there any other transplant options for the diabetic patient?

Isolated islet cell transplantation remains an experimental procedure at the time of this writing (see chapter 15). Much research has been done in recent years to refine the isolation process, determine the best mode for transplanting the isolated cells, and determine the long-term effects of islet cell transplantation. Several centers are participating in patient trials in islet cell transplantation, but candidate selection is rigid and limited at this time.

38. Are there enough donors to support whole pancreas transplantation and islet cell research?

As pancreas transplantation graft survival and patient survival continue to improve with newer immunosuppressive therapies and refined surgical techniques, the list of patients waiting for transplant has soared. With additional islet cell transplantation often requiring 2–3 donors to maintain insulin independence, the pancreas will become as scarce as livers to those in need of that life-saving transplant.

39. What alternatives are under investigation?

Currently, there is no cure for the organ shortage that exists for all organs. Experimental research on live donation and partial pancreas transplantation has had poor results. As pancreas transplantation becomes more accepted as a treatment for patients with type-I diabetes, the supply vs. demand will certainly continue to hinder progress. However, the need continues to accelerate because of the severe complications of diabetes. Whether the research is on whole organ transplantation or islet cell isolation, the need to explore alternatives for the donated organ is an ongoing quest.

BIBLIOGRAPHY

1. Danovitch GM: Handbook of Kidney Transplantation, 3rd ed. Philadelphia, Lippincott Williams & Wilkens, 2001.
2. Ginns, LC, Cosimi AB, Morris PJ: Transplantation. Malden, MA, Blackwell Science, 1999.
3. International Transplant Nurses Society: 9th Annual Symposium and General Assembly. Las Vegas, NV, 2000.
4. International Transplant Nurses Society: 10th Annual Symposium and General Assembly. Cambridge, England, 2001.
5. Greussner AC, Sutherland DER: Analysis of United States (US) and non-US pancreas transplants as reported to the International Pancreas Transplant Registry (IPTR) and to the United Network for Organ Sharing (UNOS). In Cecka JM, Terasaki PI (eds): Clinical Transplants 1999. Los Angeles, UCLA Tissue Typing Laboratory, 1999.
6. Smith SL: Tissue and Organ Transplantation: Implications for Professional Nursing Practice. St. Louis, Mosby, 1990.
7. Kuo PC, Johnson LB, Schweitter EJ, et al: Simultaneous pancreas-kidney transplantation—a comparison of enteric and bladder drainage of exocrine pancreatic secretion. Transplantation 64:933–935, 1997.
8. Shoemaker WC, Ayres SM, Grenvik A, Holbrook PR: Textbook of Critical Care, 3rd ed. Philadelphia, Saunders, 2000.
9. The Diabetes Control and Complications Trial Research Group: The effect of intensive treatment of diabetes on the development and progression of long-term complications in insulin-dependent diabetes mellitus. N Engl J Med 329:977–986, 1993.

13. LIVER TRANSPLANTATION

Bridget M. Flynn, BSN, RN, CCTC

1. How many cadaveric liver transplantations are performed each year?

In the year ending December 2001, there were 5177 liver transplantations performed in the United States. This number is somewhat above the 4478 cadaveric liver transplantations performed in 1999. Living liver donations are on the rise. (Information on living donors can be found in chapters 16 and 17.) Dr. Thomas Starzl performed the first human liver transplantation in 1963 and the first successful liver transplantation in a human in 1967. Since that time there have been significant advances made in surgical and procurement procedures and in the immuno-suppressant regimens. The advances have contributed to the increasing success of liver transplantation for those with end-stage liver disease.

2. What are the current liver transplant survival rates?

Liver transplantation has been recognized as the standard of care for treatment of patients suffering from acute and chronic end-stage liver disease. The current rates for patient survival are approximately 85% at 1 year and > 70% at 5 years.

3. Describe the main functions of the liver.

The liver is the largest and one of the most complex organs in the body. It lies just below the ribs, lungs, and diaphragm and just above the stomach and intestines. It weighs 1–3 pounds and has 2 lobes: the right, which is the larger, and the left. Along with the gallbladder and the pancreas, the liver produces substances to help digestion and use food. The liver performs over 500 different functions, which include the following:
- Storage of carbohydrates for energy
- Storage of blood sugar, iron, and vitamins for use in the body
- Removal and breakdown of harmful substances such as ammonia and toxic chemicals
- Production of bile, which is stored by the gallbladder and used to break down and use fats
- Production of proteins that are needed for normal blood clotting

4. What is the difference between acute and chronic liver disease?

Liver disease can present suddenly, or acutely, as fulminant liver failure in which the onset of liver dysfunction and encephalopathy are seen within 8 weeks of the onset of symptoms. Acute liver disease often first presents with vague symptoms such as anorexia or malaise and is described as a viral syndrome until jaundice occurs. The most common example of acute liver disease is acetaminophen toxicity, but other causes include cryptogenic, drug-induced hepatitis B, hepatitis A, Wilson's disease, acute fatty liver of pregnancy, Budd-Chiari disease, and mushroom poisoning. Acute liver failure is generally seen in young patients who were relatively healthy until the time of illness. Before transplantation, acute or fulminant liver disease was associated with a high mortality rate because affected patients often require transplantation within 24–48 hours to avoid death.

Chronic liver diseases cause liver failure by damaging the liver over a period of time. The damage is usually irreversible. Chronic disease often causes cirrhosis that develops when normal liver cells are damaged and die and are replaced by scar tissue. Cirrhosis arises from various liver diseases, including chronic viral hepatitis, primary biliary cirrhosis, and primary sclerosing cholangitis.

The complications of liver disease, rather than the disease itself, indicate when transplantation is necessary. Such complications fall into two categories: portal hypertension and reduced liver cell mass. The presence of portal hypertension may result in gastrointestinal bleeding and refractory ascites. Complications of reduced liver cell mass include coagulopathy, jaundice, impaired drug metabolism, and encephalopathy.

5. Is transplantation the only option for patients with acute liver failure?

Currently, liver transplantation is considered the best option for irreversible acute liver failure, but many patients with acute liver failure die while waiting for a suitable organ because of the severe shortage of donors. For this reason, patients with acute liver failure should be referred to centers that not only perform transplants, but also have the capability of supporting patients until an organ is available. The following are some options for hepatic support:

- Artificial liver support devices
- Bioartificial livers
- Hepatocyte transplantation
- Extracorporeal liver perfusion

6. What are the main indications for liver transplantation?

The most common indications for transplantation in the adult population are chronic hepatitis C, alcoholic liver disease, chronic hepatitis B, primary biliary cirrhosis, primary sclerosing cholangitis, and autoimmune hepatitis. Cholestatic diseases such as biliary atresia and metabolic disorders such as α_1-antitrypsin deficiency account for more than 60% of all pediatric liver transplants.

Cirrhosis and Liver Transplantation

	SPECIAL CONSIDERATIONS FOR LIVER TRANSPLANTATION (OLT)
Hepatocellular diseases	
✓ Chronic hepatitis	
• Hepatitis B	Virus should be nonreplicating (HBV-DNA negative).
• Hepatitis D	Co- or superinfects hepatitis B. Rare in the United States.
• Hepatitic C	Important to exclude alcohol as comorbid factor.
• Autoimmune	Pre-OLT medication may affect post-OLT bone disease.
• Drug-induced	Examples: nitrofurantoin, alphamethyldopa.
✓ Steatohepatitis	
• Alcohol	Abstinence and social support critical for OLT.
• Obesity	Increasing prevalence of cirrhosis. Rate of recurrence.
• Drug-induced	Example: Amiodarone.
✓ Vascular disease	
• Chronic Budd-Chiari syndrome	Acute occlusion is amenable to decompressive surgery. R/O myeloproliferative syndrome, thrombotic tendency.
✓ Inborn errors of metabolism	
• Hemochromatosis	Cardiac involvement results in increased OLT morbidity.
• α_1-antitrypsin deficiency	Lung disease is rare in the presence of liver cirrhosis.
✓ Wilson's disease	OLT for acute disease not amenable to medical therapy.
• Glycogen storage disease type I/III	Can present in early adulthood.
Cholestatic diseases	
✓ Disease of intrahepatic bile ducts	
• Biliary atresia	Kasai procedure may offer relief for a few years before OLT.
• Primary biliary cirrhosis	Bone disease can be especially problematic post-OLT.
• Drug-induced disease	Examples: Chlorpromazine, tolbutamide.
• Familial cholestasis	Byler's syndrome, arteriohepatic dysplasia.
• Cystic fibrosis	Inspissated bile syndrome leading to cirrhosis.
✓ Disease of extrahepatic bile ducts	
• Primary sclerosing cholangitis	Secondary cholangiocarcinoma may contraindicate OLT.
• Secondary biliary cirrhosis	Requires Roux-en-Y anastomosis at OLT.

HBV = hepatitis B virus, OLT = orthotopic liver transplantation.
From Stuart F, Abecassis M, Kaufman D: Organ Transplantation. Georgetown, TX, Landes Bioscience, 2000, with permission.

Liver Abnormalities Without Cirrhosis

✓ Congenital abnormalities	
• Urea cycle enzyme deficiency	Severe hyperammonemia may cause neurological deficits.
• Homozygous hypercholesterolemia	Important to assess status of coronary arteries pre-OLT.
• Primary hyperoxaluria type I	May also require renal transplantation.
• Familial amyloidotic polyneuropathy	Need to assess cardiac status. Disease may be too advanced.
✓ Developmental abnormalities	
• Polycystic liver disease	OLT indicated for symptoms from massive hepatomegaly.
• Caroli's disease	Chronic biliary sepsis can be an indication for OLT.

OLT = orthotopic liver transplantation.
From Stuart F, Abecassis M, Kaufman D: Organ Transplantation. Georgetown, TX, Landes Bioscience, 2000, with permission.

7. Are there any contraindications to liver transplantation?

The number of patients being referred for transplantation continues to rise each year, but because of the disproportionate number of donor organs available and differences among individual centers' criteria for transplantation, minimal listing criteria guidelines have been accepted as well as contraindications. Absolute contraindications include the following:

• Multisystem organ failure
• Extrahepatic malignancy
• Advanced cardiac or pulmonary disease
• Severe or uncontrolled extrahepatic infection
• Active substance abuse

Transplantation should be considered on an individual basis for patients with renal insufficiency, human immunodeficiency virus (HIV) infection, primary hepatobiliary malignancy, hemochromatosis, and noncompliance with medical therapy because these factors are associated with decreased posttransplantation survival but are not absolute contraindications.

8. What is the age limit in considerations for a liver transplant?

Different transplant centers have individual protocols with regard to the maximal age that they will consider a patient for transplantation. Most centers consider each patient on an individual basis with regard to their current and past health history rather than impose a maximal limit criterion.

9. Why are patients with alcoholic liver disease considered for liver transplantation?

Potential candidates with end-stage liver disease from alcoholic cirrhosis are currently considered suitable candidates for transplantation so long as they meet the minimal listing criteria stipulated by the United Network of Organ Sharing (UNOS). However, patients with alcoholism, or other forms of substance abuse, are often asked to meet certain center-specific requirements before being accepted for placement on waiting lists. These requirements may include ongoing psychiatric evaluation, a minimal period of abstinence set by the individual center (e.g., 6 months is often an acceptable minimal time of abstinence), random serum or urine screening, and participation in a formal rehabilitation program.

The long-standing opinion that patients with alcoholic liver disease should be subjected to a more severe selection process than nonalcoholic patients persists in general society, but has raised many medical, surgical, and ethical discussions among transplant professionals as well. Although circumstances today require that all potential candidates undergo a more thorough screening process, primarily because of the scarcity of organs, it has yet to be proven that patients with alcoholic liver disease are any less deserving of equal access to medical care for liver disease than those who have developed liver disease or failure from intravenous drug use or from ignoring medical advice regarding such practices as smoking, diet, exercise, or medications.

10. Under what circumstances would a patient with a liver tumor be considered for a liver transplant?

Patients with primary liver cancer who are not candidates for liver resection and have no evidence of metastasis outside of the liver and/or macrovascular involvement may be considered for transplantation. The evaluation should include an ultrasound; a computed tomographic (CT) or magnetic resonance imaging (MRI) scan of the chest, abdomen, and pelvis; a bone scan; and an alpha-fetoprotein level. A single nodule should be < 5 cm in size; two or three nodules should all be < 3.0 cm and in a single lobe. Those with neoplasms > 5 cm or nodules in both lobes and those with evidence of extrahepatobiliary tumor should not be considered for transplantation.

If a patient is accepted and listed for liver transplantation, a reevaluation of tumor status is done every 3 months.

11. Under what circumstances would a patient with human immunodeficiency virus be considered as a candidate for liver transplantation?

Until recently, HIV-positive patients were excluded from consideration for transplantation. Advances in the management of patients with HIV and results from a few centers that have transplanted such individuals successfully have led to broader protocols. Now HIV is an individual consideration in transplantation rather than an absolute contraindication.

In addition to meeting all of the same listing criteria as an HIV-negative candidate, the HIV-positive candidate may have to meet requirements that are specific to the HIV infection. For example, HIV-positive patients in need of liver transplantation must meet the following criteria at the University of Pittsburgh Medical Center:
- CD4 > 150
- Nadar CD4 > 50
- HIV viral load:
  - Undetectable on HIV medication regimen
  - Positive off HIV medication regimen secondary to worsening liver function tests
- No history of opportunistic infections

12. What steps are involved in the evaluation process for liver transplantation?

The evaluation process involves various tests and procedures that are carried out by the transplant team. A transplant team generally consists of a hepatologist, surgeon, coordinator, social worker, psychiatrist, financial counselor, anesthesiologist, pathologist, pharmacist, and dietitian.

Laboratory testing should include the following:
- Complete blood count (CBC)
- Prothrombin time (PT), international normalized ratio (INR), and partial thromboplastin time (PTT)
- Blood urea nitrogen (BUN), creatinine, electrolytes (including a fasting blood sugar)
- Liver enzymes (serum glutamate pyruvate transaminase [SGPT], serum glutamate oxaloacetate transaminase [SGOT]) and liver function tests (total bilirubin and albumin)
- Total protein
- Hepatitis B and C serologies, HIV, cytomegalovirus (CMV), and Epstein-Barr virus (EBV) serologies
- Antinuclear antibody (ANA), antimitochondrial antibody (AMA), ferritin, alpha-fetoprotein
- Thyroid function tests
- Cholesterol and triglyceride levels
- Drug and alcohol testing

Other tests generally included in the evaluation are the following:
- Chest x-ray, electrocardiogram (EKG)
- Doppler ultrasound of the hepatic vein and artery
- Pulmonary function tests
- Liver biopsy
- Computed tomographic (CT) scan

- Endoscopy, colonoscopy
- Echocardiogram (ECHO), multiple gated acquisition (MUGA) scan, and angiogram/arteriogram

Routine healthcare screening is also requested during the evaluation phase. Such screening includes gynecological examination, including a Papanicolaou smear and mammogram for women and prostate specific antigen (PSA) testing in men. Depending on the age, diagnosis of the liver disease, patient history, and review of the potential recipient by the transplant team, other tests may be added or deleted, as indicated.

13. When is a patient officially on the list?

Once the evaluation testing is completed, the potential candidate is presented formally to the entire transplant team for discussion of suitability for transplant. At this time, any special considerations that may affect the posttransplant phase are brought to the attention of the team, such as family support, financial situation, and psychiatric history. Then, so long as the patient fulfills the minimal listing requirements and each individual center's guidelines, a decision is made by the whole team about whether to list the patient at that time. The transplant coordinator generally informs the patient and the referring physician when the patient is activated on the waiting list.

14. What are the minimal listing criteria for liver transplantation?

The Child-Pugh score provides the minimal listing criteria for potential liver transplant candidates. The score is obtained using the Child-Turcotte Pugh (CTP) Classification, often referred to as the Child-Pugh score, to ensure that the patient's liver disease is severe enough to necessitate transplantation.

Child-Turcotte Pugh Classification

POINTS	1	2	3
Encephalopathy	None	Moderate Stage 1–2	Severe Stage 3–4
Ascites	None	Slight or controlled with diuretic therapy	At least moderate despite diuretics
Bilirubin			
For primary biliary cirrhosis or primary sclerosing cholantitis	1–4	4–10	> 10
For all other diseases	< 2	2–3	> 3
Albumin	> 3.5	2.8–3.5	< 2.8
Prothrombin time	< 4	4.6	> 6
or	< 1.7	1.7–2.3	> 2.3

A patient must have a score of at least 7 to be placed on the waiting list, which indicates a Child's Class B. Certain complications (such as refractory variceal bleeding, encephalopathy, ascites, and spontaneous bacterial peritonitis), guidelines for patients with extenuating circumstances, and quality of life exceptions (such as pruritus, metabolic bone disease, and xanthomatous neuropathy) must be reviewed on an individual basis by each center's regional review board.

Once a candidate is actively listed, he or she is given a MELD (model for end-stage liver disease) or PELD (pediatric end-stage liver disease model) score, which prioritizes patients waiting for a liver transplant. The MELD score is used for adult candidates, and the PELD score is used for pediatric candidates. These models have been designed to better identify patients, based on medical urgency, in need of transplantation and thereby decrease the number of deaths of patients awaiting liver transplantation.

The MELD/PELD scoring system replaces all previous status 2A, 2B, and 3 categories with a continuous score calculated by the MELD/PELD model. Adult patients receive a score based on objective laboratory standards of bilirubin, INR, and creatinine; scores range from 6 (less medically urgent) to 40 (more medically urgent). Pediatric patients (those < 18 years of age) receive a score based on bilirubin, INR, albumin, growth failure, and whether the child is < 1 year old. Status 1 category remains in place for both adults and pediatric candidates and is not affected by MELD or PELD. Waiting time is still used as a tiebreaker, if necessary.

15. What causes some patients with liver disease to develop ascites?

An accumulation of fluid in the abdominal cavity occurs when fluid leaks from the liver and the intestine as a result of portal hypertension, a decreased ability of the blood vessels to retain fluid, fluid retention by the kidneys, and alterations in the liver's ability to regulate bodily fluids. This accumulation is seen in patients with chronic liver diseases, such as cirrhosis, rather than in patients with acute liver disease.

16. What is encephalopathy?

Encephalopathy is a term used to describe what happens to a patient with liver disease who experiences a change in his or her mental status because of the build-up of toxic substances in the blood. When liver function is impaired, it cannot remove such substances as they pass through the liver; or, as a result of liver disease, some toxins may bypass the liver altogether. The build-up of these protein synthesis byproducts in the blood, such as ammonia, or conditions that increase the levels of protein breakdown products in the blood, such as gastrointestinal bleeding, infection, or a diet high in protein, may cause encephalopathy to occur. Changes in mental status range from mild changes in logical thinking, mood changes, and impaired judgment to drowsiness, confusion, disorientation, lethargy and coma. The degree of encephalopathy is an indication of the severity of the liver disease and is generally graded as mild, moderate, or severe.

17. What can be done for a patient with encephalopathy?

The treatment of encephalopathy consists of treating any precipitating factors, such as an infection or a drug interaction, or making dietary modifications with a protein-restricted diet. Elimination of toxic substances may be achieved with a synthetic sugar (lactulose) given orally or via a nasogastric tube. Lactulose alters the acidity of the intestines, changing the type of bacteria present, which decreases the absorption of ammonia, and it acts as a laxative to rid the body of the toxins causing the changes in mental status. Neomycin may also be used in place of lactulose. The treatments may also be given in the form of an enema. With severe encephalopathy a nasogastric tube and endotracheal intubation may be necessary to prevent aspiration. Through these interventions the encephalopathy is generally reversible.

18. What is spontaneous bacterial peritonitis?

Spontaneous bacterial peritonitis (SBP) is seen in patients with advanced liver disease and ascites. Clinically, the candidate may present with fever, abdominal pain, hepatic encephalopathy, and abrupt onset of worsening renal and hepatic function. SBP is diagnosed with paracentesis and with blood and ascitic fluid cultures. SBP is treated with antibiotics acutely and then prophylactically to prevent repeat episodes. A repeat paracentesis is necessary upon completion of the course of antibiotics because SBP is a contraindication to transplantation.

19. What is hepatorenal syndrome?

Hepatorenal syndrome is kidney dysfunction that results from persistent renal vasoconstriction, which is often present in patients with advanced liver failure. It is characterized by severe hyponatremia that does not respond to fluid resuscitation. It is documented with a rising serum creatinine of 1.5 or greater with no other known cause of renal insufficiency. Hepatorenal syndrome is generally a reversible condition following transplantation.

20. What is the possibility that a patient will die while waiting for a liver transplant?

The difference between the number of people needing an organ and the number of organ donors remains one of the toughest problems facing organ transplantation today. All efforts to increase organ donation continue to fall short of the need. Current UNOS data for the year ending on June 30, 2001, reveal that out of 18,089 patients on the list for a liver transplant, 1799 died while waiting. The statistics also currently show discrepancies in waiting times among the 11 designated regions across the United States. Patients in areas with longer waiting times have a greater risk of dying while waiting. The data reinforce why there are changes currently being made to the listing and allocation policies for livers.

21. What reasons are given for the poor rate of donation?

It is unrealistic to expect to ever have enough organs for transplantation to meet the needs of patients who are waiting; however, the rate of organ donation could be much higher than it is currently. Although the majority of the population claims to support organ donation, less than half agree to donate when approached for consent. Lack of consent has been attributed to the following identified barriers:

- Demographics, race, gender, education, and socioeconomic level
- Distrust of the medical community
- Religious beliefs
- Fear of mutilation of a loved one's body
- Concern about the actual use of the organs for transplantation versus use for research or discarded
- Lack of knowledge of the wishes of the deceased
- Misunderstanding of brain death criteria
- Family's emotional state at the time

22. What efforts are being made to address the organ shortage?

While educational programs continue to target barriers to donation, current potential alternatives to meet the liver shortage include (1) the legal requirement that all families of patients who have been declared brain dead be asked to consent to organ donation (mandatory request), (2) the assumption of consent to donate by patients who have been declared brain dead without the requirement for family consent (presumed consent), and (3) financial incentives in the form of partial financial assistance with funeral expenses paid directly to the funeral home for the donor families. Reduced-sized liver transplants, split liver transplants, and living donor liver transplants are all surgical options that have the potential to ease the donor shortage. There is also an increasing use of organs from "marginal donors" that once would not have been accepted, including livers from older donors, livers infected with hepatitis B or C, fatty livers, and livers from donors with a history of cancer.

23. Can a person who has received a liver transplant ever be an organ donor?

Yes, persons who have received a liver transplant can be a donor, so long as they meet the same guidelines as required for other donors.

24. What are the major differences among reduced liver, split-liver, and living donor transplants?

At one point, survival rates among children with end-stage liver disease were as low as 50% at some centers because of the difficulty in finding livers small enough for pediatric recipients. Then reduced-sized liver transplants were utilized. The procedure involves the transplantation of the left lobe or the left lateral segment of the liver from the donor to the recipient. Major complications include size mismatch, primary nonfunction, biliary complications, and increased blood loss.

Split-liver transplantation followed in 1988 with some success in eliminating the need to waste a portion of the reduced liver, as well as eliminating the difficult decision whether to use the organ for a child or an adult. This method was thought to be the answer to the donor shortage because one liver provides a viable organ for a child and an adult with no waste. However, because of the complexity of the procedure and postoperative complications of bleeding and biliary leaks, this option is best used only in select situations. Ideally, young, stable, multiorgan donors who have not experienced any significant compromise before harvesting the organs would be considered for splitting of the liver.

Later it was recognized that while split liver transplantation worked well in specific situations, it was not the answer to the organ shortage that it was hoped to be. Those previously opposed to living donation could no longer deny that insufficient strides were being made to increase access to organ transplantation, especially for the pediatric population. Living donation was initially performed only in pediatric patients, partially because of the technical difficulty and partially because of ethical concern for the donor. However, technically capable surgeons rapidly expanded the living liver donor pool to meet the needs of the adult patient.

Success rates with living liver donors in children are nearly 95%, even higher than with standard cadaver transplantation; and even though biliary complications are slightly higher, primary nonfunction in a living donor is rare. Early data on adult-to-adult living liver donation report 3 deaths in approximately 600 cases, a number which continues to fuel that ethical dilemma of what is an acceptable risk for the donor. Living kidney donation has an acceptable risk of 0.1–0.2%, whereas living liver donation is currently 1% (see chapters 16 and 17).

25. What factors determine whether a donor liver is a good organ for transplantation?

Local organ procurement staff do the initial evaluation. Factors include basic demographic information; the medical, surgical, and social histories of the potential donor; the actual cause of brain death; hemodynamics; laboratory data; and serologies. The liver surgeon is then given this information and makes the final decision whether to recover the liver.

Evaluation of Potential Donors by Organ Procurement Organization Staff

Demographics	Laboratory tests
• Donor age, sex, race, and cause of death	• Blood type
History	• Blood gases
• Medical	• Chemistries
• Surgical	• Liver functions
• Social	• Protime, international normalized ratio (INR)
Physical examination and studies	• Cultures of blood, urine, and sputum
• Chest x-ray	• Serologies (human immunodeficiency virus type 1
• Electrocardiogram (EKG)	[HIV1], human immunodeficiency virus type 2
• Echocardiogram	[HIV2], human T-lymphocyte virus [HTLV],
• Cardiac catheterization and/or ultrasound,	rapid plasma reagin [RPR], Venereal Disease
if specifically requested	Research Laboratory [VDRL], Hepatitis B and C)

Many factors have been studied, such as donor age, prolonged intensive care unit (ICU) stay, and cold ischemia time, to help eliminate organs that may be more likely to have primary nonfunction or early dysfunction. However, it is believed that the most accurate test to be done before recovery of the organ is the transplant surgeon's own visual evaluation. The surgeon's experience in evaluating such factors as the color, texture, sharpness of the edges, and fat content and his or her judgment based on the overall appearance of the liver are invaluable in determining probable outcome of a donor liver. For this reason many centers send their own surgical teams to perform the organ recovery.

26. How is it decided which transplant center will receive the offer when a donor liver is available?

Transplant centers are divided into 11 regions geographically. The current UNOS guidelines mandate that when an organ is identified, it is offered locally within the Organ Procurement Organization (OPO) area first, then regionally; if it is not utilized within the OPO region, it is then offered nationally. The fact that these 11 regions differ in size and number of transplant centers that they serve has led to a disparity between between OPOs. Patients with similar degrees of liver disease in different geographic areas have great differences in the amount of time they must wait for an organ. The disparity led the Secretary of State of Health and Human Services, who oversees UNOS, to mandate that initiatives be instituted that will eliminate these differences among regions while creating fairer organ sharing to allow patients who have the greatest medical need not to be penalized by geography (see chapter 1).

27. When a transplant center accepts an offer of a liver, how is it decided who will receive the organ?

When an OPO offers a transplant center an organ, it is offered for a specific patient on the active candidate list. The lists are computerized, and the liver is matched to a specific candidate based on severity of liver disease (the MELD/PELD score described earlier in question 19), blood type matching, size/weight, and, if necessary, the length of time spent on the waiting list.

28. Describe the surgical recovery and preservation of the liver before transplantation.

Once a donor has been deemed suitable, a surgical team proceeds with the recovery. Several teams may be present, each to harvest the respective organ for their center (liver, heart, lung, kidneys, pancreas, and intestines). The surgical team that harvests the liver identifies and preserves the hepatic artery, the portal vein, and the common bile duct. Rapid cooling is necessary and involves placement of a catheter into the distal abdominal aorta and cannulation of the splenic vein or the inferior mesenteric vein. The liver is then perfused with preservation solution. Once the liver is removed from the donor, it is placed on ice and transported in a cooler to the recipient's hospital. With improvements in preservation solutions, the liver may be viable for up to 24 hours, but it still should be transplanted as soon as possible. Most centers attempt to use a liver within 12 hours of preservation because livers that have been used with longer than 12-hour preservation times have been shown to be associated with higher rates of primary nonfunction, hepatic artery thrombosis, and biliary complications.

The donor surgery is done in the operating room under sterile procedure just as any other operation would be. Once the organs are recovered, the donor's body is surgically closed, and the funeral home is notified. Organ donors are treated with great care and respect; an open-casket funeral is possible.

29. What is involved in preparation of the recipient for surgery?

The recipient is evaluated for suitability for immediate surgery. The evaluation involves basic procedures, like those for any general surgery as instituted by individual hospitals, generally consisting of basic information such as height, weight, vital signs, laboratory tests, NPO, intravenous access for fluids and preoperative antibiotics, cultures for urine and blood, EKG, chest x-ray, type and cross for blood, fresh frozen plasma, and platelets, as well as anesthesia consultation and consent for surgery. The family is asked to wait in a designated waiting area and informed that the operation may last from 6–12 hours. Some operations may take longer, depending on the recipient's condition going into surgery or complications that may arise during the operation. Most hospitals have some type of system in place to give families periodic updates throughout the transplant operation.

30. Provide an overview of the actual liver transplant surgery.

After the patient is anesthetized and properly positioned for a long operation, the anesthesiologist gives the surgeons the approval to proceed with the operation. The surgeons begin by making an incision in the abdomen, which is often referred to as a "Mercedes," "peace sign," or "upside-down Y" incision. The surgeons remove the diseased liver, the hepatectomy, by locating the main liver arteries and veins and bile ducts and then clamping and protecting them while the liver is removed. This stage may be complicated by the degree of portal hypertension, which makes the liver hard and removal difficult. Portal hypertension may cause the vessels around the liver to be enlarged and bleed. Ascites causes excess fluid to be present in the abdominal cavity. Bleeding is also affected by the degree to which the liver is able to make clotting factors, and any previous abdominal surgeries will have caused scar tissue, which makes it more difficult to get through the abdominal wall and dissect the liver.

Simultaneously, another surgeon is preparing the liver on the back table for transplantation into the patient. Preparation involves inspection and repair of the blood vessels. The donor gall bladder is removed. Once the new liver is in place, the vessels are sewn together, and the clamps are removed slowly to check for any leakage. After the surgeon is satisfied with the vascular anastomoses, the bile duct is connected. The bile duct of the donor is sewn to the bile duct of the recipient over a tube, generally referred to as a biliary stent or T-tube. This type of bile duct configuration is a duct-to-duct reconstruction, or a choledochocholedochostomy. If the bile duct of the recipient is affected by the liver disease, such as with primary sclerosing cholangitis, the diseased portion is removed. The remaining portion of the bile duct is then usually too short for a duct-to-duct anastomosis; therefore, it is connected directly to the intestine in a procedure called a Roux-en-Y choledochojejunostomy. Patients with a Roux-en-Y anastomosis will not have a T-tube.

After all of the anastomoses have been completed and there are no signs of leaks or bleeding, the abdomen is closed with absorbable sutures and staples, and several abdominal drains, usually 2–3 Jackson-Pratt drains, are placed. The recipient is then taken directly to the ICU. A liver transplant recipient is usually in the ICU for 24–72 hours because of the length of the procedure itself; prolonged anesthesia; hypothermia; the potential for hemorrhage; observation of immediate graft function; large fluid resuscitations; the number of tubes, catheters, and drains; and the need for initial short-term mechanical ventilation. A patient's length of stay is often estimated by the severity of illness before surgery.

31. How soon can the team tell if the liver is working?

Liver function is one of the three most important considerations in the postoperative period for a liver transplant recipient. However, monitoring of liver function actually begins in the operating room. The intraoperative signs that are monitored include hemodynamic stability, adequate urine output, acid–base balance, coagulation normalization, regulation of body temperature, normal blood sugars, good bile production, and good texture and color of the liver.

After the patient is transferred to the ICU, liver function continues to be monitored with regard to the patient's hemodynamic stability; how quickly he or she awakens from the anesthesia; lactate clearance; continued normalization of blood sugars; normal PT, PTT, and INR; decrease to normalization of liver functions, and the amount and color of bile (if a T-tube is in place to observe the bile).

If there is evidence of liver dysfunction, it is important to determine the cause. Primary nonfunction is one of the worst postoperative complications, and early retransplantation is necessary. In addition to primary nonfunction, there are many forms of liver dysfunction. Liver, or graft, dysfunction can range from mild to severe, and retransplantation is not always necessary; however, supportive medical measures are needed.

In the presence of primary nonfunction and severe liver dysfunction, other technical complications need to be ruled out. However, once technical complications have been eliminated, the main difference between primary nonfunction and severe hepatic dysfunction is that progressive deterioration of mental status and increasing, uncorrectable protimes are seen in primary nonfunction patients.

Causes of Hepatic Dysfunction

Immediate	Delayed
1. Primary allograft nonfunction	1. Rejection
2. Primary allograft dysfunction	2. Infection
3. Hepatic artery thrombosis	3. Biliary tract obstruction
4. Portal vein thrombosis	4. Recurrent disease
5. Hepatic vein and caval thrombosis	
6. Biliary tract obstruction/leak	

From Stuart F, Abecassis M, Kaufman D: Organ Transplantation. Georgetown, TX, Landes Bioscience, 2000, with permission.

Causes of Hepatic Dysfunction

1. Failure to regain consciousness	5. Renal dysfunction
2. Hemodynamic instability	6. Rise in transaminases and bilirubin
3. Poor quality and quantity of bile	7. Acid-base imbalance
4. Increasing prothrombin time	8. Persistent hypothermia

From Stuart F, Abecassis M, Kaufman D: Organ Transplantation. Georgetown, TX, Landes Bioscience, 2000, with permission.

32. What other complications are common in the postoperative phase?

The most common complications are rejection, infection, mechanical problems, and psychological changes.

Rejection: Rejection is the natural response of the transplant recipient's immune system , which fights or rejects the new liver. Up to 70% of liver recipients have at least one episode of rejection, often occurring between the first 4–14 days after transplant and the first 3 months. Medications that specifically suppress the transplant recipient's immune response are given immediately after surgery and most likely will be taken for the rest of the recipient's life.

There are signs of rejection, but a liver biopsy is the only true way to diagnose whether a person is having rejection. One advantage in liver transplantation is that elevated liver functions are often the first sign of rejection and can be monitored easily with routine blood work before physical symptoms develop. Patients need to be informed that they can feel perfectly well and still have rejection. Most rejection is reversible if diagnosed and treated early, so patient compliance with the recommended schedule for laboratory testing is important.

The following are possible signs and symptoms of rejection:

- Elevated liver enzymes
- Fatigue
- Fever
- Tenderness or pain over the liver
- Dark-colored urine
- Yellow eyes
- Yellow skin
- Ascites
- Itching of the skin

Histopathologic confirmation can be made with the Banff scale for grading acute cellular rejection in the liver recipient:

- Indeterminate—characterized by portal inflammatory infiltration that does not meet the criteria for the diagnosis of acute rejection.
- Mild (grade I)—shows a rejection infiltrate in a minority of the triads that is confined within the the portal spaces.
- Moderate (grade II)—shows a rejection infiltrate in most or all of the triads.
- Severe (grade III)—includes the same criteria as in moderate rejection, but also shows spillover into the periportal areas and moderate-to-severe perivenular inflammation extending into the hepatic parenchyma, and is associated with perivenular hepatocyte necrosis.

Infectious complications: Most of the infections seen in the postoperative liver transplant patient are related to immunosuppressions that are necessary after transplantation. The most common are bacterial, fungal, or viral infections. In the early postoperative period, nosocomial gram-negative bacterial and candidal infections are the most common. From 1–6 months after transplantation, cytomegalovirus (CMV), Epstein-Barr virus (EBV), *Pneumocystis carinii* and *Aspergillus* are often seen; but after 6 months, the rate of infection reverts to that often seen in the general population, except for patients on high doses of immunosuppression medications.

The immunosuppressant medications that are given to fight rejection are the same ones that make it more difficult for the body to fight infections. A transplant recipient also may have additional factors that increase the risk for infections, which include disruptions in skin integrity, chronic illness, poor nutritional status, and extremely young or extremely old age. Unfortunately, the signs and symptoms are similar as well; therefore, transplant recipients need to be informed that all symptoms need to be evaluated for potential risks.

Some common signs and symptoms of infection are listed below:

- Fever/chills, especially any fever of 38.5°C (101°F), or any low-grade fever 37.8°C (100°F) that lasts longer than 24 hours
- Confusion and changes in mental status
- Cough, sputum production, and shortness of breath
- Nausea/vomiting
- Anorexia/weight loss
- Fatigue and lethargy
- Joint pain and muscle aches
- Neck stiffness
- Swollen glands
- Urinary burning, frequency, pain, or bleeding
- Drainage, redness, pain, swelling, leaks, or odor at the wound, incision, T-tube, or catheter sites

Bacterial infections are seen in as many as 50% of posttransplant patients in the form of intravenous-line, wound, biliary tract, urinary, respiratory, and blood stream infections. Patients with bacterial infections primarily present with fever and should be screened immediately whenever infection is suspected.

Mechanical problems: Arterial complications occur between 5 and 15% of the time and include hepatic artery thrombosis, stenosis, and pseudoaneurysm. Thrombosis is the most common of the three with an incidence of 1.6–8%. These complications are followed by portal vein thrombosis, which occurs with an incidence of about 2%. Stenosis or thrombosis of the hepatic vein or the inferior vena cave is rarely seen. Biliary complications have an incidence of up to 30%. Such complications include leaks, strictures, and obstruction.

33. Is it true that some transplant recipients will not need to take immunosuppressant medications for the rest of their lives?

Microchimerism, or the state by which donor and recipient cells integrate, occurs within minutes of revascularization of any whole organ transplantation. The presence of these donor cells within the recipient may lead, over time, to immunologic nonreactivity or tolerance. When a patient receives a transplant, he or she is considered to be chimeric or to have evidence of microchimerism. Chimerism itself does not determine whether immunosuppressant medications can be discontinued, but tolerance does. Tolerance is the drug-free state that has been achieved safely in some liver recipients as reported by the University of Pittsburgh Medical Center; however, there are currently no valid tests available to identify these patients accurately other than methods of trial and error. Therefore, no organ recipient should ever adjust or stop his or her immunosuppressant medications unless under the direct supervision of the physician or transplant surgeon.

34. What medications are typically used for immunosuppression after transplantation?

There are almost as many immunosuppression combinations as there are transplant centers. But the primary goal is the same for all: to prevent rejection while minimizing side effects.

Induction therapy

Purpose: To be given at the pre- or intraoperative phase with the goal of decreasing the incidence of acute rejection or delaying the first rejection incident, and/or to delay the additional use of calcineurin inhibitors because of the association of renal toxicity with these agents.

Agents: Antilymphocyte globulin (ALG)–MALG
Antithymocyte globulin (ATG)—ATGAM
Antithymocyte globulin (ATG)—Thymoglobulin
Monoclonal anti-CD3 antibodies—Orthoclone, OKT3
Basiliximab—Simulect
Daclizumab—Zenapax

Considerations: The use of induction therapy is much more accepted in the patient with renal insufficiency than in the general liver population, and although it is rapidly becoming a more accepted practice, the results are still early. However, despite the projected advantages of this practice, it needs to be weighed against the impact if may have on infection (e.g., CMV) and recurrent disease (e.g., hepatitis C virus [HCV]).

Calcineurin inhibitors

Purpose: The prevention of rejection and use for long-term maintenance therapy in organ transplant recipients through the inhibition of T-cell proliferation, inhibition of interleukin-2 production, and the the prevention of γ-interferon release.

Agents: Cyclosporine: Sandimmune—original form
                              Neoral—modified form
                              Gengraf—modified form
       Tacrolimus (Prograf)

Considerations: Although the opinion of the efficacy of cyclosporine versus tacrolimus is still largely based on the individual center's practice, one or the other remains a first-line drug in the prevention of graft loss due to rejection. However, as a result of the indisputable side effects of all immunosuppression, efforts are made to minimize side effects or to limit doses of these calcineurin inhibitors with the addition of other agents to be used for double- or triple-drug therapy. And even though toxicity, renal insufficiency, and metabolic complications are generally dose-related, too little may result in rejection and possible graft loss. The complex nature of this balancing act, along with the complexity of each liver patient's condition, has precluded development of only one acceptable immunosuppression regimen.

Corticosteroids

Purpose: To act as global anti-inflammatory and immunosuppressive agents to be used concurrently with a calcineuron inhibitor, at least in the initial postoperative phase.

Agents: SoluMedrol IV
       Prednisone

Considerations: Corticosteroids are effective against the immune system, but the immune system is not their only target. Because of the many and severe side effects of steroids and the improvement in other immunosuppressant agents, transplant centers have developed steroid-reduced or steroid-free drug protocols. Steroid-free protocols have seen an improvement in complications of hypertension, diabetes mellitus, high cholesterol, and obesity. In centers with widespread use of steroid-free protocols, the main reason for reinstituting the use of steroids was the exacerbation of autoimmune diseases such as autoimmune hepatitis.

Other agents

Azathioprine (Imuran)
Mycophenolate mofetil (CellCept)
Rapamycin (Sirolimus)

The primary use of these agents is as steroid-sparing, cyclosporine-sparing, tacrolimus-sparing agents. Although azathioprine has been used for more than 30 years, it has been used less frequently recently because of the emergence of other, more powerful agents; however, it is still used more often in the presence of autoimmune diseases. The gastrointestinal side effects of mycophenolate mofetil often self-limit its use despite the benefit in the situation of renal insufficiency. Rapamycin is also useful for its lack of nephrotoxic side effects, but its full potential has yet to be determined in the liver transplant population.

---

35. On an average, how many medications does a liver transplant recipient use immediately after transplantation?

Each patient's needs are different, but a minimum average is between 6 and 8 medications:
- Antirejection—single, double, or triple therapy)
- *Pneumocystis carinii* pneumonia (PCP) prophylaxis—Bactrim, dapsone, or pentamidine
- Herpes prophylaxis—acyclovir
- Candida prophylaxis—nystatin, clotrimazole (Mycelex)
- CMV prophylaxis—ganciclovir (Cytovene), valacyclovir hydrochloride
- Antacid—e.g., Axid, Pepcid, Prilosec, Protonix

This guide is specific to the liver transplant itself and does not include any other medications that the patient may have been taking before the transplantation or any medications needed secondary to side effects from the medications such as hyperglycemics or antihypertensives. It is important to warn transplant recipients not to take acetaminophen, aspirin, ibuprofen, or any other over-the-counter medications without checking with the transplant center first.

36. Which medications are given for rejection episodes that may occur?

Medications for the treatment of rejection are often the same medications used for maintenance therapy, only in larger doses. Liver rejection is often treated with oral or intravenous boluses of corticosteroids. Tacrolimus is an effective agent in steroid resistant rejection. A third agent such as mycophenolate mofetil or rapamycin is often added in the setting of rejection. OKT3 and Thymoglobulin have also been effective in treating resistant or recurrent rejection episodes.

37. Which fungal infections are seen most frequently in liver transplant recipients?

Candida accounts for about 75% of all fungal infections; *Aspergillus* accounts for another 20%. Fungal infections are seen more often in high-risk patients, patients with renal failure/dialysis before transplant, retransplantation, excessively long operating room time, high transfusion needs, high levels of immunosuppression, antibiotic needs, and current CMV infections. Such infections are associated with a high mortality rate. The majority of fungal infections can be avoided through use of nystatin swish and swallow or troche, generally until the prednisone dose is 10 mg or less, until the immunosuppression is believed to be at a maintenance level or as recommended by the program's protocol, which is approximately 12 weeks after transplant.

38. Which viral infections are risks to the liver transplant patient?

Cytomegalovirus (CMV) is a common virus that with which more than 50% of the population has been infected at some time in their lives. Most infected individuals probably were not diagnosed with CMV specifically because it generally presents with the same symptoms as many other viruses: fever, chills, and body aches. CMV is much more serious when it infects a patient who is immunosuppressed, and it can cause fever, pneumonia, gastrointestinal infection, hepatitis, pancreatitis, and retinitis. The CMV status of both the donor and the recipient is known at the time of the transplant, and the recipient is monitored after transplant for any signs of infection with blood and/or urine tests. CMV is most likely to occur during the first few months after transplantation when immunosuppressant-medication doses are at the highest.

The liver transplant patient at highest risk is the CMV-negative recipient who receives a liver from a CMV-positive donor. However, a latent CMV virus may occur in any immunosuppressed recipient because of other factors such as antilymphocyte antibodies or cytotoxic drugs, infection, or rejection. CMV is treated effectively with intravenous ganciclovir until the virus is cleared. Intravenous ganciclovir is also given prophylactically to patients who have the highest risk for developing the CMV virus. The majority of transplant centers believe that prevention is the best treatment for CMV and provide prophylactic treatment in the form of oral or intravenous ganciclovir or with valacyclovir hydrochloride, depending on each center's drug choice, dosage, and schedule.

39. Are there any other viruses that benefit from prophylaxis?

Herpes simplex virus infections can be practically eliminated by treatment of all posttransplant recipients with the prophylaxis of low-dose acyclovir (Zovirax) in the immediate postoperative period. The length of treatment is usually center specific.

40. What can be done for Epstein-Barr virus?

Epstein-Barr virus (EBV) occurs less frequently than CMV but is more dangerous for the immunosuppressed patient. The most common forms of EBV are hepatitis and posttransplant lymphoproliferative disorder (PTLD). EBV is usually detected by a blood test, an EBV-PCR, or on biopsy with the finding of a monomorphic mononuclear B lymphocytic infiltrate in the absence of bile duct damage. Patients respond best to withdrawal of or significant decreases in immunosuppression. Chemotherapy is a consideration if immunosuppression withdrawal fails or PTLD recurs.

41. What is *Pneumocystis carinii* pneumonia?

Pneumocystis carinii pneumonia (PCP) is a specific type of pneumonia to which transplant recipients are susceptible because of their immunosuppressed state. PCP prophylaxis is achieved with daily dosing with Bactrim or dapsone or monthly dosing with pentamidine inhalation treatments for patients with sulfa allergies. The length of treatment is center specific and may range from 6 months to lifelong.

42. What is the recurrence rate of original liver diseases?

Recurrent liver diseases such as hepatitis (B, C, nonA, nonB, nonC), primary biliary cirrhosis (PBC), primary sclerosing cholangitis (PSC), autoimmune liver disease, nonalcoholic steatohepatitis (NASH), alcoholic liver disease, and malignancy are the most common causes of late graft loss. Recurrent hepatitis B is seen in 60–90% of cases within 5-years after transplant. Hepatitis C is seen practically 100% of the time by 2 years after transplant and sometimes as early as a few weeks after transplant. PBC, PSC, and autoimmune diseases are seen in 10–30% of patients by 5 years after transplant, and alcoholic liver disease recurs in approximately 20% of patients within 5 years after transplant.

43. What can be done for patients with hepatitis B to prevent or treat recurrent disease?

Current practices require that all patients under consideration for transplantation for hepatitis B are hepatitis B early antigen (HbeAG)–negative and DNA-negative at the time of transplantation. Some patients receive treatment with lamivudine before transplantation, but recent data suggest that treatment with lamivudine should be held until after transplantation because of the high rate of mutant viruses seen with long-term treatment. However, because of the low donation rates and the unpredictability of organ transplantation, holding treatment is generally not practiced.

All liver recipients undergoing transplantation receive human hepatitis B immunoglobulin (HBIG) at a dose of 10,000 IU during the anhepatic phase and then daily for 1 week. Subsequent dosing of HBIG is given to maintain an adequate hepatitis B surface antibody (HbsAb) titer. The exact dosing and frequency of treatment with HBIG, intravenous and intramuscular, varies from center to center. Treatment with HBIG can be given alone or with lamivudine at a dose of 100–150 mg/day. Lamivudine is given as a lifelong treatment.

With the use of these treatment therapies, the retransplantation rate for recurrent hepatitis B is extremely low.

44. What treatment is available for hepatitis C?

One-third of all liver transplantations are performed because of hepatitis C. Many patients with chronic hepatitis C receive treatment with interferon and ribavirin before transplantation, but the liver disease often deteriorates to cirrhosis, at which point liver transplantation is the only option.

For liver transplant recipients with recurrent hepatitis C, the best treatment option to date is combination therapy with interferon and ribavirin; however, the response rate remains low. Much optimism exists with the use of long-acting interferon and weight-based dosing of ribavirin, but it is too early to report improved response rates at this time.

Despite the high rate of recurrence of hepatitis C, it is not yet considered a contraindication to transplantation; however, the debate continues about whether recurrent hepatitis C should be a contraindication for retransplantation.

45. After the intensive care unit, what would a typical hospitalization entail?

In addition to monitoring of liver functions, the posttransplantation patient has the same postoperative course as any other patient undergoing major abdominal surgery, which includes early ambulation, respiratory toilet, standard wound care, and diet as tolerated. Patients are educated about wound care upon discharge, medications, doses, indications, and recommendations for posttransplant follow-up care, as well as laboratory schedules. A liver transplant recipient without complications has a hospital stay averaging 7–14 days.

The "Y" abdominal incision is closed with staples that generally remain in for 3 weeks after transplantation. The Jackson-Pratt drains are removed before discharge from the hospital. If the patient has a T-tube, it is usually clamped off about 1 week after transplantation and left in place for at least 3 months. The dressing around the T-tube should be changed once a day. If an area of the wound has been left open or has opened for some reason (e.g., infection), the patient is instructed about frequency and type of wound dressing needed. A wet-to-dry dressing with sterile saline, done twice a day, is often the standard care. The patient should be instructed that showers rather than tub baths should be taken until the wound has healed completely.

46. What type of follow-up care is required after transplantation?

The transplant recipient is requested to have blood work done 2 or 3 times a week initially. The frequency is then decreased depending on how stable the liver functions are and the rate at which the immunosuppressant medications are adjusted. Generally, the frequency decreases to about once a week until the first 3 months, then every other week, and then monthly by 6 months until the first year anniversary. Various centers have different protocols for patients after more than 1 year after transplant; however, all patients are recommended to have blood work done at least 3–4 times a year for life.

Posttransplant patients are seen most frequently in the first 3 months and then with decreasing frequency throughout the rest of the first year, after which they are seen even less frequently provided that there are no complications. Some transplant centers return primary care of the transplant recipient back to the patient's referring or primary care physician after 6 months to 1 year, whereas other centers remain active in the ongoing management of the immunosuppression, working along with the patient's primary care physician indefinitely.

The use of surveillance biopsies in the liver transplant population is center-dependent; however, many centers require a surveillance biopsy at the first anniversary of the transplant. An ultrasound of the liver is also done at the first-year mark to check for vessel patency.

Other tests are recommended on the first anniversary and annually thereafter:
- Chest x-ray
- Regular routine laboratory tests
- Hepatitis B and C screens
- 24-hour urine collection for protein and creatinine clearance (to monitor kidney function)
- Uric acid (to check/monitor for gout)
- Cholesterol and triglyceride
- Bone density test (to monitor of osteopenia/osteoporosis)
- Thyroid-stimulating hormone (TSH) (to monitor thyroid functions)
- Hemoglobin A1C
- Ophthalmologic examination (to check for cataracts or glaucoma)
- Mammography
- Papanicolaou smear
- Prostate specific antigen (PSA)
- Screening for skin cancers
- Dental examination

Patients have no one specific diet that they are recommended to follow after receiving a liver transplant other than a normal healthy diet. Dietary restrictions are individualized according to each patient and to the type of diet each patient followed before transplantation. However, side effects or complications of the medications given after transplant often require some new dietary modifications for which a dietician is extremely helpful in instructing patients. It is helpful to have printed diets and materials to give to any transplant patient who requires a new modification. Because of the immunosuppressants that the patient will be taking, he or she is advised to avoid all raw seafood, raw meats, and uncooked foods such as eggs in eggnog or sauces or unpasturized dairy products.

47. What is the incidence of patients' developing kidney problems after liver transplantation?

Renal dysfunction is primarily the result of side effects of the calcineurin inhibitors, cyclosporine and tacrolimus. With transplant recipients living much longer, annual evaluation of renal function is recommended, usually with a 24-hour urine collection for protein and creatinine clearance. Although the majority of liver recipients maintain stable renal function, some patients develop progressive renal failure, even to the point of dialysis. Patients should be educated that drugs that exacerbate renal dysfunction in the presence of calcineuron inhibitors, such as erythromycin and ketoconazole, should not be taken, unless under the direct supervision of the transplant center. Other nephrotoxic agents such as nonsteroidal anti-inflammatory drugs should be avoided as well.

A small percentage of liver recipients develop end-stage renal disease, and both dialysis and kidney transplantation are viable options for them. They must undergo the same evaluation protocol as any other potential kidney candidate. Liver recipients with an original liver disease of hepatitis C are recommended to have a liver biopsy as part of the evaluation for kidney transplant because any treatment needed for the hepatitis would have to be given before the kidney transplantation. An increased incidence of renal allograft loss occurs when interferon is used after kidney transplantation.

48. Do all patients develop hypertension after liver transplantation?

Although not all patients develop high blood pressure after liver transplantation, the rate may be as high as 70%. This development is generally due to the use of corticosteroids and calcineurin inhibitors. Reduction in the use of steroids, or the current trend to wean all steroids completely, may help to reduce or eliminate the need for antihypertensives after transplant. In addition, reduction of the calcineuron inhibitors with or without the use of a calcineuron sparing agent such as imuran, mycophenolate mofetil, or rapamycin may also help in the management of posttransplant hypertension.

49. Which factors suggest that a liver recipient may develop hyperlipidemia?

As many as 40% of all liver transplant recipients experience hypercholesterolemia after liver transplantation. The percentage is slightly higher in recipients who receive cyclosporine than in recipients who receive tacrolimus-based immunosuppression. Other identified risk factors for the development of hyperlipidemia after liver transplantation include female gender, cholestatic liver disease, treatment with more than 3 boluses of steroids for rejection episodes, and pretransplant cholesterol of more than 141 mg/dl.

Patients can be managed safely with antilipid-lowering agents, along with weight and diet control and smoking cessation. Elevated liver enzymes have been seen in liver transplant recipients who have been started on lipid-lowering agents; therefore, liver function should be monitored frequently at the beginning of therapy.

50. Does liver transplantation increase the risk of osteoporosis?

Bone disease is often already present before transplantation for patients with liver disease, especially those with cholestatic disease such as primary biliary cirrhosis (PBC) and those receiving steroid treatment before transplantation, as has been seen in patients with autoimmune diseases. The degree of osteoporosis depends on the duration of liver disease, intestinal calcium malabsorption, and postmenopausal condition. Baseline bone density tests should be completed before transplantation and should be followed continually after transplantation. Baseline osteopenia is exacerbated in the early posttransplant course because of the use of high-dose corticosteroids and prolonged bedrest after transplantation. Up to 80% of patients with PBC and decreased bone densities below the fracture threshold have at least one fracture within the first 6 months after transplantation. Most of the bone loss occurs within the first 3–4 months after transplantation. Early intervention is needed in the forms of early mobilization, calcium and vitamin D supplementation, medication therapy that may include the use of calcitonin, bisphosphonates, and/or estrogen, and weight-bearing exercises.

51. What are the most common neurologic complications after transplantation?

Neurologic disorders ranging from tremor and headaches to seizure and stroke are most often due to the neurotoxic effects of cyclosporine and tacrolimus. Seizures occur more often as a result of cyclosporine or tacrolimus when they are given intravenously. Between 30 and 50% of patients receiving a liver transplant report some form of neurologic complaint. Ischemic infarcts and hemorrhage can occur after liver transplantation and are typically due to coagulopathy complications.

52. Is there an increased risk of cancer associated with immunosuppressant medications?

According to the Transplant Tumor Registry, which was formed when the Cincinnati Transplant Tumor Registry (CTTR) merged with the UNOS Scientific Registry of Transplant Recipients, which now is managed by UNOS, the risk of cancer is 3–5 times greater in transplant recipients than in the general population. The most common forms of cancer in the transplant recipient are skin and lip cancers. Squamous cell carcinomas occur more frequently than basal cell carcinomas and are more aggressive. Lymphoproliferative disorders are the second most-common forms of cancer seen, followed by lung cancer and Kaposi's sarcoma. The data specific to the liver population finds that lymphomas make up 57% of all posttransplant tumors.

Transplant centers strive for minimization of immunosuppressive therapy and educates transplant recipients to avoid direct prolonged sun exposure, use sun screens specific to UV-B rays, and schedule annual dermatology evaluation for skins cancers and prompt early evaluation and treatment of any suspicious lesions. Patients with primary sclerosing cholangitis (PSC) and ulcerative colitis should be screened annually because of an increased risk of colon cancer. These measures need to be taken in addition to routine recommended cancer screening for the general population, which includes mammography, gynecologic examination, colonoscopy, and prostate serum antibody for male transplant recipients. A healthy lifestyle, which includes abstinence from smoking, is also recommended.

53. When is it safe to resume sexual activity?

Patients may resume sexual activity whenever they feel comfortable enough to do so. A patient's sexual performance may be affected because of the length of illness and recovery time before and after transplantation, but it may also by affected by certain medications such as antihypertensives.

Even if a patient is monogamous, it is possible to transmit viruses such as hepatitis B and C because the virus is not removed from the blood by transplantation. Also, as immunosuppressed transplant recipients, patients should also protect themselves against the risk of infection or disease, especially if they are intimate with a new partner or more than one partner. Therefore, safer sex practices must be reinforced. When used properly, latex condoms can greatly reduce the transmission of sexually transmitted diseases.

54. Which types of birth control are recommended after transplantation?

Acceptable methods of birth control after transplantation are the following:
• Foam with a condom
• The sponge with a condom
• A diaphragm with spermicidal gel

Permanent methods of birth control should be discussed with the physician and/or gynecologist. Birth control pills are contraindicated in some liver transplant recipients because of the increased risk of clotting, and intrauterine devices (IUDs) are not recommended because of the increased risk of infection.

Most female liver transplant recipients do resume menstrual cycles, usually within a few months. High doses of prednisone may stop the menstrual flow, but ovulation may still occur. Therefore, it may be possible for the recipient to become pregnant before resuming normal periods. (See chapter 22 for more information about pregnancy after transplantation.)

55. When is it safe to resume driving after liver transplantation?

A transplant recipient's reflexes, judgment, and vision may be affected by the medications used after transplantation. Before recipients resume driving, it is important that they feel well enough to be safe drivers, both for themselves and for others on the road. Their mobility needs to be such that they can turn the head quickly from side to side and move their legs up to the abdomen comfortably to imitate sudden brake motion. Patients need to be reminded that if they experienced seizures after transplantation, they need to examine state laws regarding the amount of time they need to be seizure-free before resuming driving. Patients also should be reminded that seat belts not only are the law, but also are safe to wear and will not hurt the liver. A small pillow or towel can cushion a wound that is still open or tender so that the seat belt does not rub against it. All patients should have another driver with them for the first few times they drive after transplantation.

56. Can transplant recipients return to work or school?

Returning to work or school is recommended, not just for financial reasons, but for psychological well-being too. It is generally not recommended, however, that liver recipients return to work or school for the first 12 weeks during which they have the greatest risk for infections because immunosuppression is highest during the early postoperative phase. After this initial period, patients are encouraged to resume regular daily activities, including employment or school, as soon as they feel they are able. Depending on how long they were sick and the severity of illness before transplantation, patients may require additional time for physical rehabilitation; or, depending on their type of employment before transplantation, they may require vocational rehabilitation.

The only general rule of thumb is that liver recipients avoid occupations that require exposure to toxic chemicals or lifting of excessive weight in the early postoperative period, the first 3–6 months. Obviously, some jobs have higher risks than others, such as working in a daycare center or a pet store, but with some basic precautions, education, and common sense, any job is possible.

57. What are the guidelines for weight lifting after liver transplantation?

Specific guidelines for weight lifting should be obtained from the surgeon; however, a general guideline is to lift nothing heavier than an average bag of groceries (about 10 lb) for the first 8 weeks. After the first 8 weeks, weights can be gradually increased, with the understanding that heavy lifting is not dangerous to the liver but does put the patient at an increased risk of an incisional hernia, which may require an additional surgical intervention and general anesthesia. After the first 6 months, patients can increase weight lifting as tolerated.

58. What are the recommendations regarding smoking and alcoholic intake after liver transplantation?

Transplant candidates should be strongly encouraged to stop smoking before their transplantation and discouraged from smoking after transplantation. Immunosuppressed patients who smoke are at greater risk for infections and cancer. Discuss interventions to help the patient to stop smoking, such as nicotine patches and/or support groups. It is recommended that patients abstain from all alcohol because alcohol is a toxin that is metabolized through the liver.

59. Are there any special precautions that need to be taken before dental appointments or procedures?

Routine dental care should be the same as for all healthy individuals, but because of the immunosuppressant medications and increased risk of bacteremia, it is recommended that the transplant recipient alert his or her dentist of the need for antibiotic prophylaxis before appointments, including routine teeth cleaning and polishing. Most transplant centers use the guidelines set by the American Heart Association. The current recommendations are as follows:
  • Amoxicillin, 2 gm orally 1 hour before dental procedure, not to be repeated afterward
  Patients who are allergic to amoxicillin and penicillin may take the following:
  • Clindamycin, 600 mg 1 hour before dental procedure, not to be repeated afterward.
  Erythromycin is not recommended because of the interaction with cyclosporine and tacrolimus. It is the responsibility of the patient's dentist to prescribe the necessary antibiotic coverage.

60. Can liver transplant recipients receive the flu vaccine?

Because any immunocompromised patient is at higher risk for influenza, an annual flu shot is recommended. Each transplant center may differ slightly, but general guidelines include that recipients do not receive the flu vaccine within the first 3 months after transplantation because immunosuppression doses are the highest during that time. In addition, as with the general population, it is not recommended that anyone receive the flu vaccine if he or she currently has a cold, virus, or allergy symptoms or is allergic to chicken or eggs.

61. Are there any other vaccines that a transplant recipient should or should not receive?

Transplant recipients must always receive dead virus vaccines; no live virus vaccines should ever be given. Oral polio, rubella, smallpox, yellow fever, measles and mumps vaccines are types of live virus vaccines that should be avoided. Transplant recipients should avoid all contact with children who have received the oral polio vaccine for 8 weeks. If a transplant recipient is in close contact with a child who has not received the polio vaccine yet, the inactivated (Sabin) polio vaccine, which is not a live virus, can be requested.

Exposure to chicken pox, caused by the varicella virus, may result in the development of chicken pox, even if the recipient has had the virus in the past, if immunity is low. The varicella virus is contagious as early as 5 days before the chicken pox virus breaks out on an individual. A transplant recipient who has had chicken pox may also develop shingles or herpes zoster, which is caused by a reactivation of the virus, which lies dormant in the nerve roots of the body forever. Herpes zoster is treated with acyclovir, orally or intravenously. The chicken pox vaccine is a dead virus vaccine, and there are are no special recommendations with regard to exposure to a child having received this vaccine.

In addition to the flu vaccine, other types of dead virus vaccines that transplant recipients can receive safely are diphtheria-tetanus booster, tuberculosis, pneumococcal, and hepatitis A and B vaccines.

62. Are transplant recipients allowed to have pets?

Pets are acceptable after transplantation. They can provide great emotional and psychological support; therefore, it is never recommended that anyone get rid of a family pet just because he or she has had a transplant. However, it the patient does not currently have a pet, the first year is not necessarily the best time to get a new pet. Recipients with pets do need to be reminded of a few general guidelines:
- Good hand washing is and always will be the best line of defense.
- Recipients should avoid cleaning up after pets that are sick but, if necessary, should be sure to wear gloves.
- Indoor or house pets are preferable to outdoor pets.
- It is not recommended that recipients change cat's litter boxes because of the possibility of toxoplasmosis; however, if it is absolutely necessary, gloves and a mask should be worn.
- Recipients should be wary of cat scratches because they easily get infected (cat scratch fever).
- Dogs may also carry germs in their feces, so recipients should avoid cleaning up after dogs, if possible, or wear gloves.
- Birds carry many parasites and bacteria and of all pets should be avoided, if possible. Birdcages should be avoided at all costs, but if a recipient must change the papers, gloves and a mask should be worn. If a recipient does not have a bird before transplantation, do not recommend that he or she get one after transplantation.

63. Are there any special precautions if a transplant recipient has well water?

Transplant recipients may drink treated (chlorinated) tap water. Although it is not necessary for all transplant recipients to drink bottled water, it is advised that well water be boiled at a rolling boil before it is used for drinking. Immunocompromised patients are at higher risk for infections, including those carried in such sources as well water. Transplant recipients should have their water tested for at least the following 3 types of organisms:

• *Escherichia coli*-like organisms and other gram-negative organisms
• *Giardia lamblia*
• *Legionella pneumophilia*

Well water should be checked even if the patient is not drinking it because organisms may be spread in the air, as in showering. Water can be tested by contacting the local water company or the EPA Safe Water Hotline at (800) 426-4791.

64. Discuss the most common psychological issues in the liver transplant population?

Psychological issues are very different for patients who are awaiting organ transplantation than for those with other chronic illnesses. Patients waiting for a liver transplant are facing death with their only hope being that they will receive a transplant in time. Depression and anxiety are not uncommon for many recipients and their families before and after transplantation. Patients and families often have unrealistic expectations of the transplant itself. Prolonged waiting times often result in depressive symptoms. Candidates also frequently experience "over idealized thinking about the miraculous transition to full health almost immediately after surgery," which often results in disappointment, depression, and anxiety.

Symptoms of depression may include a depressed or nervous mood; loss of interest in activities previously found enjoyable; weight loss or gain without dieting; increased sleeping or difficulty sleeping; feelings of worthlessness or helplessness; irritability; difficulty thinking, concentrating, or making decisions; and frequent thoughts of death or suicide.

Transplant candidates often do not think through posttransplant issues because they are too preoccupied with the actual transplant. Disruptions in family dynamics, financial concerns, physical setbacks, and physical discomfort are several reasons that depression or anxiety may occur after transplantation. Additional issues that may complicate the posttransplant phase are psychological complications from side effects of the medications, as well as stress related to the loss of the "sick role," unrealistic occupational expectations, and even unrealistic expectations of them from their families or support systems.

The transplant patient needs psychological, physical, medical, pharmacologic, and family support throughout the entire transplant process. Patients and families should also be encouraged to explore other avenues of support, such as support groups, talking with other transplant recipients, stress management, and relaxation modalities as well.

BIBLIOGRAPHY

1. Busittil R, Klintmalm G: Transplantation of the Liver. Philadelphia, W.B. Saunders, 1996.
2. Cecka JM, Terasaki P: Clinical Transplants 1999. Los Angeles, UCLA Immunogenetics, 1999.
3. Lindor K, Heathcote EJ, Poupon R: Primary Biliary Cirrhosis: From Pathogenesis to Clinical Treatment. Dordrecht, The Netherlands, Kluwer Academic Publishers and Axcan Pharma, 1998.
4. Lucey M, Merion R, Beresford T: Liver Transplantation and the Alcoholic Patient: Medical, Surgical and Psychosocial Issues. Cambridge, Cambridge University Press, 1994.
5. Makowka L: The Handbook of Transplantation Management. Austin, TX, R.G. Landes, 1991.
6. Makowka L. Sher L: Ortho Biotech Handbook of Organ Transplantation. Georgetown, TX, R.G. Landes, 1995.
7. Molmenti E, Jain A, Marino N, et al: Pregnancy in Liver Transplantation. Clin Liver Dis 3:163–174, 1999.
8. Nolan M, Augustine S: Transplantation Nursing: Acute and Long-Term Management. East Norwalk, CT, Appleton & Lange, 1995.
9. Norman D, Turka L: Primer on Transplantation, 2nd ed. Malden, MA, Blackwell Publishers, 2001.
10. Stuart F, Abecassis M, Kaufman D: Organ Transplantation. Georgetown, TX, Landes Bioscience, 2000.
11. UPMC Health System: Liver Transplantation: A postoperative booklet for patients. UPMC Health System, Pittsburgh, PA.

WEBSITES

1. www.sti.upmc.edu
2. www.transplanthealth.com
3. www.unos.org/About/policy_policies03_06.htm
4. www.livertransplant.org/livedonorlivertransplant

14. INTESTINAL TRANSPLANTATION

Beverly Kosmach Park, MSN, CRNP

1. Why are intestinal transplants performed?

Transplantation of the small intestine is a therapeutic option for adult and pediatric patients with permanent intestinal failure due to short gut syndrome. Such patients require total parenteral nutrition (TPN) to meet nutritional needs and are at high risk for developing life-threatening complications, including TPN-induced liver disease, recurrent sepsis, and loss of venous access.

2. What is short gut syndrome?

Short gut syndrome (SGS) occurs when the patient's small intestine is unable to enterally maintain an adequate nutritional status or fluid and electrolyte balance. SGS may result in
- Malabsorption
- A hypersecretory state
- Poor growth and development
- Inability to maintain weight

SGS is classified as structural or functional depending on the cause of the disorder. Structural causes, which result in a significantly decreased length of the small intestine, result from extensive surgical resection or anatomic abnormalities. Patients with functional causes may have an adequate length of intestine, but intestinal dysfunction occurs because of absorptive, secretory, or motility disorders of various types and severity.

3. Do all patients with short gut syndrome require transplantation?

The severity of SGS varies depending on the cause of the disorder and the extent of malabsorption. Some patients may be managed on continuous enteral feedings with elemental formulas. Adequate nutrition may also be maintained through a combination of enteral and parenteral feedings, with the goal of discontinuing TPN as the bowel adapts. Surgical revision to lengthen the intestine may be helpful in some cases. Intestinal transplantation is reserved for patients with SGS who have permanent intestinal dysfunction. Such patients require parenteral nutrition with no possibility of discontinuation to maintain fluid balance and provide complete nutritional requirements.

4. Why do children require intestinal transplantation?

In children, the most common structural indications for intestinal transplantation are volvulus and gastroschisis. A volvulus results from a malrotation of the intestine around a fixed point caused by congenital or adhesive bands. It can also occur when the small intestine twists around the mesentary, resulting in vascular insufficiency. Volvulus is often diagnosed in utero or within the first 2 months of age, but it can occur at any time. Gastroschisis presents more frequently in premature infants and occurs when variable lengths of the intestine herniate through an abdominal wall defect. Other structural indications include congenital atresias and stenoses of the small intestine, necrotizing enterocolitis (NEC), and trauma.

The most common functional disorders in pediatric patients with SGS are Hirschsprung disease and chronic intestinal pseudo-obstruction (CIP). In Hirschsprung disease, a congenital absence of the intramural nerve plexuses or aganglionosis results in a functional obstruction of the intestine with a dilated colon. Patients present with abdominal distention, severe constipation, recurrent fecal impaction, anemia, and malnutrition. CIP is usually diagnosed at birth or within 1 year of age and may involve the entire intestinal tract or selectively involve the colon and other hollow viscera such as the bladder. CIP presents as an obstructive disorder in the absence of any anatomic obstruction and is caused by ineffective intestinal contractions. Patients usually present with bilious vomiting, abdominal distention, and constipation.

5. What are the indications for intestinal transplantation in adults?

The indications for intestinal transplantation in adults are quite different from those for children. Crohn's disease and vascular insufficiency are the leading indications. Crohn's disease is a chronic inflammation in the intestine that varies in extent and severity. In severe cases, it can involve multiple segments of the GI tract and requires extensive bowel resections resulting in TPN-dependence. Vascular insufficiency with thrombosis may be the result of a hypercoagulable state, a veno-occlusive disorder, or trauma. Other indications include familial adenomatous polyposis (a precancerous state involving the development and progression of intestinal polyps) and radiation enteritis due to radiation damage to the intestine.

6. When were intestinal transplants first performed?

Early attempts at intestinal transplantation began over 40 years ago, although clinical success has only been achieved in the last 10 years. From 1964 to 1972, 8 intestinal transplants were performed with the longest survival being only 6 months.[27] Technical complications, sepsis, and the inability of conventional immunosuppression to control rejection led to the failure of these early trials. Because of the disappointing results, as well as the introduction of total parenteral nutrition, interest in intestinal transplantation declined.

The introduction of cyclosporine in 1980 dramatically increased survival in kidney, heart, and liver transplant recipients. Consequently, there were renewed attempts at intestinal transplantation. Although survival improved for intestinal transplant recipients, results did not match those of the other solid organs. Extended survival of 1–5.5 years was seen in a few patients with a mean survival of 25.7 months in a series of 6 patients.[4] Immunosuppressive protocols varied and included cyclosporine, corticosteroids, azathioprine, antilymphocyte globulin, monoclonal antibodies, and recipient and graft irradiation. One patient from this era continues to survive at over 13 years posttransplant, although her primary immunosuppression was changed to tacrolimus in 1998 following an episode of rejection.[13]

7. Which factors have contributed to increased survival for intestinal transplant patients?

The introduction of tacrolimus in 1990 significantly improved patient and graft survival for all types of intestinal transplantation. Other factors that enhanced the feasibility of intestinal transplantation include the following:

- Improved surgical techniques
- The use of tacrolimus as the primary immunosuppressant
- The availability of an increased array of immunosuppressive agents
- Early detection methods and interventions for infection
- Suitable patient selection criteria

8. How many patients have received intestinal transplants?

Since 1985, information from the international experience of intestinal transplantation has been compiled through the International Intestinal Transplant Registry (http://www.lhsc.on.ca/itr/). As of May 2001, 55 intestinal transplant programs have performed a total of 696 intestinal transplants in 656 patients with 355 recipients surviving. Because many patients, particularly children, develop end-stage liver disease secondary to TPN-induced cholestasis, the combined intestine–liver transplant was the most common procedure performed (44%). Isolated intestinal transplantation accounted for 42% of cases, and multivisceral transplantation, for patients requiring other organs in addition to the liver and intestine, was the least common procedure (15%).[15]

9. What is the survival rate for these recipients?

According to the Intestinal Transplant Registry (ITR), 5-year actuarial graft survival for isolated intestine transplantation is over 45% for the total international experience. Actuarial graft survival for combined intestine–liver and multivisceral transplantation is 43% and nearly 30%, respectively. Full function of the transplanted intestine has been achieved in nearly 80% of survivors.[15]

In comparison to survival rates of the complete international experience complied by the ITR, higher graft and patient survival rates are seen at the more experienced programs with the learning curve reflecting improved outcomes. The ITR has reported a significant difference in patient and graft survival based on transplant center volume. Centers performing at least 10 transplants had significantly better outcomes than those performing less than 10 transplants.

At the University of Pittsburgh, the most active intestinal transplant center, 165 intestinal transplants have been performed in 155 patients (89 children and 66 adults). One-year, 3-year, and 5-year patient survival is 83%, 58%, and 53%, respectively.[5]

Since 1994, The University of Miami has performed 120 intestinal transplants (multivisceral, 40%; isolated intestine, 32%; liver-intestine, 28%) in 111 patients, including 64 children and 47 adults. Survival has increased considerably since 1998 with the addition of daclizumab.[17]

The University of Nebraska reports that 117 intestinal transplants have been performed in 106 patients (104 children and 13 adults). One-year patient survival following isolated intestine and combined liver–intestine transplantation was 80% and 70%, respectively. Three-year survival was 70% and 61%, respectively.[21]

The Hôpital Necker-Enfants-Malades has performed 36 pediatric intestinal transplants since 1995 with 27 survivors. The follow-up for this group has ranged from 6–76 months posttransplant. At a median follow-up of 34 months, 75% of patients have survived.[14]

10. How can an intestinal transplant center be located?

Currently, 55 transplant centers internationally perform intestinal transplants, with the majority of clinical experience being contained in a few centers. Centers located in the United States may be found through the United Network for Organ Sharing (UNOS) (www.UNOS.org). Information about each center is available and includes the number of transplants performed, survival, age at time of transplant, indication for transplant, and the number of patients on that center's waiting list. A complete listing of all international centers is provided by the Intestinal Transplant Registry (ITR) (www.lhsc.on.ca/itr).

11. What are the most common causes of death following intestinal transplantation?

Sepsis (49%) is the most common cause of death following intestinal transplantation. Other causes include rejection (10%), lymphoma (8%), technical complications (8%), and respiratory complications (7%).[15]

12. What costs are associated with intestinal transplantation?

There is great variation in the cost of intestinal transplantation. Factors that affect the cost include the following:
- The patient's pretransplant medical status
- Postoperative length of stay
- Surgical and infectious complications
- Occurrence and severity of rejection
- Center-specific protocols

Improvements in intestinal transplantation have resulted in decreased costs. Between 1990 and 1994, the average charges for intestinal transplant procedures at a large-volume center were approximately $200,000 for an isolated intestine transplant, $252,500 for a combined liver–intestine transplant, and $284,500 for a multivisceral transplant. By 1999, the average costs had decreased appreciably and were approximately $132,000 for an isolated intestine transplant, $215,000 for a combined liver–intestine transplant, and $219,000 for a multivisceral transplant.[1,2]

13. Is intestinal transplantation covered by most third-party payers?

With improved survival, more third-party payers are covering intestinal transplantation as a treatment for permanent intestinal failure. A recent landmark decision by the Centers for Medicare and Medicaid Services (CMS), formerly the Health Care Financing Administration, provides for Medicare coverage of the costs of intestinal transplantation if the procedure is performed in a

Medicare-approved facility.[2] As a result of CMS's decision, additional third-party payers may now consider intestinal transplantation as an accepted therapy. Transplant centers usually have a financial coordinator who works with the family to obtain coverage when an insurance company does not recognize intestinal transplantation as an approved treatment.

14. What are the out-of-pocket expenses for the families?

Even with adequate insurance coverage for transplant surgery and hospitalization, the patient and family may still have a significant financial burden. Costs associated with transplantation may involve relocation to the transplant center area for several months, maintaining two households with associated expenses, transportation and daily living expenses, and life-long medications that may involve significant copayments. The adult patient and/or primary caregiver are often unable to work for an extended period of time. With the added expenses associated with transplantation, families often face a decreased income if the caregiver takes family medical leave. Families may find fundraising for personal expenses to be helpful. Transplant social workers guide families to seek further services through referrals to financial assistance programs and support groups.

15. How is a patient referred to a transplant center? How does the transplant evaluation process begin?

Evaluation for intestinal transplantation usually begins with a referral by a local physician to a transplant coordinator at the transplant center. However, direct referrals by the patient or family are also common. The transplant coordinator discusses the patient's diagnosis, history, and current medical status with the referring physician and/or family. The patient's pertinent medical records, history, and current physical examination, laboratory tests, and results of procedures are requested. The information is reviewed by the transplant surgeon, and the case is discussed with the primary referring physician. If an evaluation is considered appropriate, the transplant coordinator schedules the evaluation for the earliest convenient time. Information about health insurance (private or public) must also be obtained and confirmed before the evaluation process begins.

16. What is involved in the intestinal transplant evaluation?

The evaluation process is center-specific, but is usually conducted over a 3–5-day inpatient hospitalization. Some centers conduct the evaluation on an outpatient basis over a period of several days. The evaluation includes a complete assessment of the candidate through laboratory testing and diagnostic procedures. Various consultations are obtained based on the patient's diagnosis, medical status, and complications. Services most commonly consulted include gastroenterology, nutrition, cardiology, anesthesia, infectious disease, pulmonology, neurology, occupational/physical therapy, and psychiatry or child development, if applicable. A psychosocial assessment is completed at most centers to assess family support, coping ability, compliance with care routines, and understanding of the transplant process. Although the consultants vary, the psychosocial assessment is usually completed by the psychiatrist/psychologist, social worker, clinical nurse specialist, and/or child life specialist. Transplant coordinators and/or transplant clinical nurse specialists provide detailed information for patients and family members.

17. What information is obtained during the evaluation?

The evaluation for intestinal transplantation focuses on the patient's GI tract anatomy and function, nutritional status, hepatic function, vascular patency, infection history, growth and development, and psychosocial history.

18. What is the outcome of the evaluation?

Findings and results of the physical examination, laboratory tests, diagnostic procedures, and consultations are reviewed in a multidisciplinary conference. Patients not meeting criteria for transplantation are given an alternative medical management plan to be followed by the referring physician. Patients accepted as candidates are listed for intestinal transplantation according to the United Network of Organ Sharing (UNOS) guidelines.

19. How are patients listed with UNOS?

The transplant coordinator lists the candidate on the UNOS waiting list according to blood type, weight, and specific UNOS criteria (www.UNOS.org). Status I candidates are those patients requiring an intestinal transplant in the near future because of permanent intestinal failure, poor venous access, and liver dysfunction. Status II candidates have permanent intestinal failure but have stable liver function and venous access. If intestinal transplant candidates also require a liver graft, they are also placed on the liver transplant list. The grafts are procured from the same donor, so if the patient is offered a liver, the transplant center will request the intestine as well for that patient. If the intestine cannot be procured or is offered to another center, the liver is accepted for an isolated liver recipient, and the intestine transplant candidate continues to wait for a suitable donor. Organs procured in the same region as the transplant center may be offered to that center first.

20. What happens during the waiting period for transplant?

Routine communication between the referring physician, family/candidate, and the transplant center is essential so that the patient obtains optimal medical management and is prepared for the transplant process. Any changes in health status, hospitalizations, or infections should be reported to the transplant coordinator immediately.

21. How long is the waiting period?

The waiting period may range from a few weeks to years for medically stable patients. Median waiting times for patients on the waiting list between 1995 and 1999 ranged from 151–305 days.[39]

22. Do a majority of intestinal transplant candidates receive organs?

Solid organ transplantation has become an accepted treatment for many end-stage diseases. Unfortunately, the supply of cadaveric organs does not meet the ever-increasing demand. In 2000, nearly 65,000 people were waiting for transplants, but only about 5000 patients received organs. As of March 2002, 178 adults and children were on the UNOS waiting list for an intestinal transplant, whereas only 79 patients received intestinal transplants in the United States in 2000 (www.UNOS.org). In recent years, about 100 intestinal transplants have been performed internationally each year. A study on pediatric transplant candidates revealed that about 40% of pediatric candidates died before organs were available.[7]

23. What types of intestinal transplants are performed?

The types of transplant procedures performed depend on the indication for transplant as well as other affected organs. There are three types of intestinal transplant procedures:

1. An isolated intestinal procedure

2. A composite graft of the intestine and liver for those patients with short gut syndrome as well as TPN-induced cholestasis

3. A multivisceral transplant that involves the intestine with a liver, stomach, pancreas and/or kidney.

24. What are the selection criteria for cadaveric donor grafts?

Because the intestine is very sensitive to ischemia, hemodynamically stable donors are preferred. Organs are not accepted from donors who have a history of malignancy, sepsis, cardiac arrest, resuscitation, or extended periods of hypotension. The donor and recipient must have compatible blood types; human leukocyte antigen matching is random. Preferably, the donor should be similar or smaller in size than the recipient because the available volume of the abdominal cavity is often reduced because of previous surgeries. In children, however, the donor weight may range from 50% less to 20% greater than that of the recipient. In some cases, the size of the liver graft can be reduced to transplant into a smaller child, or slightly larger organs can be used in children with abdominal distention. CMV-seropositive donors should not be considered for CMV-seronegative recipients, particularly in isolated intestine transplantation, because of the significantly higher mortality rate in this group.

25. Is the donor graft treated in any way?

Treatment of the donor graft varies by center and may include intestinal decontamination with amphotericin B, an aminoglycoside, and polymixin; administration of broad-spectrum antibiotics before and during procurement; irradiation of the donor tissue; and administration of muromonab-CD3.

26. In general, how is the intestine procured?

Procurement of the small intestine takes approximately 3 hours. The stomach is isolated with division at the pylorus, and the ileum is transected at the ileocecal valve with mobilization of the colon. The intestine is preserved in situ with University of Wisconsin preservation solution and venous bed decompression. At the back table, the intestine is separated from the composite graft, then stored in ice for transport. A cold ischemia time of less than 12 hours is recommended to avoid preservation injury.

27. What is the operative time for intestinal transplantation?

The length of surgery varies depending on the type of transplant, the number of previous surgeries, and the patient's pretransplant medical status. However, the procedure time usually ranges from 8–16 hours.

28. Describe the intestinal implantation procedure.

In an isolated intestine transplant for patients with dysmotility or dysfunctional absorption, the abdomen is exposed and the diseased intestine removed from the ligament of Treitz to the ileocecal valve or ileocolic anastomosis. In patients with functional disorders, the residual intestine is usually retained. Vascular anastomoses vary according to the patient's current anatomy, which may be altered from previous surgeries. The most common method to anastomose the vessels includes an anastomosis of the superior mesenteric artery of the donor to the infrarenal aorta and the donor superior mesenteric vein to the recipient portal vein or inferior vena cava. After the graft is reperfused, the intestine is reconstructed by an anastomosis of the donor jejunum to the recipient's residual duodenum or jejunum. The ileum is then connected to the native colon in an end-to-side fashion. An ileostomy is formed by exteriorizing the distal end of the graft and anastomosing the recipient's ileum or colon to the side of the graft below the stoma.

29. When is the ileostomy reversed?

The ileostomy is usually temporary and provides easy access for frequent endoscopic evaluations during the first 3–6 months following transplantation when rejection is most common. The timing of ostomy closure depends on the patient's history of infection and rejection. Typically, however, closure is achieved in 3 months to 1 year, depending upon center-specific protocols. Ostomy closure may not be possible in patients without a colon or in patients with certain motility disorders that affect the entire GI tract, such as long-segment Hirschsprung disease or chronic intestinal pseudo-obstruction.

30. What are the most common complications following intestinal transplantation?

Intestinal transplant recipients frequently experience multiple complications. The most common complications are related to the surgical procedure itself. Other common complications include postoperative hemorrhage, gastrointestinal bleeding, hypermotility, and complications associated with biliary reconstruction and the vascular and gastrointestinal anastomoses.

31. What are the most common surgical complications?

Although surgical complications occur in nearly 50% of intestinal transplant recipients, they rarely cause graft failure. The most common complications include postoperative hemorrhage, vascular leaks or obstructions, and biliary leaks or obstruction in patients with a composite intestine–liver graft. Other reported complications include intestinal leaks and perforations, wound dehiscence, intra-abdominal abscess, and chylous ascites.

32. What are the causes of postoperative hemorrhage?

Patients with liver dysfunction are at risk for postoperative hemorrhage secondary to pre-existing coagulopathy and/or portal hypertension. Bleeding is usually resolved following implantation of the donor liver and administration of blood products and cauterization. Postoperative intra-abdominal bleeding is often a technical problem originating at an anastomosis or from the peritoneal surface. It is usually resolved with surgical exploration and repair.

33. What vascular complications may occur?

Postoperative vascular complications are rare, but serious, events. Thromboses of the major arteries usually result in necrosis of the organs nourished by those arteries. Patients present with an acute onset of sepsis, fulminant liver failure, or pallor of the stoma with clinical deterioration. The diagnosis is confirmed through Doppler ultrasound that assesses vessel patency. Patients with isolated intestine grafts may require a graft enterectomy; however, they typically recover. Patients with composite grafts require emergent retransplantation within the setting of clinical deterioration and multisystem organ failure.

34. What gastrointestinal complications may occur?

Gastrointestinal bleeding is the most common complication following intestine transplantation and necessitates immediate assessment through endoscopy with biopsy. Because bleeding can be caused by either rejection or infection, it is essential to distinguish infectious processes from rejection so that the correct treatment can be initiated.

Leaks from the gastrointestinal anastomoses are a common complication and may occur within the first week posttransplant. Although the risk of leakage is minimized through intestinal decompression via the jejunostomy and ileostomy, leaks may still occur due to operative technique or poor wound healing as a result of immunosuppressive medications and/or malnutrition. Patients usually present with peritonitis, abdominal distention, and fever. Surgical exploration and revision with removal of the peritoneal contamination is necessary. Patients require a full course of antibiotics and/or antifungal therapy.

Hypermotility is common during the early postoperative period because the baseline motility of the denervated intestinal graft is altered. Hypermotility is usually controlled with a combination of antidiarrheal agents and fiber. Because increased output is also associated with rejection and infection, it is important to determine the etiology of the hypermotility. Rejection should always be considered in the setting of acute changes in motility that are accompanied by fever or abdominal distention.

35. Describe the focus of medical management during the first 6 months posttransplant.

Intestinal transplant recipients are predisposed to various complications related to technical problems, rejection, and infection, particularly in the first 6 months posttransplant. Medical management is labor-intensive and demands a meticulous approach with consistent, long-term follow-up care. Patients have numerous care needs and require frequent surveillance studies, routine laboratory tests, and clinical examinations. A multidisciplinary approach that includes transplant surgeons, GI specialists, infectious disease specialists, dieticians, nurses, social workers, and psychologists optimizes patient outcomes.

36. What are the most important medical management issues in the first 6 months post-transplant?

Important medical management issues include the following:
- Management of immunosuppressive agents: Maintaining a balance between administration of adequate immunosuppression to avoid rejection and prevention of infection is a challenging task.
- Routine surveillance for infectious complications: A preventive approach with attention to each patient's unique risk factors is essential.
- Maintenance of adequate nutrition and fluid and electrolyte homeostasis: Maintenance is achieved through oral, enteral, and/or intravenous methods.

Full graft function, as assessed through absorption, motility, and tolerance without infection, remains the goal of the posttransplant phase.

37. What is the major immunosuppressant used in intestinal transplantation?

Tacrolimus has been the mainstay of immunosuppression for intestinal transplantation since 1990 and has been a significant factor in the increased survival of patients. Tacrolimus is usually combined with corticosteroids and adjunctive immunosuppressants in various center-specific protocols.

Intravenous tacrolimus is administered intraoperatively at a dose of 0.15–0.2 mg/kg/day through a continuous infusion. When GI motility resumes, oral tacrolimus is usually started at 3–4 times the intravenous dose divided into 2 doses.

Whole blood trough tacrolimus levels are typically maintained at around 20 ng/ml to a maximum level of 25 ng/ml for about 3 months. Levels may remain high for up to 6 months in the presence of rejection. For stable patients, trough levels are decreased to 10–15 ng/ml within 6–12 months. Most intestinal transplant recipients at 2 or more years posttransplant can often tolerate levels of less than 10 ng/ml. Tacrolimus levels vary over time, depending on the length of time posttransplant, renal function, and the presence of infection or rejection.

The most common side effects of tacrolimus are an increased risk of infection, nephrotoxicity, and neurotoxicity.

38. Are steroids a part of the immunosuppressive protocol?

Although steroid use varies by center, intravenous methylprednisolone is usually given as an intraoperative bolus followed by a taper over 5 days from 5 mg/kg/day to 1 mg/kg/day in children or 200 mg/day to 20 mg/day in adults. Long-term immunosuppressive management has usually included tacrolimus with low-dose prednisone; however, long-term stable patients who demonstrate tolerance may be weaned from steroids.

Clinical trials with new immunosuppressive strategies, induction agents, and graft irradiation with short-term or steroid-free therapies are underway.

39. What adjunctive immunosuppressant agents are commonly used?

Adjunctive immunosuppressant agents, such as azathioprine, mycophenolate mofetil (MMF), and sirolimus, may be used when additional immunosuppression is required to maintain graft tolerance, to treat rejection, or to lessen tacrolimus-related toxicities. Induction therapy with muromonab-CD3, rabbit antithymocyte globulin, cyclophosphamide, MMF, or daclizumab has been used in some centers, with varying results.

40. Is rejection common in intestinal transplant recipients?

Because of the large quantity of lymphoid tissue associated with the intestine, acute rejection of the graft is common, with an overall incidence of 90%. One series reported a mean of 4 episodes of rejection per patient.[5] Although rejection can occur at any time, it is most commonly seen within the first 6 months posttransplant. Rejection is seen most frequently and with greatest severity in isolated intestine recipients (88%) and with lesser frequency in composite liver-intestine grafts (66%) and multivisceral grafts (75%). Because the incidence of liver rejection in recipients with composite grafts of the liver and intestine transplant is 43%, it is theorized that the liver may play a protective role when it is part of a composite graft.

41. What are the symptoms of acute rejection of the intestine?

Although serum markers may suggest rejection in liver or renal transplant recipients, there are no specific serum tests to detect rejection of the intestinal graft. Recent studies report that serum citrulline, a nonessential amino acid produced by the intestinal mucosa, may be a potential marker for rejection,[24] but at present, timely diagnosis of rejection is most reliably based on clinical presentation, the endoscopic appearance of the graft, and definitive histologic findings. Rejection may vary from a mild clinical course with minimal histologic changes to severe, intractable rejection resulting in graft enterectomy or death.

Most episodes of acute rejection occur within the first 3 months posttransplant. The most common clinical manifestation is a change in stool output. Other symptoms include fever, malaise, abdominal pain, abdominal distention, nausea and vomiting, and/or a dusky stoma. Severe rejection may also cause the following:
- GI bleeding secondary to mucosal ulceration and sloughing
- Ileus
- Septic shock syndrome
- Acute respiratory distress syndrome

Sepsis often occurs with rejection because of bacterial or fungal translocation secondary to the disruption of the mucosal barrier of the intestine.

42. How is the graft monitored for rejection?

Surveillance endoscopies through the ileostomy are usually performed twice weekly for the first 4–6 weeks following transplantation. Depending on the recipient's clinical status, rejection history, and risk factors for rejection, the interval between endoscopies is gradually increased. Stable recipients at 3 or more years posttransplant may require only an annual surveillance endoscopy.

Endoscopically, acute rejection of the intestine is characterized by a loss of the normal velvety appearance of the mucosa, edema, granularity, erythema, and/or duskiness. Peristalsis is often reduced or absent. Friable tissue with diffuse ulcerations is seen in more advanced rejection, and severe rejection is associated with ulceration, aperistalsis, and denuded mucosa with pseudomembranes.

The definitive diagnosis of rejection is made through histology. The histologic criteria for acute rejection include edema of the lamina propria with mononuclear cell infiltrates, villous blunting, crypt epithelial injury, and crypt cell apoptosis. In severe rejection, there is crypt destruction and complete sloughing of the epithelium. The ileum is most commonly affected, although changes may be seen throughout the graft.

43. What is chronic rejection of the intestinal graft?

Chronic rejection of the intestinal graft occurs following repeated episodes of acute rejection that may be partially resolved or refractory to treatment. It usually develops over a longer period of time, and patients present with chronic diarrhea, progressive weight loss, intermittent fevers, abdominal pain, and GI bleeding. Endoscopic findings may include a normal or tubular intestine with thickened mucosal folds, pseudomembrane formation, and/or chronic ulcers. Histology reveals villous blunting, focal ulcerations, and epithelial metaplasia with rare cellular infiltrates. Full-thickness biopsies from enterectomies display obliterative thickening of the arterioles.

44. How is rejection treated?

Mild-to-moderate rejection is usually treated by increasing tacrolimus levels to 20–25 ng/ml and administering intravenous methylprednisolone as a bolus dose with decreasing cycled doses over 5 days (e.g., 5 mg/kg/day, divided every 6 hours for 4 doses [max: 50 mg/dose] tapered to 1 mg/kg/day, 1 dose daily). The steroid bolus with or without a recycle may be repeated if rejection is refractory to treatment.

Adjunctive agents may also be added to the baseline immunosuppression. Muromonab-CD3 is typically used in cases of severe rejection. Muromonab-CD3 may be administered for up to 14 days; however, the duration of muromonab-CD3 therapy is determined by biopsy results. For refractory or severe rejection, rabbit antithymocyte globulin is currently being used in some centers as an alternative to muromonab-CD3.

Endoscopy with biopsy is performed up to twice weekly to assess the effect of treatment and to determine immunosuppressant management until the rejection episode resolves.

45. What can be done if treatment for rejection fails?

If rejection is refractory to all available treatment and complications related to increased immunosuppression are increasing, the only alternative may be timely graft enterectomy with retransplantation before the patient experiences life-threatening sepsis or further organ system deterioration. Survival rates following retransplantation are much lower than primary transplantation. Morbidity and mortality are increased during the waiting period because patients again require parenteral nutrition, which may result in liver dysfunction and the need for a composite graft. Additionally, the patient and family may be overwhelmed by the psychological and psychosocial impact of a second transplant.

46. What other medical management issues are of concern for the intestinal transplant recipient?

During the early postoperative period, maintenance of fluid and electrolyte balance is essential because patients commonly develop intravascular volume depletion while simultaneously retaining fluid. This condition may be caused by increased interstitial fluid accumulation in peripheral tissue, the intestinal graft, and the lungs in the setting of increasing ascites from leakage of mesenteric lymphatics. Management includes attentiveness to renal function and electrolytes and strict measurement of intake and output with precise adjustments in intravenous fluids. Fluids are usually administered at two-thirds' maintenance to maintain a central venous pressure (CVP) of 6–10 cm H_2O and a urine output of 0.5–1.5 ml/kg/hour.

As the patient and graft stabilize, fluid imbalances are associated with water, sodium, magnesium, and bicarbonate losses secondary to increased stomal output. Intravenous replacement fluids are usually required to correct dehydration, metabolic acidosis, and hyponatremia until the ileostomy is reversed and/or the older patient is able to tolerate an adequate amount of fluids by mouth.

47. Describe the early postoperative nutritional management of the intestinal transplant recipient.

Total parenteral nutrition (TPN) is used to provide full nutritional support during the early postoperative period. When GI motility recovers, usually within the first 2 weeks, a gastrograffin study is completed to evaluate the integrity of the intestinal anastomoses. If there are no anastomotic complications, enteral feedings are slowly initiated and TPN is usually weaned within 4 weeks. Although TPN is discontinued in a majority of patients, nutritional support may again be required during periods of rejection or infection. Some pediatric patients, in particular, may require intermittent partial TPN support for weight gain and growth.

48. What types of enteral feedings are used? How are they administered?

Feeding protocols are center-specific, but enteral feedings are usually begun through the jejunostomy tube (JT) within 2 weeks posttransplant if there are no postoperative complications. Enteral feedings usually consist of an age-appropriate, low-osmolality isotonic dipeptide formula containing medium-chain triglycerides and glutamine. This type of formula allows maximum absorption and use of nitrogen, and direct absorption of fat while preventing hyperosmolar diarrhea. Early feedings are half-strength concentration and are administered continuously at a low rate, usually 2 ml/hour in infants to 10 ml/hour in adults. Feedings are slowly increased to a goal rate that provides total caloric needs as TPN is weaned. When patients are able to tolerate the desired rate, the formula concentration is increased to three-quarters' strength, then to full strength over a few days. During this time, patients are encouraged to take a clear oral diet that is slowly advanced to a full diet.

The enteral route is transitioned to feedings through a gastrostomy tube (GT) when the patient tolerates full volume and concentration from jejunostomy feedings, providing additional absorption from the stomach to the duodenum. Patients, particularly pediatric recipients, who were managed nutritionally on TPN with minimal oral intake before transplantation, may initially be uncomfortable with GT feedings because they are not accustomed to a large gastric volume of feedings.

The long-term nutritional goal is for the patient to tolerate a regular oral diet without enteral or parenteral supplementation. This goal is achieved in most adult patients within 1 year and in children within 2 years.

49. How is absorption assessed?

Adequate absorption and tolerance of feedings are significant indicators of satisfactory graft function and are evaluated by assessing the following:
- Daily stomal outputs
- Serum electrolytes
- Nutritional markers,
- Presence of blood or reducing substances in the stool

Carbohydrate absorption is assessed through D-xylose testing and the presence of reducing substances. If not delayed by early surgical complications or rejection, most patients have adequate carbohydrate absorption within 1 month posttransplant with continued improvement over time. Abnormal D-xylose test results are suggestive of rejection.

Malabsorption of fats is common following intestinal transplantation and may be due to disruption of the lymphatic channels during surgery and/or postoperative pancreatitis. Fat absorption is evaluated by a 24-hour fecal fat collection and by obtaining fat-soluble vitamin levels. One study reported that fat malabsorption in intestinal transplant recipients ranged from 50–100% (normal: 0–8.5%).[36] Interventions to improve fat absorption and decrease stomal output include the use of pancreatic enzymes, a daily multivitamin containing fat-soluble vitamins, a low-fat diet, and short-term intravenous intralipids.

Stomal output, as an indicator of absorption, ranges from 40–60 ml/kg/day in children and from 1–2 L/day in adults. A low stool output and the absence of reducing substances are associated with feeding tolerance. In the absence of rejection, a high stomal output is treated with antidiarrheal medications such as loperamide, opiates, and clonidine hydrochloride. Intravenous or subcutaneous somatostatin may be used in some cases of moderate-to-severe hypermotility. Pectin, as a fiber source, is administered with enteral or oral feedings as another strategy to decrease intestinal motility and increase absorption by thickening feedings and slowing the transit time. Pectin is added in a ratio of 3–5 tablespoons/L of formula per day.

Maintenance of a stable and satisfactory tacrolimus level can also indicate adequate absorption. Unless the tacrolimus level is being adjusted during episodes of rejection or infection, a stable level is usually achieved within 1 month posttransplant.

50. How is graft function assessed?

Adequate functioning of the transplanted intestine is assessed through the absorptive capacity of the intestine, as discussed, and also by routine surveillance for rejection through endoscopy with tissue biopsy. Additionally, radiologic evaluation through barium studies is used to assess the mucosal pattern of the graft and motility. Intestinal transit time should be approximately 2 hours with a normal mucosal pattern. Rejection is indicated if a tubular intestine with mucosal edema is visualized in the setting of an increased transit time.

51. What are the caloric and nutritional requirements of intestinal transplant recipients?

Caloric requirements are based on age and then adjusted for several pre- and posttransplant factors:

Pretransplant factors:	Posttransplant complications:
• Nutritional status	• Surgical re-explorations
• Growth failure	• Repeated or extended episodes of rejection
• Weight loss	• Infectious processes
	• Pancreatitis
	• Hypergylcemia
	• Renal insufficiency
	• Growth failure

Because malabsorption is common in the early posttransplant period, vitamin, mineral, and trace element levels should be monitored routinely. Zinc levels are usually low during the first year posttransplant because of high stomal outputs. Zinc supplementation at 1.5–3 times the Recommended Daily Allowance (RDA) is suggested with monthly monitoring of zinc and albumin levels until ostomy closure. Deficiencies in red blood cell folate and copper levels have also been reported.[8,35,36]

Some centers advocate the use of L-glutamine as an additive to enteral feedings. Glutamine administration has been associated with increased villous height, villous surface area, mucosal weight, and brush border enzyme activity. The suggested pediatric and adult doses are 0.6 gm/kg daily and 30 gm daily, respectively.

52. Do intestinal transplant recipients have food allergies?

Food allergies, particularly to lactose and gluten agents, are common in intestinal transplant recipients. Radioallergosorbent testing (RAST) is completed when intestinal biopsies reveal eosinophilia. Results may range from 0 (no allergy) to class IV (high allergy). Food restrictions are advised in those patients diagnosed with class III or IV allergies. Patients with prolonged eosinophilia may also benefit from low-dose oral steroids.

53. Do patients have any eating difficulties?

Enteral supplementation, as discussed, may be necessary for some time based on the patient's ability to meet caloric needs by an oral diet alone. Following optimal recovery from transplantation, most patients are able to eat a regular oral diet and have a desire for eating. However, oral aversion is common in pediatric recipients because they usually have limited feeding experiences before transplantation. Other factors that affect oral intake include pretransplant medical and nutritional status and conditions that preclude oral feeds such as the following:
- Severe gastroesophageal reflux with aspiration
- Age at onset of short gut syndrome
- Hypergag reflex
- Hospital environment
- Parenting factors
- Behavioral issues

Occupational and speech therapy is usually necessary for young pediatric recipients, and, in many cases, child development and psychiatry consultations are also required. Inpatient feeding rehabilitation programs provide continuity with behavior modification in severe cases of oral aversion.

54. Are infections common after intestinal transplantation?

Infection is the leading cause of morbidity and mortality following intestinal transplantation and accounts for up to 70% of all deaths. Patients are predisposed to infection because they require high levels of maintenance immunosuppression, particularly in the early postoperative period. Postoperative infections are common with a median of 4 infections per patient.[15,29,31]

Other factors that contribute to infection are listed below:
- Prolonged operative time
- Severity of liver disease pretransplant
- Sepsis prior to transplant
- Transfusions
- Re-explorations due to surgical complications
- Inability to close the abdominal wall immediately after surgery
- Multiple invasive lines, catheters, and drains that alter skin integrity.

55. What are the most common infections seen after intestinal transplantation?

Following intestinal transplantation, over 80% of patients acquire bacterial infections, most commonly staphylococcal and enterococcal infections.[12] Enteric organisms are often present in abdominal wound infections, deep abdominal abscesses, peritonitis, and pneumonia. Patients may have repeat infections or require polymicrobial therapy for simultaneous infections from multiple sources. Bacterial translocation may also occur because the mucosal barrier of the transplanted intestine may be impaired as a result of preservation injury, rejection, high immunosuppressive levels, bacterial overgrowth, or disruption of the lymphatics. If the patient is febrile, without an obvious source for infection, an endoscopy with tissue biopsy should be performed.

Antibiotic prophylaxis varies by center, but broad-spectrum antibiotics may be administered for up to 5 days postoperatively. Bacterial translocation is prevented by selective bowel decontamination through enteral administration of tobramycin, colistimethate, and amphotericin B for up to 2 weeks postoperatively. Stool cultures are monitored routinely, and intravenous antibiotics are administered if cultures show more than 10^8 organisms in the presence of sepsis or rejection. Bacterial overgrowth is treated by a cyclic course of enteral bowel decontamination agents.

Because immunosuppressed patients are at risk for *Pneumocystis carinii* pneumonia (PCP), some centers recommend lifetime prophylaxis with a single daily dose of oral trimethoprim-sulfamethoxazole (TMP-SMX) 3 times per week. Patients with sulfa allergies are prescribed dapsone twice daily or pentamadine aerosol treatments monthly.

56. What are the risk factors and treatment options for fungal infections?

Risk factors that predispose intestinal transplant recipients to fungal infections include the following:

- Pretransplant clinical status
- High levels of immunosuppression to treat rejection
- Intestinal leaks and other surgical complications
- Repeated surgical explorations
- Extensive use of antibiotics
- Fungal translocation
- Intravenous–line contamination

Patients at risk for fungal infections receive prophylaxis with low-dose intravenous amphotericin B. Oral nystatin is used to prevent noninvasive candidiasis while immunosuppression is maximized, particularly in the first 3–6 months posttransplant and during treatment for rejection. Refractory candidiasis may be treated with intravenous amphotericin B or fluconazole. Because tacrolimus levels increase with the administration of fluconazole, tacrolimus levels should be monitored frequently and the dosage adjusted to maintain the desired level.

Confirmed systemic infections with candida are treated with an extended course of full-dose intravenous amphotericin B, Abelcet, or fluconazole with careful monitoring of renal function and tacrolimus levels. Aspergillosis, a rare fungal infection, has a high mortality rate.

57. What is the most common viral pathogen following intestinal transplantation?

Cytomegalovirus (CMV) is the most common viral infection. It occurs in 34% of intestinal transplant recipients and involves the transplanted intestine in 65% of cases.[12]

58. What are the risk factors for cytomegalovirus?

The most significant risk factors are a donor-recipient serology mismatch and high levels of immunosuppression. CMV-seronegative candidates who receive an allograft from a CMV-seropositive donor are at significant risk for primary CMV disease. Such patients usually have a more aggressive infection with a higher incidence of recurrence, disease persistence, and further disease involvement.

Some centers have reported that CMV-matching results in a decreased incidence in CMV and recommend that allografts from CMV-seropositive donors should not be considered for CMV-seronegative recipients, particularly in isolated intestine transplantation.[11] Intensified immunosuppression, which decreases the number of cytotoxic T lymphocytes and natural killer cells, adds to the patient's risk of developing CMV by interfering with the body's normal immunologic response to the virus.

59. How does cytomegalovirus present in intestinal transplant patients?

CMV usually occurs within the first 6 months posttransplant. Presenting symptoms are usually fever and gastroenteritis of varying severity. Other symptoms may include the following:

- Myalgia
- Arthralgia
- Malaise
- Anorexia

- Focal ulcerations of the intestine with bleeding
- Hematologic abnormalities (e.g., leukopenia, thrombocytopenia, and atypical lymphocytosis)

Although CMV usually presents in the transplanted intestine, it can also cause gastroduodenitis and colitis of the native organs, pneumonitis, central nervous system disease, hepatitis, and retinitis.

60. How is cytomegalovirus diagnosed?

Diagnosis is made by clinical symptoms and findings and confirmed by endoscopic and histologic results. A routine work-up for fever is completed with cultures of urine, blood, stool, and sputum. An endoscopy usually reveals protruding flat ulcers, aphthoid lesions with a white center, or ulcerations in the setting of normal mucosa. On histology, there are numerous CMV-inclusion bodies with inflammatory changes.

61. Describe the prophylactic and therapeutic strategies for cytomegalovirus infection.

The pretransplant serologic status of the donor and recipient is reviewed to guide prophylactic and therapeutic strategies. As stated previously, to decrease the risk of primary CMV disease, transplantation of CMV-seropositive grafts is avoided in CMV-seronegative recipients of isolated intestine grafts. Patients considered at-risk for CMV are monitored routinely by CMV-pp65 levels, a rapid diagnostic method that uses monoclonal antibodies to detect CMV-specific antigens in peripheral polymorphonuclear cells. CMV prophylaxis with intravenous ganciclovir is given for 2 weeks in some centers, but this therapy has not been effective in preventing CMV infection in intestinal transplant recipients.

Current treatment strategies for patients with a primary CMV infection are center-specific, but usually include administration of intravenous ganciclovir and/or CMV-specific hyperimmunoglobulin, routine monitoring of CMV-pp65 levels, and close monitoring of immunosuppressive levels. Therapeutic baseline immunosuppression is usually maintained during treatment and only decreased if the patient deteriorates.

62. What is the outcome following cytomegalovirus infection?

Although CMV is commonly seen in intestinal transplant recipients, nearly 90% of these patients have been successfully managed and treated with resolution of the infection.[6,29]

63. What is the significance of Epstein-Barr virus infection in intestinal transplantation?

Infection with Epstein-Barr virus (EBV) and EBV-associated posttransplant lymphoproliferative disease (PTLD) is one of the most serious consequences of immunosuppression. This virus encompasses a range of disorders from a nonspecific viral illness or self-limiting mononucleosis to more serious polyclonal or monoclonal disease, and ultimately, lymphoma. Because intestinal transplant recipients require high levels of immunosuppression as a result of the large amount of lymphoid tissue in the graft, such patients are at high risk for developing EBV infections and PTLD. PTLD is a significant cause of morbidity and mortality in intestinal transplantation, with an incidence of 20%, which is higher than in any other type of solid organ transplantation.[23,30] It occurs most often in pediatric multivisceral transplant recipients (40%) and less frequently with isolated intestine transplantation (11%). The intestinal graft is most commonly affected, but the residual native GI tract may also be involved.[23,30,38]

64. What are the risk factors for Epstein-Barr virus and posttransplant lymphoproliferative disease?

PTLD usually presents at a mean of 9 months following transplantation and is usually the result of high levels of immunosuppression.[3] Children are at greater risk than adults (30% vs. 9%) because children are usually EBV-seronegative at the time of transplant.[23,30] However, in some series, EBV seronegativity or positivity was not seen to be a significant factor in development of disease. Other risk factors include the type of intestinal graft, treatment with muromonab-CD3, and recipient splenectomy.

65. What is an EBV-polymerase chain reaction assay?

Patients at high risk for EBV and PTLD are followed routinely through monitoring the EBV-polymerase chain reaction (EBV-PCR) assay. This serologic test identifies increased levels of circulating EBV-infected lymphocytes through measurement of peripheral blood leukocytes and provides an accurate quantitative measure of the EBV viral load. Pediatric intestinal transplant recipients were reported to have viral loads ranging from 500 to greater than 25,000 genome copies per 10^5 peripheral blood leukocytes (PBL). Patients with viral loads ranging from nondetectable to 200 genome copies per 10^5 PBL did not have disease. Findings may be inconsistent, however, and some patients with elevated viral loads are asymptomatic. Although the EBV-PCR assay is a useful method to monitor high-risk patients and direct treatment, histologic confirmation is necessary.[16,33]

66. How are Epstein-Barr virus and posttransplant lymphoproliferative disease diagnosed?

Various symptoms and findings are used to diagnose EBV infection and PTLD. The intestinal recipient may present clinically with fever, lymphadenopathy, lethargy, malaise, GI complaints, diarrhea, bloody stools, and/or pain. A complete blood count (CBC) may reveal anemia, leukopenia, or atypical lymphocytosis. Computed tomography (CT) scans of the chest and abdomen are obtained to evaluate any tumors, masses, lymphadenopathy, or disseminated disease.

The EBV-PCR assay is monitored weekly to monthly in high-risk patients to obtain a quantitative measurement of the EBV viral load. Endoscopy with histology, however, provides the definitive diagnosis of EBV disease. On endoscopy, early PTLD lesions present as nonspecific, nonulcerated submucosal nodules within normal mucosa. Progressive disease reveals larger ulcers with raised margins and a necrotic base. Histologically, the tissue has lymphocytic infiltrates with a monomorphic and/or polymorphic appearance. The diagnosis is confirmed by staining through the Epstein Barr Early RNA probe (EBER-1), which labels EBV-encoded RNA in infected cells.

67. What is the treatment for Epstein-Barr virus and posttransplant lymphoproliferative disease?

The most widely accepted treatment for EBV infection and PTLD consists of restoring the body's natural immune surveillance by reducing or discontinuing immunosuppression so that EBV-cell proliferation is contained. Although this strategy may be successful in other solid organ transplant recipients, it places the intestinal transplant recipient at increased risk for rejection. The medical management dilemma of decreasing immunosuppression to treat EBV disease while intensifying immunosuppression to treat rejection leads to significant morbidity and mortality in these patients. Generally, immunosuppression may be reduced by up to 50% with the patient monitored weekly to biweekly for any evidence of rejection. If the patient develops rejection, immunosuppression is increased to the baseline level. More severe rejection may be treated with increased corticosteroids and/or adjunctive agents.

68. What other treatment strategies are used?

Intravenous antiviral agents including ganciclovir, acyclovir, hyperimmunoglobulin, cytokine therapy (interferon-alpha), and chemotherapy have also been used in some centers. Treatment with reduced immunosuppression and antiviral therapies is usually continued until resolution of the disease. Rituximab, an anti-CD20 monoclonal antibody, has recently been approved for treatment of certain CD20-positive B-cell lymphomas.

69. What is the outcome of Epstein-Barr virus-associated posttransplant lymphoproliferative disease?

PTLD is a major cause of death following intestinal transplantation with a mortality rate of up to 50%.[3,30] Preventive medical management with early detection and treatment of PTLD is necessary to decrease the morbidity and mortality of this complication.

70. What other infections are common following intestinal transplantation?

Respiratory syncytial virus (RSV), adenovirus, and parainfluenza are the most common community-acquired viruses seen in these patients. These viruses can lead to severe morbidity and mortality depending on the age of the recipient, time posttransplant, level of immunosuppression, and concurrent rejection.

71. What are the care requirements following transplantation?

Care requirements vary according to the patient's age, postoperative complications, and any concurrent episodes of rejection or infection. In the early postoperative period, patients may receive up to 20 medications daily, tube feedings, intravenous fluids, and/or intravenous medications. Routine care and maintenance of the gastrostomy tube, jejunostomy tube, ostomy, and Broviac catheter are also required. Patients are usually examined 1–2 times weekly in the transplant clinic, and endoscopies are performed 2–4 times a month. Although care requirements are quite demanding during the first 6 months posttransplant, these routines generally decrease over time as a result of ostomy closure, increased oral intake, stable graft function, and appliance removal. In a group of pediatric recipients more than 3 years posttransplant, the majority of patients had all their appliances removed with only 17% still requiring a gastrostomy tube for feedings secondary to oral aversion. In this group, patients received a mean of 7 medications daily.[20]

72. What is the quality of life for patients surviving intestinal transplantation?

Survival following intestinal transplantation has increased dramatically over the last 15 years. Many recipients have an extended survival of more than 5 years. Quality of life, as an endpoint for the effectiveness of intestinal transplantation, is currently being assessed at some of the larger transplant centers. Findings have suggested that psychiatric and psychosocial problems affecting quality of life following intestinal transplantation vary inversely with social support and are related to severity of disease, duration of postoperative TPN, length of the waiting period, and a prolonged postoperative course. A high incidence of affective disorders, such as depression and anxiety, is reported in the early postoperative period.[9,32]

Pediatric recipients are reported to have greater limitations in physical activities as a result of physical health and/or emotional problems compared with the general population and other chronic illness groups. However, clinical experience reveals that many recipients appear to have improved considerably in physical and psychosocial functioning compared with their pretransplant status.[18,19,37]

Assessing quality of life in these patients is very challenging because there is great patient variability with respect to the underlying disease, age at time of transplant, the postoperative course, long-term complications, and psychosocial factors. However, it is imperative to assess quality of life to better understand what life is like after transplant for these patients and also to use the findings to guide the transplant team in medical management decisions. Information about quality of life is also important for intestinal transplant candidates who are considering this treatment for end-stage short gut syndrome.

73. What is the future of intestinal transplantation?

Significant progress has been made in intestinal transplantation for adults and children with permanent intestinal failure. Further developments in the treatment of rejection, new immunosuppressive medications and combination therapies, infection prophylaxis and treatment, improvements in graft surveillance, and optimal patient selection will lead to increased survival and improved outcomes.

BIBLIOGRAPHY

1. Abu-Elmagd K, Reyes J, Bond G, et al: Clinical intestine transplantation: A decade of experience at a single center. Ann Surg 234:404–417, 2001.
2. Abu-Elmagd K, Reyes J, Fung J: Clinical intestinal transplantation: Recent advances and future consideration. In Norman D, Turka L (eds): Primer on Transplantation, 2nd ed. Malden, MA, Blackwell Publishing, 2001, pp 610–625.

3. Abu-Elmagd KM, Reyes J, Todo S, et al: Clinical intestinal transplantation: New perspectives and immunologic considerations. Am Coll Surg 186:512–527, 1998.
4. Asfar S, Atkinson P, Ghent C, et al: Small bowel transplantation [abstract]. Transplant Proc 28:2751, 1996.
5. Bond G, Mazariegos G, Sindhi R, et al: Pediatric intestinal transplantation: Current status [abstract 52]. Presented at the VII International Small Bowel Transplant Symposium, Stockholm, Sweden, September 12–15, 2001.
6. Bueno J, Green M, Kocoshis S, et al: Cytomegalovirus infection after intestinal transplantation in children. Clin Infect Dis 24:1078–1083, 1997.
7. Bueno J, Ohwada S, Kocochis S, et al: Factors impacting the survival of children with intestinal failure referred for intestinal transplantation. J Pediatr Surg 34:27–33, 1999.
8. Davis AM: Pediatric small bowel transplantation: A case presentation of nutrition support. J Am Diet Assoc 17:5–11, 1995.
9. DiMartini A, Fitzgerald G, Magil J, et al: Psychiatric evaluation of small intestine transplantation patients. Gen Hosp Psychiatry 18(6 suppl):25S–29S, 1996.
10. Furukawa H, Abu-Elmagd K, Reyes J, et al: Technical aspects of intestinal transplantation. In Braverman MH, Tawes RL (eds): Surgical Technology International, vol 2. San Francisco, University Medical Press, 1994, pp 165–170.
11. Furukawa H, Manez R, Kusne S, et al: Cytomegalovirus disease in intestinal transplantation. Transplant Proc 27:1357–1358, 1995.
12. Furukawa H, Reyes J, Abu-Elmagd K, Todo S: Clinical intestinal transplantation. Clin Nutr 15:45–52, 1996.
13. Goulet O, Colomb V, Jan D, et al: Virginie, ten years later [abstract 21]. Program and abstracts of the VI International Small Bowel Transplant Symposium, Omaha, Nebraska, October 6–9, 1999
14. Goulet O, Jan D, Lacaille F, et al: Intestinal transplantation in children: Results from Paris [abstract 79]. Presented at the VII International Small Bowel Transplant Symposium, Stockholm, Sweden, September 12–15, 2001.
15. Grant D: International Intestine Transplant Registry Data. Available at: www.lhsc.on.ca/itr. Accessed June 20, 2001.
16. Green M, Michaels MG, Webber SA, et al: The management of Epstein-Barr virus associated posttransplant lymphoproliferative disorders in pediatric solid organ transplant recipients. Pediatr Transplantation 3:271–281,1999.
17. Kato T, Nishida S, Mittal N, et al: Intestinal transplantation at the University of Miami [abstract 78]. Presented at the VII International Small Bowel Transplant Symposium, Stockholm, Sweden, September 12–15, 2001.
18. Kosmach-Park B: Pediatric intestinal transplantation. Prog Transplant 12(2):97–115, 2002.
19. Kosmach-Park B: Physical and psychosocial functioning as indicators of quality of life following pediatric intestinal transplantation [abstract 2]. Presented at the VII International Small Bowel Transplant Symposium, Stockholm, Sweden, September 12–15, 2001.
20. Kosmach-Park B: Current status of pediatric intestine transplant recipients: Care requirements and patient outcomes. [abstract 3]. Presented at the VII International Small Bowel Transplant Symposium, Stockholm, Sweden, September 12–15, 2001.
21. Langnas AL, Chinnakotla S, Sudan D, et al: Intestinal transplantation at the University of Nebraska Medical Center: 1990–2001 [abstract 75]. Presented at the VII International Small Bowel Transplant Symposium, Stockholm, Sweden, September 12–15, 2001.
22. Langnas AL, Sudan S, Kaufman S, et al: Intestinal transplantation: A single-center experience [abstract]. Transplant Proc 32:1228, 2000.
23. Nalesnik M, Jaffe R, Reyes J, et al: Posttransplant lymphoproliferative disorders in small bowel allograft recipients [abstract]. Transplant Proc 32:1213, 2000.
24. Pappas PA, Suudubray JM, Tzakis AG, et al: Serum citrulline as a marker of acute cellular rejection for intestinal transplantation. Transplant Proc 34:915–917, 2002.
25. Pirenne J: Advances in intestinal transplantation: Report from the VII international small bowel transplant symposium. Medscape Transplantation, 2002. Available at: http://transplantation.medscape.com.
26. Pinna AD, Weppler D, Nery K, et al: Intestinal transplantation at the University of Miami: Five years of experience. Transplant Proc 32:1226–1227, 2000.
27. Pritchard TJ, Kirkman RL: Small bowel transplantation. World J Surg 9:860–886, 1985.
28. Reyes J, Abu-Elmagd K: Small bowel and liver transplantation in children. In Kelly DA (ed): Diseases of the Biliary System in Children. Osney Mead, Oxford, Blackwell Science, 1999, pp 313–331.
29. Reyes J, Bueno J, Kocochis S, et al: Current status of intestinal transplantation in children. J Pediatric Surg 33:243–254, 1998.
30. Reyes J, Green M, Bueno J, et al: Epstein-Barr virus associated posttransplant lymphoproliferative disorders after intestinal transplantation. Transplant Proc 28:2768–2769, 1996.
31. Roberts CA, Radio SJ, Markin RS, et al: Histopathologic evaluation of primary intestinal transplant recipients at autopsy: a single center experience. Transplant Proc 32:1202–1203, 2000.

32. Rovera GM, Martini A, Schoen RE, et al: Quality of life of patients after intestinal transplantation. Transplantation 66:1141–1145,1998.
33. Rowe D, Qu L, Reyes J, et al: Use of quantitative competitive PCR to measure Epstein-Barr virus genome load in peripheral blood of pediatric transplant recipients with lymphoproliferative disorders, J Clin Microbiol 35:1612–1615, 1997.
34. Sigurdsson L, Reyes J, Putnam PE, et al: Endoscopies in pediatric small intestinal transplant recipients: Five years experience. Am J Gastroenterol 93:207–211,1998.
35. Silver HJ, Castellanose VH: Nutritional complications and management of intestinal transplant. J Am Diet Assoc 100:680–684, 2000.
36. Strohm SL, Koehler AN, Mazariegos GV, Reyes J: Nutritional management in pediatric small bowel transplantation. Nutr Clin Res 14:58–63, 1999.
37. Sudan DL, Iverson A, Weseman RA, et al: Assessment of function, growth and development, and long-term quality of life after small bowel transplantation. Transplant Proc 32:1211–1212, 2000.
38. Sudan DL, Kaufman SS, Byers WS, et al: Isolated intestinal transplantation for intestinal failure. Am J Gastroenterol 95:1506–1515, 2000.
39. United Network for Organ Sharing: 2000 Annual Report. Number of Registrations and Media Waiting Times (in days) to Transplant: Registrations added during 1990 to 1999. UNOS Web stie. Available at: www.unos.org/Data/anrpt00/ar00_table10_01_al.htm. Accessed April 2, 2002.

15. ISLET CELL TRANSPLANTATION

Lori A. Purdie, MS, RN, and Linda Ohler, MSN, RN, CCTC, FAAN

1. Is islet cell transplantation a widely available procedure?

At this time, islet cell transplantation is offered as an experimental therapy at several hospitals throughout the United States, Canada, and Europe. The first islet cell transplants were performed in the early 1990s as an alternative to full pancreas transplantation for patients with type 1 diabetes. While current outcomes of pancreas transplantation provide approximately 80% of recipients with at least 1 year of insulin independence, the complexity of the surgical procedure and resulting complications have caused physicians to look for a less invasive alternative. Because only 2% of the pancreas is used to produce insulin and control blood glucose, transplantation of islet cells continues to be an exciting option.

Before 2000, fewer than 200 islet cell transplants were reported in the United States. The International Islet Transplant Registry at the University of Geissen in Germany reported that 407 islet transplants were performed worldwide as of 1998. Early results of islet cell transplants performed between 1990 and 1998 reported insulin independence for less than 15% of recipients 1 year after the procedure. These results were certainly not encouraging; however, the less invasive procedure provided the impetus for researchers to continue pursuing this route.

2. What accounted for the poor outcomes?

In evaluations of reasons for the poor outcomes, it was determined that several drugs used to suppress the immune system, such as calcineurin inhibitors and steroids, actually had a negative impact on islet cell function. The procurement and preservation process possibly affected islet cell function.

3. What new protocols are used for islet cell transplantation?

In 2000, a group of physicians from Edmonton, Canada, employed new methods for procuring and preserving the sensitive islet cells for transplantation. In addition, the Edmonton physicians also established a steroid-free immunosuppressive regimen that uses less of the calcineurin inhibitors. The Edmonton protocol, as the new islet cell transplant procedure is commonly called, uses low-dose tacrolimus in combination with a newer immunosuppressant agent, sirolimus. Encouraging results have provided researchers with opportunities to explore long-term outcomes in multi-institutional studies throughout the United States and Canada. While the procedure remains experimental, preliminary results are better than those reported in the last decade.

4. How many islet cell transplants have been done using the procedure described by the Edmonton physicians?

Since 2000, there have been fewer than 50 islet cell transplants performed in the United States and Canada using the new procurement and preservation procedure and the immunosuppression regimen established by the Edmonton physicians. The vast majority of islets transplanted in this protocol continue to function well according to initial reports from the Canadian and NIH studies. A new collaborative islet transplant registry was established in September 2001 through the National Institutes of Diabetes, Digestive and Kidney (NIDDK) diseases at the National Institutes of Health (NIH) and can be accessed at www.citregistry.com. The registry is coordinated by the EMMES Corporation and Dr. Bernard Hering at the University of Minnesota. Members of the executive committee for this registry are from EMMES, UCLA, the University of Geissen, the University of Minnesota, the United Network of Organ Sharing (UNOS), NIDDK, the University of Alberta (Canada), and the University of Miami. Goals for the registry include compiling and analyzing data from participating islet transplant centers. Knowledge gained regarding identified risks or successes will be adapted to current protocols.

5. What is the success rate for islet cell transplantation?

Under current protocols in the United States and Canada, it is difficult to report on long-term results because there are data for only a small number of patients transplanted in the past 2 years from Canadian and U.S. centers. Most centers participating in the studies have just begun their trials in late 2001 or early 2002. Thus, it is too early to determine any long-term outcomes, although preliminary results have been encouraging: the majority of the patients studied to date remain insulin independent at 1 year. Whereas results from the 1990s reported that less than 15% of islet cell recipients were insulin independent, the new trials hold much hope for the future.

6. Does islet cell transplantation affect the functioning of the native pancreas?

In the majority of cases of pancreas and islet cell transplantation, the patient's native pancreas remains intact. Only 2% of the pancreas functions to produce insulin and control blood glucose, and the remaining 98% of the pancreas functions well in most patients. Therefore, the native pancreas, which has no role in glucose control or insulin production, continues its role of manufacturing digestive enzymes that are delivered into the intestine (so-called exocrine function).

7. Why is islet cell transplantation considered solid organ transplantation and not tissue transplantation?

Because the entire pancreas must be procured from a cadaveric donor to obtain islet cells, the transplant still is considered a solid organ transplant.

8. Is islet cell transplantation also a treatment option for type 2 diabetes?

Type 2 diabetes is caused, at least in part, by insulin resistance. Pancreatic beta cells initially respond to insulin resistance by increasing insulin secretion. Over time, the existing beta cell mass loses its ability to cope with the increased demand for insulin. In patients with type 2 diabetes, pancreatic beta cells eventually fail to keep up with the increased demand required by the insulin resistance, and when that occurs, blood glucose levels start to rise.

Current pharmacologic treatment of type 2 diabetes employs agents designed to affect endogenous sources of glucose regulation. Specifically, agents act by either promoting insulin sensitivity and insulin secretion or by decreasing glucose production. Islet cell transplantation could prove beneficial in patients with type 2 diabetes by expanding the beta cell mass and by replacing dysfunctional beta cells with normally functioning transplanted beta cells. To date, human islet cell transplantation for type 2 diabetes has been attempted in few cases. Results from pilot trials were inconclusive and sparked interest in continued research. A major factor limiting the implementation of islet cell transplantation as a treatment option for type 2 diabetes is the competition for available organs.

9. Discuss the contraindications to the procedure.

Because islet cell transplantation is experimental at this time, researchers must adhere to strict protocol guidelines for candidacy. Current protocols exclude patients under the following conditions:

- Obesity
- Evidence of cardiac or liver disease
- Residual islet cell function
- Anemia or hematologic abnormalities
- Pregnant, breast feeding, or have plans for future pregnancy
- Insulin requirements > 0.7 IU/kg/day

- Patients > 65 years old
- Patients with advanced diabetic nephropathy
- History of previous transplants
- History of malignancy
- History of non-adherence to medical regimens
- Psychological instability
- Active infection

Although these contraindications may relax in the future, research must be done in a controlled population until the limitations and long-term safety of the technique are better understood.

10. What risks are associated with islet cell transplantation?

Risks associated with islet cell transplantation include the following:

- Portal vein cannulation (similar to risks associated with percutaneous core needle biopsy and transhepatic cholangiography)
- Transplantation of allogeneic tissue
- Risks linked to the effects of long-term immunosuppression

Risks Associated with Islet Cell Transplantation

PORTAL VEIN CANNULATION	ALLOGENEIC TISSUE INFUSION	LONG-TERM CANNULATION
Gall bladder perforation	Rejection	Infections
Hepatic artery injury	Portal hypertension related to volume of cells infused	Thrombocytopenia Leukopenia
Pneumothorax	Infectious pathogens from donor	Diabetes
Bleeding	Portal vein thrombosis related to volume, rate, and impurity of islet infusion	Hypercholesterolemia Hypertriglyceridemia
Abdominal pain		Hypertension
Liver failure		Nephrotoxicity Hyperkalemia Hypomagnesemia Malignancies: 1. Skin cancers 2. Post-transplant lymphoproliferative disease (PTLD)

Rejection is a major complication and a major cause of graft failure. Fasting blood glucose levels begin to increase with advanced rejection but are not a proven indicator of rejection. It is believed that islet cells may be lost with each hyperglycemic episode.

Infection is related to the compromised state of the immune system. Patients must be followed closely because infection during immunosuppressive therapy may have life-threatening consequences.

Intraportal infusion of islet cells into the portal vein may lead to complications, including liver failure, bleeding, portal hypertension, and hepatic infarction. The potential for portal hypertension may result from the impurity of the islet graft preparation or perhaps simply from the islets placed into the liver. Some investigators believe that single-dose infusions > 5 ml of islet preparation increase the risk of portal hypertension. The volume of islet cell transfusion should be as small as possible to minimize the extent of occlusion of the portal vein and the subsequent potential risk for ischemic damage to the liver. Particles of minced pancreas are large enough to block portal venous radicals and can affect hepatic perfusion as well. An increase in liver function tests may indicate inflammation around the islets or drug toxicity associated with the immunosuppressive regimen.

11. How soon after transplantation are patients rendered insulin-independent?

Insulin requirements following islet cell transplantation must be evaluated individually. During the transplant procedure while islets are being infused, patients must be carefully monitored for insulin requirements. Studies have shown striking differences in the achievement of insulin independence after allogenic islet cell transplantation. It may take days, months, or up to a year to achieve insulin independence. To date, a small percentage of patients undergoing islet cell transplantation have achieved insulin independence.

Full metabolic success of an islet cell transplant is characterized by insulin independence. Partial success is defined as basal and stimulatable insulin and c-peptide secretion, but not sufficient to result in insulin independence. So-defined, partial success has been reported to result in better metabolic glucose control and in less frequent or no hypoglycemic episodes. It is further believed, but remains to be proved, that partial success may arrest the progression of secondary diabetic complications.

12. What is the best method for detecting rejection of islet cells?

There are no standardized markers for detecting islet cell graft rejection. The site of graft implantation and the nature of the graft itself make access for serial biopsies or diagnostic imaging methods practically impossible. Immunologic monitoring for recurrent autoimmunity further confounds the picture. Rejection is suspected when the blood glucose levels rise. It is unclear whether intervening at that time can preserve islet function. Evidence suggests that with the appearance of hyperglycemia, a significant number of islet cells may already have been lost, making rescue immunosuppressive therapy ineffective at this juncture. Researchers are working to develop techniques that will detect rejection early enough to allow rescue antirejection therapy.

13. Who are the most likely candidates for the islet cell procedure?

By virtue of the fact that the new Edmonton procedure is investigational, candidacy is strictly bound by the protocol. Candidates must have had brittle, type 1 diabetes for more than 5 years. Brittle, in this case, is limited to patients who have (1) failed intensive insulin regimens; (2) episodes of hypoglycemia unawareness; (3) more than 2 hospitalizations in the past 18 months due to poor control of blood glucose levels; and (4) secondary complications progressing despite intensive insulin regimens.

Candidates for the procedure must demonstrate that they have no islet cell function. The arginine stimulation test is being used currently to determine islet cell function and is part of every candidate's evaluation.

14. What is hypoglycemia unawareness?

Patients who are unable to sense the effects of low blood glucose until it reaches 54 mg/dl or lower are considered to have hypoglycemia unawareness. Severe hypoglycemia can lead to mental confusion or loss of consciousness, and severe episodes can be life threatening.

15. What key tests are essential to evaluate a candidate for islet cell transplantation?

Islet cell candidate evaluation includes definitive determination of the individual's inability to produce insulin. Laboratory tests include the following:
- Fasting c-peptide and HgA1c
- An arginine stimulation test
- Panel reactive antibody (PRA) and human leukocyte antigen (HLA) typing
- Cytomegalovirus (CMV), Epstein-Barr virus (EBV), and hepatitis
- Baseline complete blood cell count (CBC) and liver function tests
- Standard serum chemistries
- Prostate specific antigen (PSA) for males > 50 years
- Urinalysis, urine culture for CMV
- 24-hour urine for creatinine clearance and albumin
- Beta human chorionic gonadotropin (HCG) for females
Other diagnostic testing includes the following:
- Chest x-ray
- Electrocardiogram, echocardiogram
- Baseline mammography for women > 40 years
- Flexible sigmoidoscopy for candidates > 50 years
- An ultrasound of the abdomen to confirm portal vein patency and to rule out gallstones and liver hemangioma
- Three stool guaiac samples
- Colonoscopies for those with positive guaiac specimens

16. Describe the process for finding islet cells for a patient.

Once a candidate has successfully completed the transplant evaluation, the patient's name is added to the waiting list through the United Network for Organ Sharing (UNOS), a computerized system for allocating organs and tissues. Candidates are listed and matched with potential donors according to blood type. Although blood work evaluating the recipient's tissue type is drawn, prospective HLA matching is not performed for islet cell transplantation. Data from HLA retrospective analysis may prove to have a role in islet cell transplantation for the future, but at this time tissue matching is done only for ABO blood type. Blood is drawn from the recipient for PRA testing to ensure that there are no preformed anti-HLA antibodies. If preformed anti-HLA antibodies are found, such patients are excluded because the antibodies increase the risk for an acute or hyperacute rejection (see chapter 4).

The pancreas is allocated to the patient highest on the waiting list of the same or compatible blood type. Size matching may enter into the allocation process because larger donors are likely to yield more islet cells. In any case, there is no guarantee that the volume of islet cells procured will be sufficient for the recipient or that the quality of the procured islets will reach transplantation standards. The quality of the islets procured is also a strong consideration in this procedure. A candidate may be admitted several times for a transplant only to be discharged without receiving islets because of insufficient volume or poor quality. Patients awaiting islet cell transplantation need to be prepared for these potential disappointments and frustrations. Most patients require 2 or more islet cell infusions to achieve full insulin independence, although occasional recipients achieve insulin independence following a single islet infusion. Each time, the islet cells will be from different donors

17. Are there donor criteria for islet donation?

Human pancreatic tissue from cadaveric donors between the ages of 15 and 65 years are accepted. Most centers exclude organs procured from donors dying from methanol toxicity, CO toxicity, or from organs suffering warm ischemia > 15 minutes or cold ischemia > 12 hours. In addition, donors with positive serology to human immunodeficiency virus (HIV) or hepatitis B or C are also typically excluded.

18. What are the crossmatching requirements for islet cell transplantation?

Potential islet cell transplant recipients and the pancreas donor must be ABO blood group compatible. Prospective crossmatching is obtained only if the recipient has an elevated PRA. Because the research protocols do not permit an individual with preformed antibodies (elevated PRA) to participate in the study, retrospective analysis for final crossmatch is obtained following the transplant.

19. How are islet cells procured?

Islet cells are procured and prepared for transplantation through a process called islet isolation. Islet cell preparation consists of several phases: isolation and digestion, purification, washing, and culturing. The isolation process is an automated procedure in which a whole pancreas is loaded into a digestion chamber. Through an enzymatic digestion process, islets are progressively released from the surrounding connective and exocrine tissue. During the purification phase, islets are further separated from nonendocrine tissue via centrifugation on density gradients. The purification phase is critical because it reduces the volume of tissue that will be implanted. Current thinking is that the volume of islet cells infused should be as small as possible to minimize the potential effect on portal vein blood flow and the subsequent risk of ischemic damage to the liver. It is believed that infusions of greater than 5 ml per islet preparation increases the risk of portal hypertension and hepatic infarction. At this point, islets may be held in a culture medium for a period of time while patients are prepared for the transplant procedure. Many transplant centers immediately transplant the islets thinking that islet loss may occur during the culture process. Other centers now test whether islets can be safely maintained in culture before transplantation.

20. How are islet cells transplanted?

Under radiological guidance, the portal vein is cannulated via the percutaneous transhepatic route. Islet cells are infused slowly into the patient's portal vein. Normal blood flow then carries the islets cells into the liver where they become lodged in the distal portal vein capillaries.

21. How many islet cells are required for transplantation?

The average human pancreas weighing 70 gm contains between 300,000 and 1.5 million islet cells. Although the precise number of islets required to establish insulin independence is not known, several factors are taken into consideration. These factors include the following:
- Cellular stressors encountered during islet cell preparation and after infusion
- Recurrence of anti-islet autoimmunity
- The diabetogenic effects of immunosuppressive regimens

During islet cell preparation, islet cells are exposed to noxious insults, including hypoxia, proinflammatory cytokines, and other nonspecific inflammatory mediators that may impair islet cell function and even islet survival. Clinical evidence also indicates that immunologic memory against beta cells is life-long and that, unless immunosuppression is employed, disease will recur. The recurrence of autoimmunity obviously would be deleterious to the fragile, newly transplanted islets and could result in their demise in the same way that an individual's native islet cells were originally affected to cause diabetes. Making matters worse, commonly used immunosuppressive agents are known to be toxic to beta cells and result in reduced insulin secretion and peripheral insulin resistance. All of these factors potentially affect transplanted islet viability and function. Most believe that in order to achieve insulin independence, a patient needs approximately 6,000–10,000 islets/kg recipient body weight. Given current islet isolation techniques, multiple donor organs are often necessary to obtain sufficient islet mass for transplantation. Most patients require more than one islet infusion before insulin independence may be achieved.

22. What is the optimal site for islet cell implantation?

The optimal site for islet cell transplantation has not been determined. The ideal transplantation site for islet cells would be easily accessed to allow for implantation and biopsy, have a rich vascular supply so that the islets can be well perfused, and represent minimal risk for the recipient. Although the liver does not meet all of these criteria, it is currently the preferred site for islet cell transplantation for several reasons. Access to the portal vein is relatively simple and inexpensive and does not require an open surgical procedure. As a result, an extended hospital stay is not necessary, and patient recovery time is lessened. Other potential sites are currently under investigation to optimize islet engraftment. Sites under investigation include the peritoneal-omental pouch, the omental pouch, the perihepatic omental pouch, and the submucosal space of the upper gastrointestinal tract.

23. Do islet cells remain in the liver forever?

Transplantation of islets into the liver is a relatively new and still experimental procedure. Although it has not been well demonstrated that islet allografts survive for long periods of time, intact islets have been found in the liver of a patient 5 years after transplantation. Once infused into the liver, islet cells appear to function as they did in the pancreas. Long-term outcomes are still under investigation.

24. Describe the process of preparing the patient for the actual transplant.

Patients are notified to come to the transplant center once a potential donor pancreas has been identified. The process for procuring the pancreas and then isolating the islet cells may take 8–12 hours. The patient is admitted to the transplant unit and placed on an insulin drip in preparation for the transplant. Blood glucose levels are monitored hourly by the nursing staff. Preoperative blood work is done including a prothrombin/partial thromboplastin time (PT/PTT) test, chemistry, lipid panel, blood type and screen, and CBC with differential. Viral tests such as CMV and EBV are repeated at this time. Patients are often anxious during as they wait for word regarding islet quantity and quality. Once the donor cells are determined to be of adequate quantity and quality, intravenous doses of each of the following medications is given:

- Cephalosporin   • Sirolimus
- Tacrolimus   • Daclizumab

The primary nurse, who monitors vital signs and blood glucose levels throughout the procedure, remains with the patient in radiology. Patients may have an immediate response to the islet infusion and often require titration of the insulin drip.

25. What are the patient care requirements in the immediate postprocedure period?

Patient care requirements in the immediate postprocedure period center on the evaluation of the overall clinical presentation and the assessment, prevention, and prompt intervention of potential complications.

Maintenance of normoglycemia: During the period immediately after the procedure, one of the major patient-care requirements is maintenance of normoglycemia. Insulin is administered prophylactically postprocedure to protect and rest the islets while they establish a foothold in the recipient's liver. Blood glucose levels must be maintained strictly, usually between 70 and 120 mg/dl. Management of the patient during this period includes vigilant blood glucose monitoring and monitoring closely for signs and symptoms of hypoglycemia or hyperglycemia. Blood glucose levels must be monitored at least once every hour for the first 24–48 hours.

Monitoring for complications: Vital signs must also be monitored closely at a minimum of once every hour. Changes in vital signs may be an indication of internal bleeding. Measures must be initiated immediately to prevent and detect infection. Patients must be assessed for signs and symptoms of infection and potential entry sites for pathogens. If central venous access is maintained, sterility must be preserved. Patients must be instructed to report promptly any onset of any unusual symptoms such as abdominal pain. The sudden onset of abdominal pain may be a sign of portal vein thrombosis or internal bleeding. Assessment priorities in the postprocedure period also include monitoring hematological parameters, serum chemistries, liver function tests, coagulation profiles, and c-peptide levels. Other patient care priorities include the administration of prophylactic antibiotics and the initiation of routine immunosuppressives. Septra/Bactrim and ganciclovir may be administered to prevent pneumocystis and CMV infections, respectively.

26. Describe the events leading to the second islet infusion.

Timing between the first and second infusion of islet cells is determined by donor availability. Durine the period before the second infusion, requirements for insulin are usually decreased, but the patient must continue monitoring blood glucose levels and must be monitored for trough levels of tacrolimus and sirolimus. The transplant team and principle investigator follow islet recipients closely. For the first few weeks after the first infusion, patients are seen twice a week, decreasing to weekly and then every other week if glucose levels are stabilized and immunosuppressive agent trough levels are maintained within an acceptable range. As with other transplant recipients, patients are monitored for infection and rejection. Because rejection signs and symptoms are not easily detected, glucose monitoring and changes in body temperature or other vital signs are closely observed and reported. For evaluation of beta cell function, c-peptide testing is done at regular intervals or if the patient's status changes

Preparation for the second infusion of islet cells is similar to that for the first. Patients may be admitted several times before islet quantity and quality are deemed acceptable for transplantation. Once the cells are determined to be acceptable, the patient is placed on an insulin drip, and daclizumab is given intravenously. The patient is taken to radiology for the infusion and is observed for potential complications, as described with the first infusion. Patients are usually discharged within 24 hours if there are no complications. Daclizumab is given every other week for a total of 5 doses. Some patients may need to continue small amounts of insulin during the next few days or weeks, whereas others may become insulin dependent after the second infusion. Some are never able to discontinue insulin therapy completely.

27. What are the important aspects of patient and family education to promote self-care?

The most important step in patient education occurs in the first meeting with the patient and family. Most patients entering these trials have a good understanding of diabetes and self-monitoring. The nurse must ascertain whether patients have a clear understanding of what it means to participate in research. Informed consent should be established through a team approach whereby the principle investigator explains the trial, including the risks and benefits, and the nurse clarifies key concepts in the informed-consent document. Patients may believe the procedure will make them totally insulin independent as soon as the islets are infused. This misconception requires teaching, with the patient and family present to hear the same message. All risks must be clearly explained. The various drugs used to decrease rejection must be described to patients, including the need for trough levels. Most patients do not understand the concept of drug trough levels. Explaining this concept may take several reminders.

Self-care monitoring is something many diabetic patients are quite comfortable with in terms of blood glucose levels. However, monitoring for subtle signs of rejection and infection or drug toxicity are all new content areas for islet cell recipients. Patients should be taught which events require a call to the transplant center or a visit to an emergency room. Slide presentations with the patient and family present usually are well received and appreciated. A paper copy of the slide presentation will serve as a reference for self-care monitoring at home. Because this procedure is relatively new, with few islet cell transplants having been performed, few patient-education materials are available. Nurses at established islet cell transplant centers are often willing to share their patient-education materials. This information can form the basis to adapt center-specific materials for patient education. Topics that should be addressed in education programs for islet cell transplantation are included in the table below.

Topics for Patient and Family education About Islet Cell Transplantation

RESEARCH	EVALUATION	THE PROCEDURE	FOLLOW-UP CARE
Role of patient as a research participant	Laboratory tests	Time it takes to process the islets	Frequency of clinic visits
Risks and benefits	Diagnostic tests	Hospital routine while islets are being processed	When to call the coordinator
What is a clinical trial?	Consultations	Intravenous medications	Trough levels of drugs
Informed consent	Team decisions	Blood work before the procedure	Self-monitoring
Inclusion/exclusion criteria	Listing for transplantation	Potential complications	Preparing for second infusion
Current findings	Waiting for a suitable donor	Length of stay in the hospital	Determining islet functions with repeated arginine stimulation tests
	Notification of a potential donor	Medications to suppress rejections	Medications
	Causes of cancellation of the procedure	Signs and symptoms of infection and rejection	Role changes Coping styles
		Purpose of abdominal ultrasound	Quality of life

28. Does gender or race affect the success of the procedure?

Many solid organ transplant centers have reported increased rejection rates among women and African Americans. Studies have demonstrated that African-American patients require higher doses of immunosuppression to control rejection after transplantation and have poorer graft survival than Caucasians. Increased rejection rates have been reported in women and African

Americans for heart, kidney, and liver transplants. There are no current reports of gender or race differences in islet cell transplantation in terms of rejection rates or graft survival. The lack of data may, in part, be due to the low number of islet cell transplants performed to date and the lower incidence of type 1 diabetes in the African-American population.

29. If someone had a failed pancreas transplant, is islet cell transplantation an option?

Under the current protocols being tested in the United States, patients undergoing islet cell transplantation cannot have had a previous transplant of any organ. The rationale is, in part, due to the fact that a previous transplant could potentially produce preformed antibodies that may contribute to increased rejection rates in the islet cell recipient. This factor would add an unpredictable variable to the research in terms of monitoring and controlling rejection. Once islet cell research has sufficient data to determine the efficacy of islet cell transplantation as a standard treatment for type 1 diabetes, physicians may consider using it in previously transplanted individuals.

30. Is simultaneous kidney/islet cell transplantation an option?

There have been reports of simultaneous kidney/islet cell transplants in the 1990s. However, with the poor results of islet cell transplantation, the procedure was not performed with great frequency. Many of the antirejection medications used in transplantation have been shown to adversely affect islet cells, especially steroids and calcineurin inhibitors. During the 1990s, most transplant centers used an immunosuppression regimen called triple therapy. This treatment most often used steroids, a calcineurin inhibitor, and azathioprine. In the latter portion of the decade, newer agents were becoming available to allow transplant physicians to take a more individualized approach to immunosuppression.

Simultaneous renal/islet cell transplantation is a very attractive goal. Although this procedure would be a preferred intervention for diabetic patients with end-stage renal disease, the reality lies in the outcomes of current trials on islet cell transplantation. If islet cell transplantation is proved to be a safe and effective treatment for type 1 diabetes, the addition of a second organ to the regimen will have more potential

BIBLIOGRAPHY

1. Angelico MC, Alejandro R, Nery J, et al: Transplantation of islets of Langerhans in patients with insulin-requiring diabetes mellitus undergoing liver transplantation—the Miami experience. J Mol Med 77:144–147, 1999.
2. Berney T, Ricordi C: Islet transplantation. Cell Transplantation 8:461–464, 1999.
3. Bretzel RG, Brendel M, Brandhorst D, et al: Islet transplantation: Present clinical situation and future aspects. Exp Clin Endocrinol Diabetes 109:S384–S399, 2001.
4. Budinger JM, Donnelly SS: Nursing care protocols for the kidney/islet cell transplant recipient. ANNA J 21:123–128, 1994.
5. Calafiore R: Perspectives in pancreatic and islet cell transplantation for the therapy of IDDM. Diabetes Care 20:889–896, 1997.
6. Drachenberg CB, Klassen DK, Weir MR, et al: Islet cell damage associated with tacrolimus and cyclosporine: Morphological features in pancreas allograft biopsies. Transplantation 68:396–402, 1999.
7. Efrat S: Prospects for treatment of type 2 diabetes by expansion of the β-cell mass. Diabetes 50:S189–S190, 2001.
8. Hering BJ, Ricordi C: Results, research priorities, and reasons for optimism: Islet transplantation for patients with type 1 diabetes. Graft 2:12–27, 1999.
9. Hering BJ, Ricordi C, Sutherland D, Bluestone JA: Pancreatic islet cell transplantation. In Norman, D, Turka L (eds): Primer on Transplantation. Mount Laurel, NJ, American Society of Transplantation, 2001.
10. Kenyon NS, Harlan DM, Alejandro R, et al: Islet cell transplantation. In LeRoith D, Taylor SI, Olefski JM (eds): Diabetes Mellitus: A Fundamental and Clinical Text. Philadelphia, Lippincott Williams & Wilkins, 2000.
11. Kenyon NS, Fernandez LA, Lehmann R, et al: Long-term survival and function of intrahepatic islet allografts in baboons treated with humanized anti-CD 154. Diabetes 48:1473–1481, 1999.
12. Kenyon NS, Ranuncoli A, Masetti M, et al: Islet transplantation: Present and future perspectives. Diabetes Metab Rev 14:303–313, 1998.

13. Kenyon NS, Alejandro R, Mintz DH, Ricordi C: Islet cell transplantation: Beyond the paradigms. Diabetes Metab Rev 12:361–372, 1996.

14. Kirk A: Immunology of transplantation. In Norton J, Bollinger LR, et al (eds): Surgery: Basic Science and Clinical Evidence. New York, Springer-Verlag, 2001.

15. Pick A, Jameson JL: Advances in islet transplantation: Use of glucocorticoid-free immunosuppressive regimen. Harrison's On Line 2000; McGraw Hill Companies. Available at: www.medscape.com. Accessed January 23, 2002.

16. Mathieu C: Current limitations of islet transplantation. Transplant Proc 33:1707–1708, 2001.

17. Patient Referral Information Package. Multicenter Trial of the Edmonton Protocol for Islet Transplantation. Available at: www.immunetolerance.org. Accessed March 23, 2002.

18. Pileggi A, Ricordi C, Alessiani M, Inverardi L: Factors influencing islet of Langerhans graft function and monitoring. Clin Chim Acta 310:3–16, 2001.

19. Ricordi C, Alejandro Angelico MC, Fernandez LA, et al: Human islet allografts in patients with type 2 diabetes undergoing liver transplantation. Transplantation 63:473–475, 1997.

20. Robertson RP: Pancreatic islet cell transplantation: Likely impact on current therapeutics for type 1 diabetes mellitus. Drugs 61:2017–2020, 2001.

21. Robertson RP, Davis C, Larsen J, et al: Pancreas and islet transplantation for patients with diabetes. Diabetes Care, a journal of the American Diabetes Association. Available at: www.InsulinFree.org/articles/dev23_lp112htm. Accessed March 23, 2002.

22. Rosenberg L: Clinical islet cell transplantation. Int J Pancreatol 24:145–168, 1998.

23. Rossini AA, Mordes JP, Greiner DL, Stoff JS: Islet cell transplantation tolerance. Transplantation 72:S43–S46, 2001.

24. Shapiro J, Lakey R, Ryan E, et al: Islet transplantation in seven patients with type I diabetes mellitus using a glucocorticoid-free immunosuppressive regimen. N Engl J Med 343:230–238, 2001.

25. Sharp DW: Clinical feasibility of islet transplantation. Transplant Proc 16:820–825, 1984.

26. Thomas FT, Ljung T, Henretta J, et al: Reversal of type II (NIDDM) diabetes by pancreas islet transplantation: An emerging new concept in pathophysiology of an enigmatic disease. Transplant Proc 27:3167–3169, 1995.

27. Thomas T, Badget L, Gray D: Islet cell transplantation for insulin dependent diabetes mellitus from the present and prospects for the future. Expert Reviews in Molecular Medicine, 2000. Available at: www-ermm.cbcu.cam.ac.uk/00001861h.htm. Accessed February 10, 2002.

28. White SA, Nicholson ML: Islet cell transplantation and type I diabetes mellitus. Diabetic Med 18 (Suppl 1):1–14, 2001.

29. Villagomez E: Pancreas transplantation. Crit Care Nurs Q 17:15–26, 1995.

16. NURSING CARE OF THE LIVING RENAL DONOR

Elizabeth Ann Sparks Ford, BSN, RN, *Mary E. Leshko*, RN, BSN, CCRN, CNN, *and Jacqueline M. Corsini*, MS, ANP, CCRN

1. What is a *living renal donor*?

A *living renal donor* is any person, friend, or relative who donates a kidney to one in need of a renal transplant and who meets physiological and psychological criteria before donation. A living renal donor can be related or unrelated to the recipient of the organ.

2. Is there a difference between a living-related and living-unrelated renal donor?

A living-related donor is biologically related to the recipient (i.e., a parent or child). A living-unrelated donor is not biologically linked to the recipient (i.e., a spouse, friend, or altruistic donor).

3. How does one become a living donor?

The potential living donor must first express an interest in renal donation and then contact the transplant center where the recipient is listed. Most transplant centers maintain strict policies whereby hospital personnel do not contact a potential donor on behalf of a recipient. Once the donor contacts the transplant center, education regarding the advantages and disadvantages of living donation is provided.

The potential living donor must undergo a thorough evaluation process that provides the transplant team with the necessary medical and psychosocial information to determine the donor's eligibility for donation. The individual must be between the ages of 18 and 65 years and meet all other eligibility criteria established by the transplant center. The donor must not be coerced in any way to undergo an evaluation. The potential donor needs to be informed that a decision to withdraw from the evaluation at any time or choice not to donate a kidney will be respected and upheld by the transplant team.

4. Describe the predonation process.

The predonation process may be broken down into three phases: screening, evaluation, and medical work-up. The potential living donor goes through initial screening (usually over the phone) to rule out any high-risk markers of renal disease such as hypertension, diabetes mellitus, or polycystic kidney disease. Many institutions test for ABO compatibility as part of the screening process before moving forward with an evaluation and complete work-up. The process of determining ABO compatibility varies from institution to institution, but generally patients may provide a sample of their blood to check blood type. Once blood type is determined, it is compared to the blood type of the recipient to see if the two blood types are compatible. If the blood types are compatible, the donor may then immediately proceed with the evaluation and medical work-up.

Traditionally, if the recipient's identified donor did not have a compatible blood type, the recipient had to go on the cadaveric list, and the living donor would simply not donate. Today, however, some organ procurement organizations offer options such as **paired donor exchange** (two incompatible donor and recipient pairs swap donors, creating two compatible pairs) and **living donor/cadaveric exchange** (an incompatible living donor and recipient pair has the living donor donate to the waiting list, placing the recipient at the top of the cadaveric list). With these alternatives in donation, transplant communities are able to use as many living donors as possible. If the incompatible living donor is agreeable to donating to someone other than the originally identified recipient, the living donor process may still move forward despite ABO incompatibility.

The potential living donor who has successfully completed the screening phase then undergoes an initial evaluation by the surgical and nephrology teams to determine the donor's general health status and eligibility to donate. This process is either followed by or done in conjunction with the full medical work-up to determine the kidney function and health status of the potential living donor. The medical work-up should also rule out any renal disease–related risk factors.

The medical work-up consists of a comprehensive history and physical examination, psychosocial assessment, and laboratory and diagnostic tests (see table below). Consultations are obtained based on specific medical need(s) before clearance for surgery. Once the work-up has been completed, a spiral computed tomography (CT) scan, magnetic resonance angiography (MRA), or intravenous pyelography and angiography are performed to evaluate the individual's renal anatomy. This evaluation assists the surgeon in determining which kidney to procure at the time of the nephrectomy.

Donor Medical Work-up

HISTORY	
Hypertension	Malignancies
Diabetes mellitus	Medication use
Cardiovascular disease	Substance abuse
Chronic obstructive pulmonary disease (COPD)	Systemic diseases with implications for renal
Renal disease	involvement

FAMILY HISTORY	
Hypertension	Renal disease
Diabetes mellitus	

PHYSICAL ASSESSMENT	
Body systems	Infections
Evidence of organ dysfunction	Height and weight
Malignancies	Body mass index

PSYCHOSOCIAL ASSESSMENT	
Motivation and willingness to donate	Coping style
Relationship to recipient	Emotional stability
Expectations regarding donation	Psychiatric stability
Methods of dealing with stress	

LABORATORY STUDIES	
Screening	
Chemistry panel	Sedimentation rate
Lipid panel	Serum human chorionic gonadotropin (HCG),
Liver function studies	if female
Thyroid function studies	Prostate-specific antigen (PSA), as indicated
Beta-$_2$ microglobulin	Toxicology screen
Complete blood count (CBC) with differential	Urinalysis
Prothrombin time/partial thromboplastin	Urine culture
time (PT/PTT) tests	24-hour urine for protein and creatinine clearance
Immunological	
Blood type	Crossmatching (repeated before transplantation)
HLA tissue typing	
Infectious disease	
Viral studies—cytomegalovirus (CMV)	Hepatitis B virus
Human immunodeficiency virus (HIV)	Tuberculosis—purified protein derivative (PPD)
Rapid plasma reagin (RPR)	Varicella
Epstein-Barr virus	Hepatitis C virus

(Cont'd. on next page.)

Donor Medical Work-up (Continued)

DIAGNOSTIC TESTS	
Chest x-ray	Oral glucose tolerance test if positive family
Electrocardiogram (EKG)	history of diabetes mellitus
Stress test, as indicated	Papanicolaou smear for females
Renal ultrasound	Mammogram, as indicated
Flexible sigmoidoscopy, as indicated	

CONSULTATIONS	
Nephrologist	Cardiologist, as indicated
Surgeon	Gynecologist, as indicated
Transplant coordinator	Pulmonologist, as indicated
Social worker	Psychologist, as indicated

5. List some potential medical contraindications to becoming a living donor.

Potential donors are not considered for donation if they are at high risk of developing renal disease or are considered a surgical risk. Some contraindications include the following:
- Glomerular filtration rate < 80 ml/min
- Abnormal urinalysis results, such as proteinuria or hematuria
- Structural abnormalities in the donor's kidneys that render the organs unsuitable for transplantation.
- Presence of comorbidities such as
  - Significant cardiopulmonary disease
  - Diabetes mellitus
  - Hypertension
  - Human immunodeficiency virus (HIV), Hepatitis B, or Hepatitis C
  - Morbid obesity
  - Psychiatric or emotional instability (e.g., substance abuse)
  - Thromboembolic disease
- History of recurrent nephrolithiasis
- History of significant systemic disorders (e.g., recent malignancy)
- Positive crossmatch between the donor and recipient
- Age younger than 18 years or older than 65 years

6. What ethical guidelines are in place to maintain the safety of the donor?

The physician who evaluates the donor should not be the same as the physician who is caring for the recipient. This guideline prevents a conflict of interest between donor and recipient advocacy. Once the donor evaluation is complete, the case is reviewed in a multidisciplinary forum to ensure that the donor's health is not jeopardized, the decision to donate is voluntary, and the recipient not only will benefit from the donation, but also has the ability to provide self-care post-transplantation, which minimizes the risk of graft loss.

An ethics consultation should be obtained in any case that poses an ethical question, such as one in which donor motivation or ability to provide informed consent is questionable.

7. List topics that should be covered in the preoperative education of a patient who is scheduled to undergo a donor nephrectomy.

Informed consent
- Operative
- Blood

Preoperative routine
- Rationale for diagnostic tests
- Routine blood and urine collection

- Visits with the surgeon and the anesthesiologist
- Nothing-by-mouth (NPO) status
- Shower and scrubs with antimicrobial soap
- Removal of jewelry, dentures, and nail polish
- Bowel preparation
- Intravenous (IV) line
- Foley catheter insertion
- Application of thromboembolic disease (TED) stockings, sequential compression devices
- Preoperative medications (sedation, antibiotic)

Intraoperative routine
- Transport to holding area via stretcher
- Safety precautions (side rails up, hands inside stretcher)
- What to expect in the operating room (attachment to monitors, cold environment, room bright and noisy from monitoring equipment)
- Induction of anesthesia
- Approximate length of surgery
- Family waiting area where surgeon will speak with family

Postoperative routine
- Transport to postanesthesia care unit (PACU)
- Attachment to monitors
- Possible extubation, oxygen mask
- Invasive lines (IV, Foley, possible epidural)
- Expected sensations (cold, blurred vision from ophthalmic ointment, dry mouth, possible sore throat from endotracheal tube, pain at incision site)

Pain relief
- Pain rating scale (1–10)
- Type of pain medication typically used after surgery
- Name, dose, frequency
- How long it takes to start working
- How long it lasts
- Side effects
- Importance of requesting pain medication, as required (PRN), before pain becomes unmanageable
- Realistic expectations about pain medication (all pain may not be eliminated)
- Instructions for use of patient controlled analgesia (PCA) pump if ordered

Postoperative exercises: Give rationale for, demonstrate, and ask for return demonstration; discuss repetitions and frequency to be done for the following:
- Deep diaphragmatic breathing to improve lung expansion and oxygen delivery
- Incentive spirometry to reinflate collapsed alveoli and remove airway secretions
- Controlled coughing while splinting incision to remove retained secretions in airway
- Turning to mobilize pulmonary secretions and increase perfusion and ventilation to lungs
- Leg exercises, early ambulation to improve blood flow and decrease venous stasis and potential clot formation

8. Name the three surgical methods available for living donor nephrectomy.

The three surgical methods available for living donor nephrectomy include open, laparoscopic, and hand-assisted laparoscopic donor nephrectomy.

9. How is an open nephrectomy performed?

The surgical procedure for each of the techniques described vary slightly from center to center depending on the preferred technique employed by the individual surgeon. Open nephrectomy is generally performed by placing the patient in the lateral position on the operating table, with flexion to extend the flank. The flank incision is created just above or below the 11th or12th rib and may include taking a portion of the rib. Care is taken to remain outside the pleural and peritoneal cavities. Once the renal vessels are ligated and divided, the kidney is removed.[1,10]

10. Explain how the laparoscopic nephrectomy is different.

The patient is placed in a lateral decubitus position on the operating table while the table is flexed at midpoint to maximize flank surface area. The abdominal cavity is inflated with carbon dioxide gas, and 3–4 ports are created through small incisions in the abdominal wall. A video camera is placed through one of the ports; the other ports are used to pass through and manipulate the surgical equipment.[1,2,10] Visualizing the procedure by watching the video screen, the surgeon identifies the renal vessels and ureter. The vessels and ureter are isolated and dissected; then the kidney is slipped into a plastic bag and removed through a small abdominal incision just large enough for removal of the bagged kidney.[1]

11. What is hand-assisted laparoscopic nephrectomy?

Hand-assisted laparoscopic nephrectomy is performed much the same way as the laparoscopic procedure. The patient position and table position are essentially the same with the placement of ports for the camera and surgical equipment. In the hand-assisted procedure, a small abdominal incision is created for the surgeon to place a hand through a pneumosleeve. The pneumosleeve is used to maintain the pressure created by the carbon dioxide to inflate the abdomen, as in the laparoscopic procedure. To remove the kidney, the pneumosleeve is inverted, creating a bag for the kidney.[1,10,14]

12. Describe the benefits of laparoscopic nephrectomy versus hand-assisted and open nephrectomies.

Open nephrectomy has a good record of removing a donor kidney safely and in good condition, providing excellent early graft function and minimal warm ischemic time. However, it leaves the donor with a long postoperative course that includes a 6–8 week recovery time and a long surgical incision.[1,10]

Laparoscopic nephrectomy has been associated with a shortened hospital stay (1–2 days vs. 2–4 days with the open nephrectomy), decreased need for pain medications during the hospital course and into the convalescent phase, as well as a quicker return to preoperative activities of daily living. The disadvantages to the laparoscopic procedure lie in its increased operative and warm ischemic times, which have been associated with graft damage and a potential for impaired early graft function. The learning curve is steep for both the donor surgeon and recipient surgeon because of difficulties in the removal of the organ and a tendency for the graft to have shorter renal vessels.[1,2,3,10,14]

Potential financial advantages, such as decreased donor costs, have been identified in the shorter hospital length of stay. Unfortunately, the costs of the equipment used in the laparoscopic procedure and increased operative time offset the savings achieved by the decreased length of stay.[3,10]

The hand-assisted procedure rests in the middle of the two procedures, with decreased operative and warm ischemic times compared with those in the fully laparoscopic procedure. The abdominal incision is usually larger to accommodate the size of the surgeon's hand, and the recovery is slightly longer with slower return of bowel function than that of the fully laparoscopic procedure.[10,14]

13. What happens when the center where the recipient is listed does not offer the laparoscopic nephrectomy and this procedure happens to be the donor's surgery of choice?

Today, patients and donors alike have wide enough access to the information available to research transplantation, the surgery, and the recovery fully. Donors and recipients often discuss the multiple surgical options and identify the best option for both of them. Frequently, recipients are listed with a transplant center before the identification of a living donor is made. On occasion, the recipient moves to another transplant center so that the donor may have the laparoscopic surgery.

14. What differences should the nurse be aware of when caring for the donor who has had a laparoscopic nephrectomy versus an open nephrectomy?
The major differences between the laparoscopic nephrectomy versus the open approach include degree of postoperative pain, location and type of surgical incisions, and potential complications.

15. What are the potential short-term complications resulting from living renal donation?
The literature identifies a perioperative mortality rate of 0.03%,[1,6,7,10] which according to Kasiske and colleagues[7] is similar to the risk of dying in a motor vehicle accident in 1 year in the United States. Nevertheless, as with any surgery, there are risks and potential complications. The most common short-term risks include atelectasis, pneumonia, pneumothorax, pulmonary embolus, hypotension, thrombophlebitis, urinary retention, urinary tract infection, wound problems, bowel dysfunction, splenic injuries, and deep vein thrombosis. Most of the complications are reversible by the time of discharge.[1,6,7,10]

16. What are the potential long-term complications resulting from living renal donation?
The long-term risks of renal donation appear to be low and associated with the risk of having only one kidney. Some studies report serum creatinine levels 20% higher than predonation levels and creatinine clearance 20% lower than predonation clearance. There appears to be an increased risk of low-grade proteinuria, with no increase in the incidence of hypertension. Despite this finding, the occurrence of renal disease in donors appears to be well within or lower than the risk expected in the general population.[1,7,12] Morris[10] reports that there is no convincing evidence to support the concern over the development of hypertension and renal dysfunction.

17. Describe some common complications following donor nephrectomy, assessments that the nurse should make, and possible interventions/treatments.

COMPLICATIONS	ASSESSMENT/DIAGNOSIS	INTERVENTION/TREATMENT
Atelectasis, usually related to anesthesia and/or immobility	Adventitious breath sounds, increased respiratory effort, inability to maintain oxygen saturations > 94% on room air, abnormal chest x-ray	Aggressive pulmonary toilet with use of incentive spirometry, coughing and deep breathing Increased mobility/ambulation
Hypoxia/hypoventilation (more common immediately postoperatively and related to anesthesia and/or narcotic	Decreased respiratory rate and effort, oxygen desaturation, increased supplemental oxygen requirements, somnolence, decreased PaO_2 and/or increased $PaCO_2$	Decrease or stop narcotic. Consider use of reversal agent such as Narcan. Elevate head of bed to improve lung expansion.
Fever, typically related to atelectasis but may be secondary to infection (wound, Foley catheter)	Elevation in temperature (usually > 38.5°), signs and symptoms of infection, abnormal chest x-ray, positive culture and sensitivity results (blood, urine, sputum wound)	Identify source and sensitivities of organism. Pulmonary toilet Consider antibiotic therapy. Administer antipyretic for comfort.
Hypotension, typically related to fluid imbalance, narcotic or bleeding. Rarely sepsis	Sustained systolic blood pressure < 90 mmHg, weak pulses, decreased capillary refill. Output > intake Signs/symptoms of bleeding—decreased hematocrit	Administer IV fluid challenge per order and note response. Monitor vital signs frequently until stabilized. Consider colloid or blood transfusion if indicated.

(Cont'd. on next page.)

COMPLICATIONS	ASSESSMENT/DIAGNOSIS	INTERVENTION/TREATMENT
Tachycardia, typically related to fluid imbalance, pain, or anxiety	Sustained heart rate > 100 bpm, subjective complaints of palpitations or racing heart	Administer IV fluids and note response. Administer pain medication and note response. Consider EKG if suspect unstable rhythm. Reassure patient.
Pneumothorax (surgeon inadvertently may have nicked pleural space)	Decreased breath sounds on the affected side, decreased oxygen saturation, hyper-resonance over affected area Diagnosed by chest x-ray.	A small pneumothorax typically resolves on its own. Patient may require a chest tube to re-expand lung.
Nausea/vomiting, usually anesthesia- or narcotic-related	Decreased peristalsis, amount and type of emesis, and medication/anesthesia side effects. If persists, consider abdominal x-ray to rule out ileus or obstruction.	Maintain NPO status, and provide fluid and electrolyte replacement via IV. Advance diet slowly, as tolerated. Administer antiemetics. Nasogastric tube rarely required.
Thrombophlebitis, typically related to immobility	Pain, redness, swelling, positive Homans sign in lower extremities. If suspected, Doppler ultrasound may be indicated.	Antiembolism stockings and sequential compression devices should be applied in OR and worn until patient is OOB and ambulating several times a day. May need to consider anticoagulation therapy.
Wound infection, caused by bacteria. May delay healing and result in scarring and development of hernia.	Postoperative dressing is typically removed 24–48 hr postoperatively. Redness, swelling, pain, drainage, healing. Culture any drainage.	Treat with antibiotic therapy specific to organism.
Constipation/gas pain, related to narcotics, immobility, CO_2 gas used during laparoscopy	Decreased peristalsis Abdominal discomfort/distension Lack of bowel movement once diet resumed	Administer stool softener and/or laxative with narcotics. May require an enema. Encourage ambulation and adequate fluid hydration.
Poor pain control, related to incision, immobility, anxiety	Inability to get pain level below a "5" with prescribed medication	Try different pain medication, dose, or delivery route. Consider anesthesia or pain management team consultation.

EKG = electrocardiography, IV = intravenous, NGT = nasogastric tube, NPO = nothing by mouth, OOB = out of bed, OR = operating room.

18. What is the immediate postoperative care of the donor nephrectomy patient?

Immediate postoperative care generally takes place in the postanesthetic care unit (PACU) and lasts approximately 1–2 hours. Upon arrival to the PACU, the nurse does a rapid assessment of the patient's respiratory and cardiovascular status while the patient is attached to an electronic monitoring device (cardiac monitoring, continuous pulse oximetry, and automatic blood pressure monitoring). Once the initial vital signs are taken, the nurse obtains a detailed report from the operating room nurse regarding the following information:

- Surgical procedure
- Review of anesthetic gases and medications given
- Allergies
- Intravenous fluids and blood products given
- Invasive lines and drainage devices
- Incisions, dressings, and surgical complications.

Any variation from the expected outcomes may indicate the onset of postoperative complications. After report, the nurse performs a more focused assessment and continues to monitor vital signs frequently. The nurse may assist the anesthesiologist with extubation if it has not already been done in the OR, and applies oxygen via a facemask. Once the assessment is completed, the nurse orients the patient to the surroundings, reassures him or her that the procedure is over, and attempts to remedy any complaints that may be offered.

19. Explain the discharge criteria that must be met before a living donor (post nephrectomy) is discharged from the PACU.

A patient with hemodynamic instability or respiratory compromise is either kept in the PACU until the condition improves or transferred to a surgical intensive care unit/step-down unit where he or she can be monitored more closely. The large majority of patients can be transferred from the PACU to a surgical floor that is skilled in caring for donor nephrectomy patients. A few centers that are performing the laparoscopic nephrectomy may transfer the patient to a same-day surgery unit and allow him or her to be discharged the same day. The following criteria should be met before a patient is transferred to a surgical floor or same-day surgery unit:

- Vital signs are stable and near patient's baseline.
- Airway is patent with good inspiratory effort and is able to maintain oxygen saturations > 95% with supplemental oxygen.
- Patient is arousable and oriented to person, place, time, and situation.
- Protective reflexes (cough/gag) have returned, and patient is able to move all extremities.
- Intravenous line is patent, and intake and output are essentially balanced.
- Foley catheter is patent and with good urine output.
- Surgical wound dressing is intact with minimal drainage.
- Postoperative pain is under control with the use of intravenous analgesic.
- Postoperative chest x-ray and blood work (serum electrolytes, complete blood cell count) are obtained, if ordered, and are reviewed by the surgeon and/or anesthesiologist.

20. What type of postoperative orders can the surgical nurse anticipate when admitting a living donor (postnephrectomy)?

- Monitoring vital signs a minimum of every 15 min × 4, every 30 min × 2, every hr × 4 then every 4 hr if stable
- Parameters to notify physician for vital signs, urine output
- NPO, advance diet as tolerated
- Intake and output Q shift.
- Foley catheter to straight drainage
- Respiratory orders—oxygen delivery, incentive spirometry, pulseoximetry
- Activity orders—out of bed 12 hr after surgery and ambulate
- Pain medications
- Laboratory work ordered

21. How is pain managed following a donor nephrectomy?

Most patients experience some degree of pain postoperatively, which can affect their ability to be mobile and do their pulmonary exercises. For this reason, it is important that patients obtain satisfactory pain control. The best way to accomplish such control is through the administration of narcotics or opioids such as morphine or fentanyl. There are several delivery methods: intravenous boluses administered by nurse, intravenous patient-controlled anesthesia (PCA), and epidural PCA. PCA is the preferred method of delivery because it gives the patient control over the pain, is not dependent on nurse availability, and gives more sustained pain relief. Epidural PCA has the additional benefit of numbing the spinal nerves if a local anesthetic is added to the narcotic. Typically, patients are changed to an oral narcotic when they are tolerating oral fluids and medications.

After 2 weeks, patients may have incisional discomfort but are able to transition to nonnarcotics or NSAIDS for pain control. Studies have shown that patients who have undergone a laparoscopic nephrectomy have fewer complaints of pain and transition off narcotics sooner.

22. What should be included in a living donor nephrectomy patient's discharge instructions?
- Review of discharge medications (names, indications, dose, frequency, side effects)
- Follow-up appointment—schedule and give date and time if possible
- Reporting of abnormal or unexpected signs and symptoms—fever, uncontrolled or new onset of pain, prolonged nausea and vomiting, difficulty voiding
- Contact numbers of the physician, transplant center, transplant coordinators
- Incision care (staples, sutures, steri-strips)
- Monitoring for signs and symptoms of infection (fever, redness, swelling, drainage)
- Instructions to resume normal diet—reminder to stay well hydrated (8 glasses of fluids/day)
- Advance activity as tolerated (walking, climbing stairs)
- Women are generally discouraged from becoming pregnant for 1 year after kidney donation because of the potential stress to the kidney. Donation does not affect fertility or the ability to conceive.
- Activity restrictions:
  - Instructions to avoid lifting anything heavier than 10–20 pounds for a period of 6 weeks (minimize development of incisional hernia)
  - Instructions that patient may shower and get incision wet by postoperative day 4, but should avoid tub baths and swimming for 2 weeks
  - Instructions to avoid driving an automobile for at least 3 weeks (patients should be encouraged to check with individual insurance company; some prohibit driving for up to 6 weeks after a major operation). Driving prohibited if patients are taking a narcotic
  - Instructions to avoid returning to work for 2–6 weeks depending upon occupation. If fatigue persists, patient may be advised to go back to work part-time at first.
  - Instructions to avoid extreme contact sports (such as football or karate), which may injure the remaining kidney

23. What type of follow-up is required after a living donor has been discharged from the hospital?

Typically, the surgeon who performed the nephrectomy sees the patient within 1 month after discharge. At that time, the patient is assessed for wound healing, any outstanding problems or complaints, and general emotional well-being. If recovery has been uneventful, the patient is often discharged from the surgeon's care and referred back to his or her primary care provider to be seen on an annual basis. CBC, blood urea nitrogen (BUN), creatinine, electrolytes, and urinalysis reports may be obtained. Because of the donor's slightly higher risk of developing high blood pressure and proteinuria, the surgeon may recommend that the primary care provider monitor blood pressure readings, serum creatinine, and 24-hr urine collections for creatinine clearance and protein excretion on an annual basis.

24. When should the living renal donor expect to return to baseline activities of daily living?

Recovery time differs depending on whether a patient undergoes an open nephrectomy or a laparoscopic nephrectomy. Laparoscopic nephrectomy patients have reported the ability to return to work; return to an exercise routine; begin driving, grocery shopping, and caring for their homes significantly sooner than open nephrectomy patients. A patient who has undergone a laparoscopic nephrectomy can expect a convalescence of 2–4 weeks. A patient who has undergone an open nephrectomy can expect a convalescence lasting 6–8 weeks.

25. How is the donor compensated for lost time and wages from work?

The living donor receives no compensation for income or time lost from work related to the donation. The living donor's medical evaluation before the transplant procedure and hospitalization postprocedure are generally covered by the recipient's insurance.

26. Describe what happens when a former living renal donor requires a renal transplant.

In the event that a former living donor requires a renal transplant later in life, he or she is given points on the United Network for Organ Sharing (UNOS) waiting list in addition to other category points. According to UNOS policy 3.5.9.6 November 17, 2000, a patient is assigned 4 points if he or she has donated a vital organ or a segment of a vital organ for transplantation within the United States.

27. What does a living renal donor experience when the recipient experiences rejection or organ failure?

The living donor may experience disappointment, sadness, depression, anger, or guilt when the recipient experiences graft rejection or kidney failure post-transplantation. Although it is not well documented in the literature, it seems that some donors go through a grieving process immediately following donation and once again following the loss of the graft in the recipient. Donors who are not biologically related may be more likely to experience dissatisfaction if the outcome of the transplant is poor. Donors should be provided resources for psychological support, as needed.

28. Name some ways by which the transplant team can recognize and acknowledge the renal donor's gift of life.

Living donors are the heroes of transplantation. A good time to acknowledge the donor is during rounds when most of the transplant team are in the patient's room. The surgeon usually shares with the donor some positive aspect of the recipient's recovery (e.g., drop in creatinine, good urine output, and freedom from dialysis). It is appropriate for someone from the transplant team to verbally acknowledge the donor's selflessness and generosity. Feedback from the transplant team can help the donor feel good about the decision to donate, especially in the immediate postoperative period. Pain and an altered body image may be part of recovery.

Other ways that transplant centers acknowledge the donor is through small gifts (e.g., t-shirts, tote bags, and buttons ordered in bulk from catalogues), having a party when the donor is discharged, and sending the donor a thank-you card after discharge signed by members of the team.

BIBLIOGRAPHY

1. Danovitch GM: Handbook of Kidney Transplantation, 3rd ed. Philadelphia, Lippincott Williams & Wilkins, 2001.
2. Flowers JL, Jacobs S, Cho E, et al: Comparison of open and laparoscopic live donor nephrectomy. Ann Surg 226:483–490, 1997.
3. Hiller J, Sroka M, Holochek MJ, et al: Functional advantages of laparoscopic live-donor nephrectomy compared with conventional open-donor nephrectomy. J Transpl Coordination 7:134–140, 1997.
4. Hiller J, Sroka M, Weber R, et al: Identifying donor concerns to increase live organ donation. J Transpl Coordination 8: 51–54, 1998.
5. Jacobs C, Johnson E, Anderson K, et al: Kidney transplants from living donors: How donation affects family dynamics. Adv Renal Replacement Ther 5: 89-97, 1998.
6. Johnson EM, Remucal MJ, Gillingham KJ, et al: Complications and risks of living donor nephrectomy. Transplantation 64:1124–1128, 1997.
7. Kasiske BL, Ravenscraft M, Ramos EL, et al: The evaluation of living renal transplant donors: Clinical practice guidelines. J Am Soc Nephrol 7:2288–2313, 1996.

8. Kercher K, Dahl D, Harland R, et al: Hand assisted laparoscopic donor nephrectomy minimizes warm ischemia. Urology 58:152–156, 2001.
9. Kerr SR, Gillingham KJ, Johnson EM, Matas AJ: Living donors >55 years: To use or not to use. Transplantation 67:999–1004, 1999.
10. Morris P (ed): Kidney Transplantation: Principles and Practice, 5th ed. Philadelphia, W.B. Saunders, 2001.
11. Nolan MT: Ethical dilemmas in living donor organ transplantation. J Transpl Coordination 9:225–231, 1999.
12. Norman D, Turka L (eds): Primer on Transplantation, 2nd ed. Malden, MA, Blackwell Publishers, 2001.
13. Parker J (ed): Contemporary Nephrology Nursing. Pitman, NJ, American Nephrology Nurses Association, 1998.
14. Ruiz-Deya G, Cheng S, Palmer E, et al: Open donor, laparoscopic donor and hand assisted laparoscopic donor nephrectomy: A comparison of outcomes. J Urol 166:1270–1273, 2001.

17. CARE OF LIVING LIVER DONORS

Marian O'Rourke, RN, CCTC

1. What is living donor liver transplantation?

Living donor liver transplantation (LDLTx) is a surgical procedure that involves the removal of a recipient's native liver and its replacement with a portion of a live donor's liver.

2. When was the first LDLTx performed?

Raia in Brazil performed the first LDLTx in 1987 from an adult to a young child. The transplantation established the technical feasibility of the procedure although the recipient did not survive. Strong and colleagues reported the first successful LDLTx in 1987 in Brisbane, Australia. However, the first large series employing LDLTx was done in the United States in Chicago in 1990. Tanaka also applied this surgical technique in Japan at Kyoto University, where cadaver organ donation was not available. Following the successful application of this procedure, it became a widely accepted treatment modality for pediatric patients awaiting liver transplantation throughout the world. The first left lobe adult-to-adult LDLTx in the US was performed in 1991 at the University of Chicago. The first right lobe adult-to-adult LDLTx in the United States was performed at Washington University. This treatment modality is now being offered at many liver transplant centers in the United States and throughout the world. In 1990, there were 14 living donor liver transplants performed in the United States, all in children. In 2000, more than 340 live liver donor transplants were performed in the United States.

3. Why is LDLTx performed?

LDLTx is a surgical technique that was developed because of the shortage of cadaver donors. The number of patients awaiting liver transplant has increased 15-fold in the last 10 years, but the number of donor organs available for transplant has increased only threefold. Based on the 2000 Scientific Registry of Transplant Recipients (SRTR) and Organ Procurement and Transplant Network (OPTN) Annual Report, the median waiting time for a liver transplant in the United States increased from 43 days in 1990 to 517 days in 1998. The number of deaths among patients on the liver transplant waiting list has increased in the same time frame from 382 to 1756. The number of patients on the United Network for Organ Sharing (UNOS) waiting list for a liver transplant has increased from 1237 to 14,707 from 1990 to 1999; however, the number of cadaver organs transplanted during the same time period has remained almost stagnant; 4509 organs recovered in 1990 and 5849 recovered in 1999. The lack of available organs has led to the exploration of different technical developments such as split liver transplant, reduced-sized grafts, and living donor liver transplant.

4. Who can be a living liver donor?

Living liver donors should be young, healthy adults who have the ability to understand the procedure and its possible complications. They should have an emotional or genetic relationship with the recipient and be able to comply with the short- and long-term follow-up required. The definition of "healthy" varies somewhat from center to center, but, in general, the donor should have no medical, emotional, or psychological condition that could potentially increase the risks of this surgery. There are three different types of living liver donors:

1. **Living related donor**—genetically related person such as a sibling, parent, or child

2. **Living unrelated donor**—person who has an emotional relationship with the recipient such as a spouse, friend, or colleague

3. **Good Samaritan donor**—a person unknown and unrelated to the recipient who has offered to donate a portion of his or her liver to a patient needing a transplant

The vast majority of living liver donors are either related or unrelated. Although rare, there have been reports of Good Samaritan living liver donors.

5. What is the criterion for age for living liver donation?

In general, living liver donors should be between the ages of 18 and 55 years, although there are reports of donors more than 55 years old. However, older donors have an increased risk of occult medical problems that may compromise their safety. There is also concern that livers from older donors may not have the same capacity to regenerate or sustain a postsurgical complication.

6. Does a donor need to be the same blood type as the recipient?

As in cadaver donor liver transplantation, living liver donors need to have compatible blood types. Type O donors can donate to all ABO type recipients, and a blood type AB recipient can receive a liver from a donor of any blood type. There are reports of incompatible living donor liver transplants, but this surgery is usually performed only in an emergency.

7. List some of the absolute and relative contraindications to being a living liver donor.

Absolute and Relative Contraindications to Living Donor Liver Transplantation

ABSOLUTE CONTRAINDICATIONS	RELATIVE CONTRAINDICATIONS
Human immunodeficiency virus (HIV)–positive	Controlled hypertension
Hepatitis C virus (HCV)–positive	Diet or oral drug-controlled diabetes
Hepatitis B virus (HBV)–positive	Mild asthma
Age < 18 years	Mild anemia with known cause
Obesity	Mild psychiatric disorder (e.g., anxiety)
Cancer in recent 5 years	Controlled hyperlipidemia
Significant medical condition	Age > 50 years
Excessive active alcohol use	
Moderate to severe psychiatric disorder	
Pregnancy	
Hypercoagulable disorder	
Idiopathic thrombocytopenic purpura (ITP) or significant hematologic disorder	

It is important to remember that this field of organ transplant will continue to evolve in the coming years. More experience and longer follow-up times on the impact of donation will help to identify factors that affect the safety of this procedure for both donors and recipients.

8. What are the advantages of LDLTx to the recipient?

There are a number of potential benefits to the recipient receiving a LDLTx, the most significant of which is timely transplantation and the reduction in waiting time to transplant. The availability of a living donor means the transplant can be performed before the recipient becomes too sick for surgery, thus improving post-transplant morbidity and mortality. A particular patient population who may receive significant advantage is that with hepatic malignancy who may develop metastasis during the long wait on the cadaver waiting list and thus not be a candidate for transplant. LDLTx is usually an elective procedure, which allows optimization of the recipient's condition before surgery. Surgery is performed during the day with a rested surgical team. Ischemia times are dramatically decreased because the portion of liver can be implanted almost immediately. These factors may lead to better post-transplant outcomes. Furthermore, a liver from a live donor is most likely of better quality than a liver from a cadaver donor. A liver from a healthy living donor has been spared the physiologic changes that brain death induces and the possible ensuing damage to organ function. The live donor undergoes extensive testing to rule out any medical problems that could affect the function of the liver graft.

9. Does LDLTx benefit the community at large?

There is a significant benefit to the liver waiting list as a whole. Every recipient who receives a liver from a live donor decreases the waiting list for cadaver livers and improves the opportunity for another patient to receive a cadaver organ.

10. Are there benefits to the donor who donates a portion of his or her liver?

One of the essential motivating factors governing LDLTx is altruism. There is significant enhancement of self-esteem for the donor through his or her role in restoring a loved one's health and saving a life. There is also the knowledge of having helped the transplant community at large by removing a patient from the cadaver waiting list. Another benefit may be the very thorough medical evaluation that the potential donor undergoes. Many potential health risks have been identified and corrected either by medical intervention or lifestyle adaptations by the potential donor. For example, many potential donors who smoke experience a very motivating goal to discontinue this habit. Asymptomatic medical conditions such as hyperlipidemia, hypertension, and cardiac disease are just some of the conditions that have been diagnosed as a result of the thorough donor evaluation.

11. Discuss the potential risks of the living donor surgical procedure that are explained to the donor.

An important component of the evaluation process is the education of the donor and his or her family about the possible risks and complications of living liver donor surgery. This multistep process involves disclosure of information in a manner that is understandable to the specific donor and family.

Disclosure of Potential Risks and Complications of LDLTx for the Donor

- Procedure-associated mortality and morbidity—center, national, and international data
- Possibility of acute liver failure or chronic liver dysfunction requiring liver transplant
- Complications of general anesthesia, intubation, line placement, deep venous thrombosis (DVT), pulmonary embolism (PE)
- Risk of transfusion-related reactions or transmission of infection
- Complications of abdominal surgery: wound infection, dehiscence, intestinal obstruction, ileus, hernia, adhesions, impact on complexity of future abdominal surgery
- Complications specific to hepatic resection: bleeding, biliary leaks, bilomas, strictures, hepatic artery thrombosis, portal vein thrombosis
- Potential long-term sequelae of right or left lobe resection
- Complications of gall bladder removal
- Inability to be a living liver donor a second time
- Impact on future health and availability of life insurance
- Impact on employment status, period of disability
- Potential effect of scar on physical appearance
- Postoperative pain
- Impact of significant and debilitating fatigue
- Period of hospital stay, short-term follow-up, and long-term follow-up

12. What are the reported risks of living liver donor surgery?

Donor complications can be categorized into those related to general anesthesia, general surgical complications, and complications directly related to hepatic dysfunction. The overall incidence of donor complications has been estimated at about 15–20%, including major and minor complications. The most commonly reported serious complications in donors are biliary, at a rate of approximately 4–5%. These include bilomas and bile leaks, usually from the cut surface of the liver. The complications usually resolve spontaneously over time and are most often managed without additional surgery. Wound infections have been reported at an incidence of 2–8%. LDLTx is considered a clean-contaminated case because the bile duct is transected. Wound infections usually require conservative treatment with antibiotics and local wound care only. Miller and colleagues reported 3 cases of intestinal obstruction in a series of 109 LDL transplantations, two of which required laparoscopic lysis of adhesions. There have also been reports of pleural effusions, atelectasis, and ileus. Todo and colleagues reported one portal vein thrombosis that was rescued surgically.

13. Is irreversible liver damage or dysfunction possible?

There are unofficial reports of at least 2 donors worldwide who presumably sustained irreversible liver damage that required liver transplantation in the immediate perioperative period. There have been no reports of late complications affecting liver function in left lateral segment donors. There are no long-term data available however on the outcomes of living liver donation, particularly for right lobe liver resections. This is an area that requires further research and analysis of outcomes and long-term results.

14. What is the risk of donor death as a result of living liver donation?

Of paramount importance is donor safety. Because of concerns for donor safety, this treatment modality was initially reserved for pediatric patients. There is an actual increased risk to the donor as the extent of liver resected from the donor increases. This is due to the increased risk of bleeding and potential damage to the vasculature or biliary anatomy during a more extensive parenchymal dissection and, more importantly, the risk of leaving the donor with insufficient hepatic volume. When the left lateral segment is used, the risk to the donor is believed to be less. However, there are risks involved in any surgery. Miller and colleagues mention at least five donor deaths in the international experience of approximately 2,500 LDL transplantations reported either in the media or at conferences. To date, only one of these donor deaths has been formally reported. It is thought that one donor death was a result of a pulmonary embolus, one was related to anesthesia complications , and three were related to technical complications and dysfunction of the remaining portion of the liver. More recently, another donor death was reported in the United States with the cause of death reported as emphysematous gastritis due to clostridial infection of the stomach. One aspect of living liver donation of critical concern is the lack of a central national or international database to monitor and report accurate donor outcomes. It is hoped that this database will be constructed in the near future, enabling transplant centers to report more accurately the potential risks and rate of complications to potential donors.

15. How does donation affect the donor's ability to work?

The recovery time for this type of surgery varies, but most donors are advised that they will require up to 3 months before complete recovery of normal health and activity. The donor's rate of recovery and job responsibilities are both factors that determine his or her ability to return to work. If a donor has a physically demanding job that requires heavy lifting, the period of disability usually is at least 3 months to allow for complete healing of the abdominal muscles.

16. What are the financial considerations for the living liver donor?

The donor should not incur any out-of-pocket expenses as a result of being evaluated for or being a living liver donor. Most recipient insurance carriers cover the expense of a donor evaluation, donor surgery, hospitalization, and early postoperative expenses related to follow-up or complications requiring medical intervention. They usually do not cover simultaneous evaluations of more than one donor but cover sequential evaluations if the original donor is not cleared to donate or decides not to proceed.

What is not clear is the period of coverage that a donor can expect from the recipient's insurance carrier for complications that are related to the procedure. This factor must be considered in the long-term follow-up protocol established by the transplant center. The author is aware of one insurance carrier that terminated donor coverage for medical care related to the donation process within 1 month of surgery. There are also some insurance carriers that require the donor's insurance to be billed first. Once an explanation of denial of benefits is issued by the donor's insurance carrier, the recipient's insurance will consider covering the donor evaluation. This process is cumbersome for the donor and the providers to follow. It often leads to undue stress on the donor.

Some transplant centers have established a system within their respective institutions that allows all donor evaluation and donation expenses to be covered by the organ acquisition fee for the recipient surgery. The transplant community must be proactive on these issues and advocate on behalf of the donor. Although the concept of payment for donation is illegal and considered unethical, a system needs to be put in place to help defray the miscellaneous costs of the donor evaluation and donation process, such as travel, pain prescriptions, and earnings lost as a result of disability.

17. What are the goals of a living liver donor evaluation?

The primary goal of the evaluation process is to ensure donor safety. It is important to determine the general health of the donor; rule out any emotional, psychological or psychiatric dysfunction; rule out any liver disease; and assess any anatomical variants that may preclude safe donation. Ascertaining the motivating factors guiding the patients' desire to be a donor and ruling out any component of coercion or financial incentive to be a donor are also important. In addition, the evaluation should determine whether the donor has any infectious or other medical condition that could be harmful to the recipient. During the evaluation process, at least one member of the evaluating team is designated as the donor advocate and should not be involved in the recipient's care. This person may be the physician, the clinical social worker, or the clinical coordinator.

18. What are the first steps in the donor evaluation process?

The exact sequence of testing and components of the evaluation may vary from center to center. The central goal of identifying a donor who is in excellent emotional and physical health and who is volunteering without evidence of coercion or financial incentives should remain central to any evaluation process. A donor should initiate the first step to proceed with an evaluation after the option of LDLTx has been explained. Usually, the first step is to administer a brief health questionnaire (see table). Important considerations at this time are ABO status of the donor and recipient; the body mass index (BMI) of the donor; his or her general medical, surgical, and psychiatric health; history of smoking, alcohol, and other illicit or recreational drug use; current medication use; the relationship of the donor to recipient; and what is motivating the potential donor to consider being a living donor.

Many centers require a potential donor to read relevant educational material about the procedure, evaluation process, risks, possible complications, financial and employment considerations, and short- and long-term follow-up. Many donors may be ruled out during this step. Insurance coverage for the donor evaluation is discussed before proceeding. A review of the current status of the potential donor's recipient should be conducted at this time as well, to rule out any contraindications to LDLTx. Size matching and consideration of the recipient's liver disease are important issues to discuss with the donor in the evaluation process.

Common Components of Screening Questionnaire

Characteristics	Age, gender, height, weight
Relationship to recipient	Genetic, emotional, none
Source of knowledge about LDLTx	Recipient, family member, media, transplant center
Medical history	Known illnesses, current medications, past hospitalizations, history of blood clot formation
Surgical history	Prior surgery
Social history	Marital status, number and ages of children, alcohol use, smoking history, illicit drug use
Family medical history	Significant cardiovascular, liver, cancer or hematological disorders
Employment status	Relative to availability of disability pay and job security
Psychiatric	Medications, hospitalizations, need for counseling/therapy

19. What is the next step for the donor to complete an evaluation?

The next step is a detailed medical evaluation and laboratory blood testing (see tables). Usually the physician responsible for the medical evaluation is a member of the transplant team but is not involved in the recipient's care, or the physician may not be part of the the transplant team. If a donor passes this step, a psychosocial evaluation is conducted either by a clinical social worker, psychologist, or psychiatrist. A surgical consultation is done to discuss the surgical procedure, reinforce the risks and possible complications, and further discuss the recovery period as well as the period of absence from work. An assessment of the donor's cardiovascular health is also completed and may consist of an electrocardiogram (EKG), echocardiogram, and stress test, depending on the age of the donor and the presence or absence of risk factors for heart disease. A routine chest x-ray is performed. Radiologic imaging studies of the liver are performed to determine the anatomy of the portal vein, hepatic veins, hepatic artery, and biliary drainage system. An arteriogram may be required, depending on the magnetic resonance imaging (MRI) or computed tomography (CT) technology available at the specific center. The MRI or CT modality also provides volumetric measurements of the lobes of the liver and assesses for the presence of steatosis.

Laboratory Studies

Complete blood count	Autoimmune markers
Chemistries	Serum protein electrophoresis
Liver function tests	Alpha fetoprotein
Thyroid function tests	Human immunodeficiency virus
Coagulation profile	Cytomegalovirus
Alpha$_1$-antitrypsin level	Epstein-Barr virus
Ceruloplasmin	Herpes simplex virus
Iron studies	Syphilis test
Lipid Profile	Hepatitis C virus
Urinalysis	Hepatitis B virus
Pregnancy test	Hepatitis A virus

Components of Standard Living Donor Evaluation

TYPE OF TEST OR CONSULTATION	ALL DONORS	DONOR- OR CENTER-SPECIFIC
Confirm ABO compatibility	X	
Screening health questionnaire		X
History and physical exam	X	
Laboratory testing	X	
Chest x-ray	X	
EKG	X	
Surgical consultation	X	
Social work consultation		X
Echocardiogram		X
Stress test		X
Psychiatric consultation		X
CT or MRI of abdomen	X	
Arteriogram		X
Liver biopsy		X

EKG = electrocardiogram, CT = computed tomography, MRI = magnetic resonance imaging.

20. Is a liver biopsy required on all donor evaluations?

Some centers do liver biopsies routinely on all donors. However, many centers only do a liver biopsy if steatosis is identified on imaging studies or if the donor has hyperlipidemia, a history of significant alcohol use, or is overweight. It is important in these circumstances to differentiate between volumetric and functional graft volume. Technology is developing rapidly, improving the diagnosis and quantification of steatosis without invasive percutaneous liver biopsy.

21. Is tissue typing or donor/recipient crossmatch necessary?

Historically, tissue typing has not been beneficial in cadaver liver transplant. LDLTx may provide a basis for reconsideration of tissue typing because many donors are genetically related to their recipients. There may be a benefit of reduced immunosuppression with certain HLA matches. As research develops in this area, HLA-typing may possibly assist in identifying recipients of an LDLTx who can be successfully withdrawn from immunosuppressive therapy. This identification may add a significant benefit to the recipient receiving an LDLTx by eliminating the long-term complications of immunosuppressive therapy. The author is aware through personal experience of at least two cases of LDLTx in identical twins performed without any immunosuppressive therapy. Crossmatching between donor and recipient is center-specific, and it is unlikely that a positive crossmatch would preclude living liver donation. It may, however, affect the type of induction immunosuppressive therapy used because the risk of rejection may be greater.

22. Is there a need to discuss the recipient's disease with the donor?

Paramount to ensuring the informed consent of the donor, in addition to the discussion of risks and potential complications, is the need for the donor to have realistic expectations about the success of the transplant. An essential component of the donor's motivation to be a living donor is the hope that he or she will save the life of the recipient. Success or failure of the transplant is, in part, due to the pretransplant condition of the recipient, the presence or absence of co-morbid conditions, and the cause of liver disease. Some liver diseases can recur in the graft, such as HCV, HBV, and hepatocellular carcinoma (HCC). It is of particular importance to the donor that full disclosure of the recipient's condition, the possibility of recurrent disease, and the impact of this on quality of life and life expectancy be divulged, particularly when a liver transplant is indicated because of HCC and HCV.

Liver transplantations in HIV-positive recipients have been reported and may potentially become more common in the future. Short- and long-term outcomes in HIV-positive recipients are unclear at this time. Therefore, fully informed consent of the donor must include disclosure of this factor, obviously with the recipient's consent. This situation is unique in medicine because it requires the disclosure of one patient's medical information to another patient, which the recipient should be made aware of in the discussion about the option of living liver donation.

23. Should the size of the donor and recipient be considered?

The size of the donor and recipient are of less significance in pediatric liver transplant candidates. Usually, the left lateral segment from an adult is of sufficient size for a child. Indeed, in some cases, the left lateral segment of a large male donor may be too big for some smaller babies. The size of the donor and the recipient are important considerations in calculating the optimal functional graft for adult recipients and calculating the residual liver volume for the donor. The potential living liver donor should ideally be of similar height and weight as the recipient. A donor who is larger or is at least ¾ the size of the recipient is likely to have sufficient liver volume to be able to donate. However, for recipients who have well preserved liver function without significant portal hypertension, such as some recipients with HCC, the size comparison may be of less significance.

24. What is the minimum volume of functional graft required to support a recipient?

In cadaver liver transplantation, it is generally accepted that graft size 40–50% of the recipient's expected liver volume is the lower limit to have initial graft function on implantation.

Emond and colleagues suggested that 50% of the recipient's ideal liver volume was the minimum volume required to provide adequate functional liver mass in a series of 25 living donor liver transplants reported in 1996. Successful adult-to-adult LDLTx cases have been reported using 25% of the recipient's ideal liver volume, although the authors did report complications related to graft function.

25. How is the minimum functional graft required calculated?

A number of formulas can be used to aid the physician in determining the minimum volume of functional graft required to support the metabolic needs of a recipient. Research has indicated that 40–50% of the recipient's expected liver volume is the lower limit to ensure immediate graft function. Graft volume of the donor can be calculated before surgery using CT or MRI computerized measurement of segmental liver volume. Standard liver volume or optimal liver mass in recipients can be calculated from a formula using their body surface area:

$$\text{Standard liver volume (ml)} + 706.2 \times (\text{body surface area [M2]}) + 2.4$$

The first method estimates the ratio of the graft volume to standard liver volume (GV/SV ratio). Kawasaki and colleagues reported good recipient outcomes in a series of cases in which the GV/SV ratio ranged from 31–54%.

Another method estimates the graft weight/recipient's body weight ratio (GRWR). In a large series of 276 LDL transplantations reported by Inomoto from the Kyoto group, the survival rate of recipients with a GRWR of < 0.8% was poorer than that of recipients with a GRWR of 0.8–1.0%. Marcos and colleagues reported a graft-to-recipient body weight ratio (GRBW) range from 0.76–1.7 in a series of 25 adult-to-adult right lobectomy LDL transplantations reported in 1999.

26. Are there other factors in addition to graft volume that may affect the success of LDLTx?

As the degree or severity of illness increases, the metabolic demands placed on a liver graft increase. In a retrospective study conducted by Tojimbara and colleagues, disease severity assessed by UNOS status and Child-Pugh classification was greater in patients who died within 4 months after LDLTx, implying that disease severity is a factor predictive of mortality after LDLTx. For this reason, in the United States, LDLTx in adults had been used primarily in the status 2B category of the UNOS classification system based on the Child-Turcotte-Pugh (CTP) scoring system. There was concern that patients with a UNOS status 2A category in the CTP scoring system may have been too sick to receive a LDLTx. However, selected cases have been reported, but careful calculation of the required functional hepatocyte mass is more critical in these patients, and the degree of the recipient's illness in addition to GRWR needs to taken into consideration. It remains to be seen how the new liver disease severity scoring system—Model for End-stage Liver Disease (MELD)—will help to define a recipient's severity of liver disease relative to the appropriateness of LDLTx. The degree of portal hypertension in recipients needs to be considered in cases with borderline GRWR ratios.

Portal vein thrombosis, although not an absolute contraindication to LDLTx, may be a relative contraindication, depending on the extent of the thrombosis and the experience of the surgeon. Other factors such as coexistent medical comorbid conditions, obesity, marginal psychosocial function, and retransplantation are reported as relative contraindications to LDLTx by some centers. As experience is gained with this procedure, like the advances made in cadaver liver transplantation, similar relative barriers will most likely be overcome in the future.

27. What is the role of the clinical transplant coordinator in the living liver donor process?

The role of the clinical transplant coordinator in living donor liver transplantation is relatively new and is evolving as the field of live donor transplant grows and evolves. The living liver donor coordinator may be the same person who manages the recipient's care or may be the donor advocate at some centers. Factors that determine the exact role the clinical coordinator will play in this process vary depending on program size, volume of donor evaluations, and internal structure. The primary responsibility of the living donor coordinator is donor advocacy, donor safety, and donor and family education. As transplant programs begin to offer this treatment modality, the clinical co-ordinator will be intimately involved in establishing protocols and criteria that maintain the primary focus of donor safety. The coordinator will also be primarily responsible for donor and recipient education about this treatment modality and for developing appropriate educational material.

Another primary responsibility of the living donor coordinator is to maintain confidentiality of the donor during the evaluation process. Details of the evaluation must not be revealed until such time as the donor is cleared to donate and has made a decision to proceed. An option for the donor to withdraw gracefully should always be maintained until the donor has clearly expressed a desire to proceed. As the situation is one of high anxiety for the recipient and family, this responsibility can be challenging for the clinical coordinator.

28. Who makes the decision about the candidate's suitability to be a living liver donor?

Once an evaluation has been completed, the multidisciplinary living donor team reviews each component of the evaluation, determining the donor's emotional and physical health, moti-vation to donate, relationship to the recipient, liver size, and anatomical variants of the liver. A thorough review of the recipient's case is completed ,and a decision is made on the donor-to-re-cipient size matching and liver volumetric requirements. The donor is informed of the team's de-cision before any communication with the recipient.

29. Once a donor is cleared, is the transplant scheduled?

Whenever possible, it is best for a period of time to elapse between notification of the donor's candidacy and the actual date of surgery. This passage of time allows the donor to con-sider all the information, to discuss the decision with his or her family, and to explore disability benefits and sick leave. It is extremely important that the donor make a fully informed and unco-erced decision. The donor is reminded again of the opportunity to withdraw as a candidate should there be a change of mind. Commonly, donors are offered a "medical out" throughout the evalua-tion and waiting period. It is important, however, not to fabricate any medical problem or condi-tion that would become part of the donor's medical record. The date for the surgery is then based on the availability of the transplant teams, the recipient's condition, and the donor's preference.

In cases of fulminant hepatic failure (FHF) in which an expedited work-up and review of the case is necessary, more careful attention must be directed to the emotional and psychological state of the donor. The urgency of the situation dictates a short period of time for the donor to consider the risk/benefit ratio. The dynamics of the situation also put an additional strain on the transplant team to ensure the expedited process of informed consent and disclosure is executed appropriately with donor safety not compromised. Many programs will not consider living donors for emmergent transplants, particularly in adult recipients.

30. How can the liver be divided while maintaining the function of both portions?

On gross examination, the liver is divided into 2 lobes: a right lobe and a left lobe. The left lobe comprises approximately 40% of total liver volume, and the right lobe comprises approxi-mately 60% of total liver volume. Functionally, however, the liver can be divided into 8 segments (see figure) that essentially correspond with the portal vein anatomical blood supply and the bile duct system. This anatomical struc-ture allows surgical division of the liver while preserving portal blood flow and biliary drainage to all segments of the liver. It is ex-tremely important to remember, however, that not everyone has this classic anatomy of the liver; because liver anatomy is highly variable, the surgery is technically challeng-ing and must be individually tailored for each case.

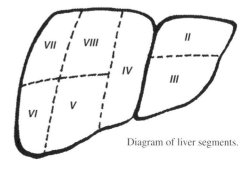

Diagram of liver segments.

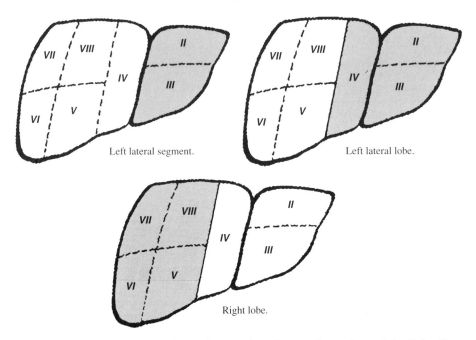

Left lateral segment.

Left lateral lobe.

Right lobe.

31. Name the different types of hepatic resections that can be performed for living liver donation.

Essentially, four different procedures can be performed that reflect the segments of the liver that are removed. In a left lateral segmentectomy, segments II and III are removed (see figure, above left). These segments account for approximately 20% of the total liver volume. In a left lobectomy (see figure, above right), segments II, III, and IV are removed. These segments account for approximately 40% of the total liver volume. In a right lobectomy (see figure, middle), segments V, VI, VII, and VIII are removed, accounting for approximately 60% of the total liver volume. In the standard right lobe resection, the surgical plane is to the right of the middle hepatic vein. However, there are reports of an extended right lobe resection—segments IV, V, VI, VII, and VIII—in which the surgical plane is to the left of the middle hepatic vein.

32. Does each portion of the divided liver regenerate?

The liver has the capacity to regenerate, and the regeneration starts immediately. Early reports suggested that most of the regeneration takes place within the first few weeks and certainly within the first 2–3 months. Marcos and colleagues reported an increase in recipient graft size of 87% on postoperative day 7. There are now some reports, however, that liver regeneration may continue up to 1 year after resection. The graft in the recipient and the remnant liver in the donor grow to a normal volume for each individual, but the shape of the liver is not normal. The abnormal shape precludes a donor from donating a portion of the liver a second time.

33. How has the surgical technique evolved to the current state of application?

LDLTx is the latest development in the continuous evolution of liver transplantation surgery because of the increasing numbers of patients awaiting this life-saving procedure. Segmental liver transplantation was initially introduced in the mid-1980s in response to the significant mortality of pediatric patients awaiting liver transplant. Split liver transplant was the next stage in this evolution and then living donor liver transplantation using the left lateral segment from a live donor for a pediatric patient in the early 1990s. The left lateral segment is used for the vast majority of pediatric recipients, but because of the its small volume, this segment is too small to use for adults. The left lobe also has limited application in adults because of functional size requirements.

Because of concerns over donor safety, the use of the right lobe has been extended to adult patients awaiting liver transplant only in the past 3–4 years. This advance in liver transplantation would not have taken place except for the severe disparity that developed between the number of patients in need of liver transplantation and the number of cadaver donor organs available.

34. How much of the donor liver is removed?

Which of the four different procedures is used determines how much of the donor's liver is removed. The size of the recipient is one of the main determining factors in deciding which procedure will be done. For pediatric recipients, the left lateral segment of the liver is used. The left lobe can be used in some large adolescents or smaller adult recipients. The right lobe of the liver is applied in the majority of adult-to-adult living donor liver transplants. The perceived risk to the donor is believed to increase relative to the amount of liver volume removed. Thus, the extended right lobe resection is potentially of greatest risk to the donor, with the standard right lobe resection next, followed by the left lobe resection, and the left lateral segment.

35. How long is the donor surgery?

The actual surgery time for a standard right lobe resection is approximately 2–3 hours. However, the average duration of a right lobectomy for an LDLTx surgery is approximately 4–8 hours, depending on the timing of the recipient's hepatectomy to limit total ischemic time. The operative time for a left lobe or left lateral resection is usually less.

36. Do donor and recipient surgeries occur simultaneously?

One major advantages for the recipient of a living donor liver transplant is the significantly shorter ischemic time. To maximize this benefit and for overall safety of the donor and recipient, most centers have two teams of surgeons and two operating rooms running simultaneously. If the recipient requires an exploratory laparotomy first to rule out metastatic HCC, the recipient's surgery begins before the donor's surgery. Otherwise, the donor's surgery commonly starts slightly ahead of the recipient's, to allow for intraoperative assessment of the biliary anatomy, or it starts simultaneously with the recipient's surgery. However, at some centers where two teams of surgeons are not available, the donor's surgery is completed first and is followed by the recipient's surgery.

37. Is a blood transfusion required during the donor surgery?

The incidence of donor blood transfusions is low. However, to limit the potential complications of a blood transfusion, most centers store 1 unit of the living donor's blood before surgery for autologous transfusion. Blood loss during the surgery is recovered with cell salvage as well. In a series of 109 LDLTx cases, Miller and colleagues reported only 2 donors who received a single unit of blood each from the blood bank in addition to their one autologous unit.

38. Do all living liver donors have the gallbladder removed?

It is common practice to remover the gall bladder when resecting the right lobe of the liver or the left lobe of the liver for living liver donation.

39. Discuss the early postoperative management of a living donor.

The donor is usually admitted the morning of the surgery. Following a final review and confirmation of the donor's desire to proceed, prophylactic intravenous antibiotics are administered and continued usually for 24 hours postoperatively. Living liver donors require standard post-anesthesia recovery care that emphasizes assessment of respiratory and mental status, assessment of renal function and liver function with careful observation for postsurgical bleeding, and appropriate pain management. Reintroduction of oral fluids and diet, which begins after bowel function has returned, should progress gradually to a normal diet over a period of days. Usually an H_2-blocker is given until normal oral intake is restored. Aggressive mobilization of the patient is extremely important in preventing DVT, pneumonia, and other sequelae of prolonged anesthesia and abdominal surgery. Liver function is assessed by daily monitoring of a hepatic panel and basic chemistries and international normalized ratio (INR). Assessment of the donor's mental status is also important in determining overall recovery and identifying overuse of narcotic pain medication.

Postoperative Daily Laboratory Monitoring

• Complete blood count	• Renal function: blood urea nitrogen (BUN), creatinine
• International normalized ratio (INR)	• Liver function: aspartate aminotransferase (AST),
• Electrolytes	alanine aminotransferase (ALT), bilirubin

40. Discuss the role of the nurse postoperatively.

In addition to the routine postoperative care, the nurse pays careful attention to the mental status of the donor and must identify decreased mental status due to possible overuse of narcotic medication or mental status changes secondary to compromised hepatic function. The nurse plays a vital role in ensuring the early mobilization of the donor and prevention of complications such as DVT, PE, pneumonia, and prolonged ileus. Because pain is significant after this surgery, attention to optimal pain management strategies enables donors to begin to mobilize early and prevents such complications. The emotional well-being of the donor and concern for his or her recipient should also be considered during the recovery period. Living donors pose unique challenges to the health care team because they were perfectly healthy and normal individuals who otherwise would not require surgery or be in the hospital. These patients experience the recovery from this surgery much differently than do patients recovering from a medically necessary surgery.

41. Pain is significant after a partial hepatectomy. What strategies can be used to minimize the donor's pain?

Pain management is an important factor in the care and safe recovery after this surgery. Most donors report significant pain in the early postoperative period, many reporting it to be much more severe than they expected. A complicating factor in appropriate management of postsurgical pain in this circumstance is the impaired ability of the decreased functional liver mass to metabolize narcotic medication. Excessive narcotic administration or inadequate breakdown and excretion can lead to depressed mental status, depressed respiratory status, prolonged ileus, and hypotension, which can lead to the development of pneumonia, DVT, PE, or other serious complications. These findings may also be due to liver dysfunction secondary to a surgical or functional complication of the resection. The goal in pain management postoperatively is to provide adequate pain control, which allows the donor to perform breathing exercises and begin walking, without causing the detrimental side effects of narcotic use that may be more pronounced in a patient with decreased functional hepatocytes. Most centers use a combination of intravenous patient-controlled analgesia (PCA) and epidural administration of pain medication. The goal is to switch to oral pain medication and no narcotic medication as quickly as is feasible.

42. What is the average hospital stay for a living liver donor?

Most donors are hospitalized for 5–7 days after surgery. During the first postoperative day, the donor is usually monitored in a step-down or postanesthetic-care-unit (PACU) environment before being transferred to the transplant unit. The incision staples are usually removed about 7–10 days postoperatively.

43. Because bile leaks are a commonly reported complication after this surgery, discuss the signs and symptoms that may suggest a bile leak.

Classic signs and symptoms of a bile leak include new onset of fever, leukocytosis, abdominal pain, and persistent or increased bile leakage from the surgical drain. Such signs may all warrant further radiological imaging studies to rule out a bile leak, formation of a biloma, or other intra-abdominal collections.

44. What is the treatment for a bile leak?

The most common site of a bile leak is from the cut surface of the liver. A bile leak is usually treated conservatively with drainage via the drain placed at the time of resection if the patient is not clinically septic. It usually resolves over time and does not warrant surgical intervention. Percutaneous drainage may be required to treat bilomas or abscesses. Resolution of the cut-surface leak is usually identified when drainage has ceased, and the drain can then be removed. Surgical intervention may be required for more serious bile leaks.

45. Discuss other common complications or symptoms the donor may experience after surgery.

Severe and debilitating fatigue is very common for the first 3–4 weeks in addition to the pain and discomfort. Wound infections can occur but are usually minor. It is important that donors be taught the signs and symptoms of a wound infection before discharge. Minor gastrointestinal symptoms are also common. Donors commonly report dyspepsia, early satiety, bloating and gas, constipation or frequent bowel movements. The cause is unclear but may be related to the removal of the donor's gall bladder or to the manipulation of the colon into the upper right quadrant to prevent twisting or torsion of the remaining portion of liver. The symptoms usually resolve within the first 3 months after surgery. Also common are a feeling of tightness in the abdominal wall and numbness of the abdomen below the surgical incision, which usually resolves within 3–6 months after surgery although some donors report more long-term decreased sensation.

46. What activity guidelines are donors advised to follow after discharge from the hospital?

All donors are encouraged to continue a program of daily exercise such as walking or using a stationary bicycle after discharge. The goal is to build up stamina and endurance gradually over the coming weeks. Donors are advised to not lift, push, or pull objects weighing more than 15–20 pounds for the first 4 weeks. Gradual increase in activity over the next 8 weeks is suggested. Donors are advised to report any adverse reactions to increased activity to the transplant center. It is common for donors to require encouragement to pursue an exercise regimen either secondary to fear of damaging the liver or secondary to pain and discomfort. Continued attention to the donor's emotional well-being during this time is important.

47. What is the usual follow-up required of the donor?

Follow-up varies from center to center, but usually the donor returns to the transplant center within a week for a wound check, assessment of pain control, general recovery status, and staple removal. Weekly to biweekly checkups based on the patient's symptoms and rate of return to normal activity are usual. Most centers require radiologic imaging of the liver with MRI or CT within 3 months of the surgery to assess volumetric regeneration of the liver. Routine laboratory blood testing is also common, including a complete blood count, chemistries, and liver function tests. A complete evaluation of the health status of the donor and review of the test results are usually performed and discussed with the donor.

Long-term follow-up requirements of the donor vary considerably from center to center and are a subject for further debate and clarification as this field evolves. It is advisable for liver donors to have a complete medical evaluation with their primary care physician annually and to report any abnormalities to the transplant center. Transplant centers commonly plan a way to honor living donors for their courage and heroism, often through donor recognition ceremonies.

48. What is the role of the transplant coordinator in the postsurgical care of the donor?

It is important for the transplant coordinator to remain an available resource and contact for living liver donors after surgery and to maintain continuity of care throughout the whole process, including postsurgery. Many donors need ongoing reassurance and support during the difficult recovery period, particularly when their recipient has a poor outcome. The transplant coordinator continues to monitor recovery and ensure close follow-up of the donor, assisting with disability applications and clearance for returning to work, education and guidance regarding diet, activity, and management of pain and discomfort, in addition to monitoring for the development of complications. This role is challenging for the transplant coordinator because the dynamics involved in caring for a healthy individual through this medically unnecessary surgery are varied and unique. The care of living donors after surgery focuses primarily on their emotional well-being and support.

ACKNOWLEDGEMENT

The author is grateful to Dr. Sander Florman for his input.

BIBILOGRAPHY

1. Authors for the Live Organ Donor Consensus Group: Consensus statement on live organ donor. JAMA 284:2919–2926, 2000.
2. Cheng YF, Chen CL, Huang TL, et al: Single imaging modality evaluation of living donors in liver transplantation: Magnetic resonance imaging. Transplantation 72:1527–1533, 2001.
3. Emond JC, Renz JF, Ferrell LD, et al: Functional analysis of grafts from living donors. Ann Surg 224:544–554, 1996.
4. Inomata Y, Uemoto S, Asonuma K, et al: Right lobe graft in living donor liver transplantation. Transplantation 69:258–264, 2000.
5. Kawasaki S, Makuuchi M, Matsunami H et al: Living related liver transplantation in adults. Ann Surg 227:269–274, 1998.
6. Marcos A, Fisher RA, Ham JM, et al: Liver regeneration and function in donor and recipient after right lobe adult-to-adult living donor liver transplantation. Transplantation 69:1375–1379, 2000.
7. Marcos A, Fisher RA, Ham JM, et al: Right lobe living donor liver transplantation. Transplantation 68:798–803, 1999.
8. Marcos A, Ham JM, Fisher RA, et al: Single-center analysis of the first 40 adult-to-adult living donor liver transplants using the right lobe. Liver Transplant 6:296–301, 2000.
9. Miller CM, Gondolesi GE, Florman S, et al: One hundred nine living donor liver transplants in adults and children: A single-center experience. Ann Surg 234:301–312, 2001.
10. Renz JF, Roberts JP: Long-term complications of living donor liver transplantation. Liver Transplantation 6:S73–S76, 2000.
11. Schiano TD, Kim-Schluger L, Gondolesi G, Miller CM: Adult living donor liver transplantation: The hepatologist's perspective. Hepatology 33:3–9, 2001.
12. Testa G, Malago M, Broelsch CE: Living-donor liver transplants in adults. Langenbecks Archiv Surg 384:536-543, 1999.
13. Todo S, Furukawa H, Jin MB, Shimamura T: Living donor liver transplantation in adults: Outcome in Japan. Liver Transplant 6:S66–S72, 2000.
14. Tojimbara T, Fuchinoue S, Nakajima I, et al: Factors affecting survival after living-related liver transplantation. Transplant Int 13:S136–S139, 2000.
15. Trotter JF: Selection of donors and recipients for living donor liver transplantation. Liver Transplant 6:S52–S58, 2000.

18. PSYCHOSOCIAL ISSUES OF LIVING DONORS

*Linda Wright, MHSc, MSW, Brenda McQuarrie, BScN, RN(EC),
and Jeanie Haines, BScN, RN*

1. Who can be a living organ donor?

The generally accepted guideline is that any healthy individual between the ages of 18 and 65 years can be assessed as a potential living donor. There are usually additional specific criteria, depending on the organ to be donated and the individual transplant program. For example, the maximum age of acceptable lung donors is usually younger, and they have to be nonsmokers. By contrast, although potential kidney and liver donors are encouraged to stop smoking before surgery and may require additional assessment, they are not be automatically excluded. All donors undergo individual program- and organ-related assessments to ensure that they are suitable donors.

2. To whom can donors donate?

The majority of programs require that the donor be a relative or have a close emotional relationship with the recipient. Therefore, family members, friends, and colleagues of recipients are considered as possible living donors. This requirement is being challenged by innovations such as nondirected donation and indirect and paired exchanges (see question 9).

3. Which organs can be donated from living donors?

Kidneys, liver lobes, and, more recently, lung lobes can be donated. Transplants of pancreas and small bowel segments have met with limited success.

4. What are the requirements for being a living organ donor?

Living donor transplants can take place when three criteria are satisfied. First, potential recipients must be suitable for transplant; i.e., they must meet the criteria of the transplant program, such as being free of infection and being able to undergo anaesthetization safely. Second, donors must satisfy the assessment criteria for the individual organ and program in terms of their physical and mental health. Third, the matching criteria for the specific organ and recipient–donor pair must be satisfied. For all organs, matching includes being blood group compatible. Kidney donors and their recipients must have a "negative crossmatch," which is a blood test in which the blood of the two individuals is mixed to be certain the recipient has no preformed antibodies to the donor's tissue. Liver and lung donors must have a lobe graft that is an adequate size for the specific recipient.

5. Describe the long-term effects of organ donation on a donor's health.

Kidney donors have been followed for as long as 30 years. Research to date does not demonstrate any long-term effects on their physical health, but there is evidence of depression in some situations (see question 29). Because liver and lung donations are newer, the duration of follow-up has been much shorter, but to date there have been no long-term effects of concern. There is, however, the potential for short-term effects if donors develop postoperative complications such as a wound infection or pneumonia.

6. What would motivate a person to donate an organ?

Living donors are generally motivated by altruism to help to improve the length and quality of life of someone whose wellbeing is important to them. The offer to donate is generally based on a personal value system that considers helping others to be very important. For example, by donating a liver or lung lobe, a living donor may be saving the life of the recipient and thus may prevent nephews and nieces from growing up without a parent.

Additional benefits may accrue to some donors (e.g., when a wife gives a kidney to her husband, she may find that there are advantages for herself from her husband's being dialysis-free, such as greater freedom to travel, more time together, or greater economic stability through his returning to work).

Sometimes a donor may hope that donation will have other effects as well. It may be a means of trying to atone for past difficulties, conflicts, or indiscretions. A donor may hope that donation will change the recipient's behavior (e.g., a mother who believes that donation will make a son become more compliant to treatment because of guilt or appreciation for the organ). These expectations may be unrealistic and are addressed during the predonation assessment process. It is vital that the donor be prepared for the likely effect of donation on his or her relationship with the recipient and accept the possibility that it may not alter after donation.

Transplants from living donors have good outcomes compared to those from cadaveric donors. In addition, the surgery can be planned, which may decrease stress and disruption for the family.

7. Do people ever sell organs?

Although the sale of organs is illegal in most countries, the media often report a black market, mostly in the Third World. Ethical objections to organ trade are that it further disadvantages the poor, increases the possibility of coercion and the level of risk for the donor, removes altruism as a motivation for donation, reduces trust in the medical profession, and cannot be controlled. Where profit is a motive in organ donation, it is more difficult to ensure standards of practice in the care of both the donor and the recipient. These issues have been challenged, and it has been suggested that a regulated sale of organs would ease the organ shortage and that some people may want to sell their organs for altruistic reasons (e.g., to pay for medications for a family member).

8. Can children be living organ donors?

For decisions regarding children as living organ donors, the same ethical principles are used as with adult donors. Children are rarely used as organ donors, but the question may arise when they risk losing a close relative who is very important to them. At issue is the child's ability to appreciate the risks and benefits of donation well enough to fulfill the requirements of informed consent. One important factor to consider is the likelihood that the child would give consent if he or she were of age. The consent of both the child and the parents is needed for pediatric living donation, but such consent may not suffice. In order to establish an objective view of the child's position, everyone involved might benefit from consultation with an independent patient advocate such as an ethicist or ethics committee.

9. Describe innovations in living donation.

Sometimes an individual is willing to donate but is not a match for the intended recipient. Several innovative methods of organ donation have been proposed to address this situation. They are in the early stages of debate and development.

Paired exchange occurs when two separate willing living kidney donors are unable to donate to their intended recipients because of ABO blood type incompatibility. In a simple exchange, donor 1 donates a kidney to recipient 2, with whom he or she is ABO compatible, and donor 2 donates to recipient 1, with whom he or she is ABO compatible. The pairs do not necessarily know each other before being matched by the transplant center.

Indirect exchange occurs when a willing living kidney donor is not blood compatible with an intended recipient. The donor donates to a matched person at the top of the waiting list for a cadaveric kidney. The donor's intended recipient moves to the top of the cadaveric waiting list. This method allows an extra living donor transplant to occur.

Nondirected donation occurs when a living donor gives a kidney to a transplant center without knowing who the recipient will be. This person is sometimes referred to as a *Good Samaritan* donor. After a thorough assessment process, the transplant center assigns the organ to the most suitable recipient at the top of the cadaveric waiting list. A nondirected donor is motivated by altruism. Nondirected donation is being implemented at a few transplant centers in the United States, but it is still fairly rare.

10. What are the financial implications of being a living organ donor?

Living donation often incurs costs for the donor during the assessment phase and at the time of donation and recovery. The costs may include loss of income, travel and childcare expenses, and cost of accommodation and meals near the transplant center. There may be financial loss if the donor is self-employed and does not have benefits or if the employer does not support a paid leave of absence.

It is acceptable for donors to be recompensed for out-of-pocket expenses, either from fundraising or direct reimbursement. Recently, the U.S. government decided to provide 30 days paid leave for its employees for the purpose of organ donation. Some state governments have followed suit. Furthermore, in 2001 the U.S. House of Representatives passed bill HR624, which offers help to living donors with nonmedical expenses related to donation such as travel and accommodation. The bill is now before the Senate. Most countries, including Canada, do not make financial provisions for living donors. The lack of government support leads to inequities because living donation is more attainable for the wealthy than for the poor.

Life insurance for kidney donors generally is not affected by donation. Most often, donors are able to obtain and keep life insurance without the rates being changed because of the donation.

11. How soon may donors expect to return to work after donating?

The length of time that donors are unable to work varies from 2–12 weeks and is influenced by three main factors. The first is the surgical procedure that they undergo. A kidney donor who has a laparoscopic nephrectomy often returns to work after 2 weeks, whereas the traditional open flank procedure usually requires 6 weeks of recuperation. Lung donors and liver lobe donors are usually off work a minimum of 6 weeks and often require 12 weeks of recuperation. The second factor which influences the recovery period is the type of work that donors do. If the work involves heavy lifting, they need at least 6–8 weeks of recuperation to ensure that their muscles have healed before they resume lifting. Donors who have relatively sedentary work often return to work sooner. The third factor which influences the return to work is whether there are any postoperative complications. For example, a liver donor who has a bile leak after surgery may need additional recuperation time while the leak is treated.

12. Does donating an organ effect a donor's sexuality?

A donor's sexuality should not be affected by organ donation other than in the recovery period. The libido of all individuals having any type of surgery is temporarily diminished by the discomfort and fatigue experienced during recovery. Potential donors, especially men who are contemplating kidney donation, are often concerned about their sexuality, for they associate their kidneys and sexuality as a result of shared organ function.

13. Describe how a recipient may show appreciation to the living donor for the organ.

How a recipient shows his or her appreciation is a personal matter between him or her and the donor. Donors need to feel that their gift of an organ is appreciated. Many are satisfied simply to know that this is the case, whether it is stated or implied. Some people find it hard to find words that are adequate to express their thankfulness appropriately and have concerns that they may minimize the extent of their appreciation. Recipients may wish to show their thanks in tangible ways. It is important that this be a token rather than an attempt to repay the donor for the organ. Some donors say that seeing the recipient with restored health is the greatest reward.

14. Explain the role of the transplant center in living donation.

The role of the transplant center is to provide quality health care and perform transplants safely. The process involves assessing the suitability and safety of living donors and recipients for the procedure, performing the operations, and providing appropriate follow-up care for recipients and donors. In order to accomplish this goal in cases involving living donors, the center is required to ensure that the benefit, which is mostly to the recipient, outweighs risk to the donor. The center must ensure that donation will be safe for the donor and will do no harm. The requirements of informed consent must be fulfilled; i.e., living donors must understand the risks and benefits of the procedure, know the treatment options for the recipient, and acknowledge that they are acting voluntarily. It is the responsibility of the transplant center to provide the necessary information to the donor for informed consent to be attained.

If testing of the potential donor finds a medical problem, the center arranges for the donor to have appropriate care. The transplant center provides follow-up care for the donor after donation to ensure that the donor experiences no ill effects from the donation. Donors may need reassurance about the state of their health. It is appropriate for transplant centers to acknowledge the courage of donors. This emotional support may help to validate the decision-making process for both donors and their families. Transplant centers employ multidisciplinary teams of health care professionals to provide care to potential donors and recipients. The teams include physicians, transplant surgeons, psychiatrists, nurses, social workers, physiotherapists, and dieticians.

15. Does the hospital give the donor and recipient information about each other?

Information about the donor and recipient is treated confidentially. The transplant center does not give the donor and recipient information about each other. The process of assessment for donation and need for confidentiality should be explained at the outset of testing. It is up to the donor to inform the recipient about results of his or her testing if he or she so wishes. Most transplant centers help donors to provide such information if they so wish.

16. Name the ethical principles that apply in living organ donation.

- Autonomy: Self-determination of the donor and absence of coercion are primary concerns.
- Beneficence: The goal of medical intervention is patient wellbeing.
- Nonmaleficence: Physicians will "first do no harm."
- Justice: Patients are treated equally.

The principle of autonomy recognizes that decisions about medical procedures rest in the donors' hands. To make autonomous decisions, donors must be capable of understanding the benefits and burdens of the alternative courses of action available to them; they must be fully informed about the burdens and benefits; and they must be free of pressure or coercion in making a decision to donate.

The principle of beneficence requires health care providers to act in the best interests of their patients. It may require providers to refrain from offering or recommending treatments that are more likely to do harm than good to patients.

The principle of nonmaleficence is a contemporary restatement of the imperative to do no harm.Health care providers must ensure that procedures offered to patients are accompanied by the least possible degree of harm.

Considerations about justice are used to help make decisions about the allocation of scarce resources among patients in a fair way. Justice-based decisions ensure that patients are treated equally unless there are morally relevant differences (such as need or medical efficiency) among them.

The risk to the donor is only justified by the benefit that accrues to the recipient. Transplantation from a living donor is performed only after the physicians are satisfied that they may expect minimal risk to the donor and after they are sure that donor is acting acting voluntarily.

17. Define the term *informed consent*.

Informed consent is a process that has four components. They are competence to understand the information, disclosure of the appropriate facts, understanding of the information by the patient, and voluntary consent to the procedure. The purpose of informed consent is the advancement of the principle of autonomous choice.

The health care team discloses to the potential living donor the information necessary to make the decision to donate. It consists of the risks and benefits involved in living donation at time of surgery and in the long term. It should ensure that the potential living donor is aware of all treatment options and likely outcomes for the recipient. Also, it should include the outcomes of the proposed surgery at the hospital in question as well as national statistics.

18. What is coercion to donate?

External coercion refers to the use of force to make a person do something against his or her wishes. In living donation, coercion applies to a situation in which a donor is threatened with sanctions such as the withdrawal of a parent's love or the danger of being outcast by a family or of being removed from a parent's will if potential donor does not agree to donate an organ. Pressure on a donor may increase if he or she is the only family member who is ABO compatible or is singled out by the family to be the donor because of being the only sibling without dependents. Essentially, coercion prevents a donor from acting autonomously.

Internal coercion refers to a person's feeling of obligation to donate due to internal factors such as religious or cultural beliefs. The sense of obligation may conflict with other issues in the donor's life. For instance, a young mother may feel a strong duty to donate to a sibling because she places high value on family members' helping each other, while simultaneously feeling that her husband and children would be negatively affected by her absence from the home during surgery and recuperation. It is essential that potential donors clarify their feelings and resolve the conflicts before deciding whether they wish to donate.

19. Describe how coercion may be addressed by a transplant center.

The transplant center must take all possible steps to ensure that a living donor's offer to donate is made freely and voluntarily. This necessity should be clarified with recipients and potential donors at the beginning of the assessment process. Donors should be interviewed alone and assured that the transplant center's role is to help the potential donor decide whether he or she is willing to donate, rather than to persuade the donor to donate. Assessment of donors and recipients by separate health care teams reduces conflict of interest for health care professionals, promotes confidentiality, and enhances the donor's ability to withdraw if concerns for self arise.

20. Who decides if a potential donor is suitable to donate?

First, the recipient must agree to transplantation from the potential donor. Second, the donor must convince the transplant assessment team that he or she is acting voluntarily. Third, the transplant team must review the potential donor's test results to establish whether donation is likely to have a negative effect on the donor's health, both currently and in the future. The donor physician acts as an independent donor advocate and makes the final decision on the acceptability of the donor. Donor approval is specific to time and to person; i.e., the individual donor is approved to donate to the individual recipient at this particular time.

21. Which factors are addressed during the psychosocial assessment of living donors?

The assessment focuses on donor motivation; informed consent; ability to cope with stress; psychological health; expectations about donation; the nature of the relationship between the donor and recipient; family support; attitudes about donation; and issues of employment, financial concerns, accommodation, and childcare. It is important that the donor's expectations be realistic (e.g., that the donor has considered the possibility of a poor outcome or disease recurrence in the recipient). The donor's feelings around these issues should be explored during the psychosocial assessment.

22. What are the psychosocial contraindications to living donation?

The psychosocial assessment of potential living donors must address certain concerns that could have a negative impact on transplant outcomes:

- Evidence that the donor is not fully informed or is unable to understand the risks and costs of donation
- Cognitive impairment

- External coercion placed on the donor by family or social affiliations such as religion
- Serious psychiatric illnesses that are not well controlled
- Pathological behaviors
- Lifestyle behaviors such as substance abuse which put the donor at risk
- Anxiety, fear of the surgery, obsessional indecision, or ambivalence
- Inadequate social support such as lack of financial resources
- Serious concerns and objections to donation by the donor's immediate family
- Difficulties in the relationship between the donor and recipient
- Indication that the donor was nominated to donate by the family, which may suggest collusion

23. How does living donation affect the donor's family?

The effect on the donor's immediate family is considerable because the donor is a healthy person undergoing an unnecessary major surgery and risk by giving away a part of his or her body. Family members may be concerned about pain and discomfort for their loved one. They may feel resentment over the intrusion in their lifestyle caused by the surgery and recuperative period. The partner or other family member will have to take on some of the duties of the donor and may experience a sense of being overwhelmed. For some time, the healthy partner may have to carry the responsibility of being the caregiver for the donor as well as continuing to work and look after children and household. If there is a history of illness in the family, the need to donate to another member may arise in the future. Then the donor must decide to which family member he or she feels the most obligation, and the family may have to address the possibility of other possible donors.

24. Is it important that a living donor's family be supportive of the decision to donate?

Family support is important for two reasons. On a practical level, families will be touched by issues such as loss of income, disruption of family life at time of surgery, anxiety about the success of the operation, and the need to care for the donor after discharge. Lack of support for donation could lead to conflict over these issues within the family. Donation involves risk. Medical complications or death has far-reaching effects on family members.

Second, donors usually need emotional support. If the outcome of donation is poor (e.g., the organ is rejected or the donor has complications), it is particularly important that the donor's family had supported the decision to donate so that they may be better able to cope with the disappointment themselves, to help the donor emotionally, and to avoid negative repercussions towards the recipient or the transplant center.

Just as family support is important, it is essential that the donor's partner be interviewed during the assessment process to evaluate his or her level of commitment to the proposed donation and that of other family members. Where there is a lack of family support for donation, it is important to explore the reasons. They may include fear for the donor's health, a poor relationship with the recipient or the recipient's family, or a belief that the recipient is not worthy of the donation or may not take care of the organ. Such issues need to be addressed before donation. The interview is generally conducted by a social worker, psychiatrist or psychiatric nurse.

25. How do people decide if they want to donate?

Simmons et al. described two social, psychological donor decision-making models. One is the **moral model**, which is based not on weighing the costs and benefits of donation but on norms that govern behavior such as family and social values. The decision is usually spontaneous and impulsive. The second model is the **rational or deliberative model**, which includes several steps specifically dealing with becoming informed and evaluating the alternatives. The second model gives credence to the potential donor's concerns about his or her physical and psychological wellbeing.

26. What happens if a potential living donor is uncertain about becoming a donor?

The goal of the transplant team is to help donors arrive at a decision that is best for them and to help them cope with any discomfort which their decision may cause. Donor need to be given adequate time to come to a decision. They should be asked at the beginning of testing and again during the testing process if they are unsure about donating, and they should be reassured that it is acceptable to withdraw at any time. Donors should be seen alone and helped to separate their own needs from those of the recipient and encouraged to do what feels best to them. The nurse, social worker, psychiatrist, and physician provide the opportunity for patients to explore concerns. Donors should not be encouraged to make any particular choice regarding donation but should be helped to arrive at their decision through a process of problem solving.

27. If a potential donor decides not to donate, how does he or she deal with consequent feelings about the decision?

The donor may need to examine his or her other responsibilities and obligations and put the role of donor in the context of personal, family, and career interests. The donor should be made aware of other treatment alternatives for the recipient. Attitudes about his or her decision not to donate should be nonjudgmental. Not everyone can emotionally handle undergoing voluntary major surgery. Nondonation may have a negative effect on the relationship with the recipient and family of origin. Staff members need to help the donor understand that there are several ways of caring for the recipient, and these alternatives need to be explored.

28. How is the recipient informed when a potential donor decides not to donate?

Transplant centers vary in how they handle a potential donor's decision not to donate. The goal is to respect confidentiality while helping the recipient and the potential donor deal with such a decision and how it affects their relationship. The recipient and the donor are informed in the beginning that there are many factors involved in becoming an acceptable donor. The person being tested may not be suitable for many reasons, including physical, social, and psychological. When it is determined that a donor wishes to withdraw, he or she will be assisted by the team to decide the most truthful and acceptable reason possible.

Staff may divulge donor information to the recipient only with the consent of the donor. Theoretically, the donor need only say that he or she is not a suitable donor. However, families may not be satisfied with this answer. They may fear a health problem or ask for more details.

The transplant social worker or nurse should ask the potential donor how he or she would like the recipient to be informed and whether there are other people who should be informed (e.g., children, parents, and siblings). The donor may need time to consider the best way of telling the recipient and may need the help of staff in making this decision. Some people benefit from help in choosing which words to use and determining where and when to tell the recipient. If the donor wishes, a member of the team will inform the recipient that the donor is not suitable; then the weight of the decision rests with the professionals. Both the donor and recipient should be offered counseling, as needed, during the period after the decision has been communicated.

29. Do many people regret having donated an organ?

Few follow-up studies have been done. In a study by Simmons and colleagues, 31% of living donors reported depression after donation; 14% had concerns for their own health; 16% had concerns about sexuality; and 26% were concerned with their appearance. Some donors felt that their altruistic offering was not adequately appreciated. Finally, 8–35% of donors report that they never returned to their previous state of health or that they feel that donation permanently harmed them.

There is the danger that the donor's generosity will be forgotten or not acknowledged sufficiently after donation. This lack of acknowledgment may leave some donors feeling unneeded or unimportant or that they have been taken advantage of. Some may feel that their pain, discomfort and significant inconvenience are forgotten too soon. Attention may focus on the recipient, who is followed by the transplant team after the donor's medical care has ended. This emphasis may cause friction between the donor, recipient, and their families.

30. What are the psychosocial advantages of organ donation for a living donor?

Living donors come from a wide range of social, religious, and family backgrounds. Some immediate positive feelings are associated with offering to be a donor, such as the recipient's gratitude, family support and recognition, and society's approval. Donors report a 70% sense of increased self-esteem, an increase in a general feeling of happiness, increased self-worth, and a better quality of relationship with the recipient. These positive feelings tend to last for years. Most donors do not suffer lasting negative physical or psychosocial consequences.

31. What are the psychosocial outcomes for a living donor when the recipient has a poor outcome?

If the transplant is not successful or the recipient dies, the donor may feel partially responsible and be distressed by grief. He or she may be lost to follow-up and left to deal with troubled feelings alone. What starts out as a shared commitment between the donor and recipient may end with a donor feeling abandoned and possibly abused. Donors may need support or professional intervention such as counselling to cope with a poor outcome of donation.

BIBLIOGRAPHY

1. Abecassis M, Adams M, Adams P, et al: The Live Organ Donor Consensus Group: Consensus statement on the live organ donor. JAMA 284:2919–2926, 2000.
2. Beauchamp TL, Childress JF: Principles of biomedical ethics. In Beauchamp TL, Childress JF (eds): Principles of Biomedical Ethics, 4th ed. City, Oxford University Press, 1994, pp 142–146.
3. The Council of the Transplantation Society: Commercialization in transplantation: The problems and some guidelines for practice. Transplantation 41:1–3, 1986.
4. Daar AS: Paid organ donation—the grey basket concept. J Med Ethics 24:365–368, 1998.
5. Matas A, Garvey C, Jacobs CL, Kahn JP: Nondirected donation of kidneys from living donors. N Engl J Med 343:433–436, 2000.
6. Olbrisch ME, Benedict SM, Haller DL, Levenson JL: Psychosocial assessment of living organ donors: Clinical and ethical considerations. Prog Transplant 11:40–49, 2001.
7. Ross LF: Justice for children: The child as organ donor. Bioethics 8,105–126, 1994.
8. Simmons RG, Klein SD, Simmons RL: The Gift of Life: the Social and Psychological Impact of Organ Transplantation. New York, Wiley Interscience. 1977.
9. Simmons RG, Marine SK, Simmons RL, et al: The Gift of Life: The Effect of Organ Transplantation on Individuals, Family and Societal Dynamics, 2nd ed. New Brunswick, NJ,. Transaction Books, 1987.
10. Spital A: Ethical and policy issues in altruistic living and cadaveric organ donation. Clin Transplant 11: 77–87. 1997.
11. Spital A, Kokmen T: Health insurance for kidney donors. Transplantation 62:1356–1358, 1996.
12. Switzer, GE, Simmons RG, Dew MA: Helping unrelated strangers. J Appl Social Psychol 26:469–490. 1996.
13. Terasaki PI, Cecka JM, Gjertson DW, Takemoto,S: High survival rates of kidney transplants from spousal and living unrelated donors. N Engl J Med 333:336–336, 1995.
14. Woodle ES, Ross LF: Paired exchanges should be part of the solution to ABO incompatibility in living donor kidney transplantation. Transplantation 66:406–407, 1998.
15. Wright L, MacRae S, Gordon D, et al: Ethical Guidelines for the Care of Living Donors. Submitted for publication 2001.
16. Zenios SA, Woodle S, Ross LF: Primum non-nocere: Avoiding harm to vulnerable wait list candidates in an indirect kidney exchange. Transplantation 72:648–654, 2001.

19. PEDIATRIC SOLID ORGAN TRANSPLANTATION

Lisa S. *Pearlman*, RN, MN, ACNP

RENAL TRANSPLANTATION

1. Explain why renal transplantation is the preferred option for pediatric patients with end-stage renal disease.

Renal transplantation is the treatment of choice for the majority of children with end-stage renal disease (ESRD) because of improved physical, psychological, and social rehabilitative outcomes associated with transplantation. All forms of dialysis and renal replacement therapy lead to a deceleration of growth and are associated with noncompliant behavior due to strict dietary and fluid restrictions. Following transplantation, children are better able to attend school and to develop normally, thus improving their overall quality of life.

2. Name the most common cause of end-stage renal disease in children.

The most common cause of ESRD in children varies significantly with age. Children under the age of 5 years are more likely than older children to develop ESRD as a result of aplastic, hypoplastic, or dysplastic kidneys and obstructive uropathy. After age 6 years, focal glomerulosclerosis becomes a primary cause of ESRD. The primary difference in the cause of ESRD between children and adults is that children have a higher incidence of congenital, urologic, and hereditary diseases and rarely develop diabetic nephropathy.

3. When is the optimal time to refer children with end-stage renal disease for renal transplantation?

There is no straightforward answer to this complicated question. In pediatric transplant centers, all children progressing to ESRD who require dialysis are considered candidates for transplantation. The ambiguity lies in the definition of ESRD, which remains controversial. In some transplant centers, ESRD is equated with patients who are dialysis-dependent, but this classification does not capture the ever-growing group of patients who receive preemptive transplantation without ever receiving dialysis.

4. Is Wilms' tumor a contraindication to pediatric renal transplantation?

Wilms tumor is the primary malignancy causing ESRD in children. Currently, many pediatric renal transplant centers will transplant children with Wilms' tumor who have been disease-free for 1 year. Earlier transplantation has been associated with the development of recurrent or metastatic disease. There are also reports that premature renal transplantation for Wilms' tumor patients has been associated with overwhelming sepsis, likely related to a combination of chemotherapy and immunosuppressants.

5. What are the most common causes of morbidity and mortality after pediatric renal transplantation?

Actuarial patient survival rates at 1, 2, and 5 years after pediatric renal transplantation are 96.5%, 95.6% and 92.7%, respectively. Short- and long-term graft and patient survival is improved for live donor recipients, particularly the youngest recipients. Live donors offer recipients improved HLA matches, shorter cold ischemia time, and lower acute rejection rates.

The use of infant donors under the age of 2 years was originally thought to be most appropriate for infants and young pediatric recipients, considering that the transplanted kidney has been shown to grow over time. However, it has been found that infant donor grafts have a high incidence of vascular thrombosis and graft loss.

Patient survival is lowest in the patients under 6 years old, especially with cadaveric donor kidneys. Other factors affecting graft survival include presensitization with repeated blood transfusions, graft dysfunction within 30 days of transplant, black race, underlying renal diseases, including oxalosis, congenital nephrotic syndrome, and Denys Drash syndrome.

Graft dysfunction, graft thrombosis, acute tubular necrosis, and rejection occur more frequently in children than adults. Children younger than 2 years old present the highest risk for graft failure after renal transplantation. North American Pediatric Renal Transplant Cooperative Study (NAPRTCS) provides data suggesting that young children may be at a higher risk for graft rejection than older children and may require more aggressive immunosuppression. Vascular anastomosis is more time consuming in a uremic infant or toddler with small vessels, thereby increasing the risk of urinary obstruction and leaks associated with impaired graft function.

According to the NAPRTCS, infection is the major cause of death followed by cardiopulmonary events, malignancy, and hemorrhage. Infection is the second most common cause of hospitalization in pediatric renal transplant patients. Urinary tract infections (UTIs) caused by *Staphylococcus aureus* or *Escherichia coli* and respiratory infections are prevalent in the first month after transplantation. Patients are prescribed trimethoprim-sulfamethoxazole to reduce the incidence of UTIs and to prevent *Pneumocystis carinii* pneumonia. The herpes virus infections are discussed below.

In pediatric renal transplantation, recurrence of the primary disease accounts for 5–15% of graft losses. Hyperoxaluria and focal segmental glomerulosclerosis (FSGS) are known to recur very rapidly in the renal allograft. The recurrence of oxalate deposits in the allograft eventually leads to graft failure. In children, the optimal strategy to prevent systemic oxalosis is to perform a combined liver and kidney transplant, which improves patient survival. FSGS has a recurrence rate of 20–60%. Other diseases affecting morbidity and mortality include membranoproliferative glomerulonephritis, IgA nephropathy, Henoch-Schönlein purpura, hemolytic uremic syndrome, and membranous nephropathy.

Pediatric patients experience hypertension after transplantation. The cause and pathogenesis are multifactorial and thought to occur as a result of corticosteroids, calcineurin inhibitors, rejection, renal artery stenosis, renin output from native kidneys, and urinary tract obstruction. Studies have indicated an association between the use of antihypertensive medications and graft failure.

6. Describe the clinical presentation of acute rejection in the pediatric renal transplant patient.

Rejection continues to be problematic for pediatric renal transplant patients and can occur within minutes following the reperfusion of the graft (hyperacute rejection) to weeks and months later (acute rejection). Pediatric renal transplant patients may present with decreased urinary output, increased urea and creatinine, fluid retention and weight gain, graft tenderness, fever, anorexia, and malaise.

The challenge for practitioners is to distinguish rejection from infection and calcineurin nephrotoxicity. Urinalysis and urine cultures are performed to determine the presence of proteinuria, leukocytes, and other cells in the sediment. A renal ultrasound identifies any structural abnormalities and obstructions. A renal scan identifies delayed excretion of the tracer by the kidney, which is suggestive of rejection. Acute rejection is confirmed through percutaneous renal biopsy.

HEART TRANSPLANTATION

7. What are the primary indications for pediatric heart transplantation?

Infants and children with complex congenital heart disease whose condition is refractory to medical management and surgical palliation represent the majority of patients (75%) less than 1 year of age referred for transplantation. The second group, the cardiomyopathies, account for approximately 65% of all pediatric heart transplants in children greater than 1 year of age. A smaller percentage of patients with viral myocarditis, benign cardiac tumors, and advanced Kawasaki disease are referred for heart transplantation.

8. When is the optimal time to refer pediatric patients for heart transplantation?

In the majority of cases, pediatric patients are referred for heart transplantation when there is evidence of progressive deterioration of ventricular function, ongoing requirements of continuous inotropic support, progressive pulmonary hypertension, malignant arrhythmias that are unresponsive to medical management, growth failure, and a poor quality of life.

9. What are the contraindications to pediatric heart transplantation?

The majority of children with end-stage cardiac failure are candidates for heart transplantation. Patients with cardiomyopathies require careful assessment to determine the genetic and metabolic implications following transplant. Children with irreversible central nervous system, lung, renal, or liver disease may be excluded following the transplant work-up.

Children with high HLA titers require prospective crossmatching with the donor prior to transplantation to avoid hyperacute rejection related to HLA-antibody destruction of the allograft.

10. What are the most common causes of morbidity and mortality after pediatric heart transplantation?

Graft survival is estimated to be approximately 80% at 1 year following pediatric heart transplantation. The most common causes of morbidity and mortality include rejection, infection, graft coronary artery disease (CAD), pulmonary hypertension, and malignancy. Infants and young children are at a high risk of developing moderate-to-severe tricuspid regurgitation as a result of injury to the valve leaflets from repetitive endomyocardial biopsies (EMBs). Atrial arrhythmias are not uncommon. Electrocardiogram often reveals a right bundle branch block.

Viral agents cause the majority of infections, followed by bacterial agents. Viral infections are discussed below. Bacterial infections are found most often in the lungs, followed by the blood, urinary tract, and sternal wound. In addition to the bacterial agents responsible for infection following conventional cardiac surgery, pediatric transplant recipients are at risk for fungi (*Candida*, *Aspergillus*, *Cryptococcus*) and protozoa (*Pneumocystis carinii*).

CAD, or graft atherosclerosis, is a manifestation of chronic rejection in heart allografts. It is a progressive process that leads to graft loss. The precise cause of CAD remains unclear, although it is thought to be a form of immunologically mediated vessel injury, leading to coronary artery narrowing and intraluminal proliferation and thickening. Unlike native coronary atherosclerosis, posttransplant CAD is a diffuse process with a significant degree of distal vessel involvement.

Incidence of CAD is reported in between 10 and 50% of children. CAD must be considered in pediatric patients who present with syncope. Because the heart is denervated, it is rare for patients to experience angina during ischemic episodes, even in advanced disease. Unfortunately, sudden death may be the first presentation of coronary vasculopathy in the pediatric patient.

Factors associated with the development of CAD include acute cellular rejection, prolonged corticosteroid use, the administration of cytotoxic B-cell antibody, hypertension, dyslipidemia, and recurrent cytomegalovirus (CMV) disease. CAD may be detected by coronary angiography done every 1–2 years. Many centers are adopting the use of the dobutamine stress echocardiogram as a noninvasive procedure to determine the functional status of graft coronary arteries.

Pediatric patients are now being treated with calcium channel blockers such as diltiazem to prevent or delay the onset of CAD and with HMG-CoA reductase inhibitors (pravastatin, atorvastatin) to reduce the risk of both CAD and rejection.

11. Describe the clinical presentation of acute rejection in the pediatric heart transplant patient.

The incidence of acute rejection is greatest within the first 3 months after transplantation and decreases markedly thereafter. The majority of patients experience a minimum of one episode of acute rejection in the first year of transplant. Most pediatric patients are asymptomatic because rejection is often not associated with symptoms until it is progressive and severe. Clinical signs and symptoms such as fever, fatigue, irritability, nonspecific abdominal complaints, vomiting, poor feeding in infants, and diaphoresis are difficult to distinguish from infection.

Tachycardia, a gallop rhythm, dysrhythmia, and hepatomegaly raise the index of suspicion for further investigation. There are no blood tests that are currently predictive of acute rejection. Chest radiograph may indicate an enlarged cardiac silhouette, and the electrocardiogram may demonstrate decreased voltages of Q, R, and S waves. Echocardiography may demonstrate wall thickening and decreased diastolic or systolic ventricular function.

Endomyocardial biopsy (EMB) is considered the gold standard for detecting acute rejection in children, yet there is controversy about the necessity and frequency of such an invasive procedure after the first year following transplantation. Some transplant centers base clinical progress using a regular surveillance echocardiogram protocol to detect changes in heart function, without the regular use of surveillance endomyocardial biopsies. Other transplant centers condone EMB as the primary diagnostic test to guide all clinical decisions. In these centers, EMB may be performed as often as every 1–4 weeks during the first 3–6 months after transplantation. Following a rejection episode, a repeat biopsy is usually obtained in several weeks.

The greatest risk of performing EMB is cardiac perforation, although incidence is low. A limitation to relying on the EMB to diagnose rejection includes sampling error in the case of obtaining poor quality specimens and the lack of inter-rater reliability in accurately identifying grades of rejection. Lastly, the EMB has a limited ability to account for the presence of vascular rejection, which is not demonstrated by acute cellular pathology.

12. Why are neonates and infants at lower risk of rejection than older children?

The neonate is born with an underdeveloped immune system that matures postnatally throughout childhood and adolescence. This offers neonates the opportunity for improved outcomes after heart transplantation because of a lower number of mature and killer T cells present in conjunction with a lower cytokine production profile, which are important processes of rejection.

Recent evidence supports that neonates and infants under 6 months of age do not make antibodies to blood group antigens, making ABO-incompatible heart transplantation a reality for patients in this age group. Early studies reveal that rejection patterns of ABO-incompatible recipients are similar to those of infants transplanted with blood type-compatible donor hearts, thus expanding the donor pool for this unique patient population.

LUNG TRANSPLANTATION

13. What are the primary indications for pediatric lung transplantation?

The most common diseases leading to end-stage respiratory failure in children are cystic fibrosis (CF), primary pulmonary hypertension, idiopathic pulmonary fibrosis, and obliterative bronchiolitis. Infant lung transplantation has been performed for pulmonary vascular disease and severe parenchymal lung disease.

14. When is the optimal time to refer pediatric patients for lung transplantation?

Pediatric lung transplantation is indicated for patients who are expected to have a poor prognosis with a life expectancy of less than 1 year. Specific markers of disease progression include the following:

- FEV_1 of less than 30% of predicted values
- Frequent pulmonary exacerbations leading to hospitalization or intravenous antibiotic therapy
- Poor exercise tolerance
- Poor nutrition
- Pulmonary hypertension
- Increasing microbial resistance

15. Are ventilated pediatric patients considered candidates for lung transplantation?

There is no straightforward answer to this controversial question. In some transplant centers, mechanical ventilation is an absolute contraindication to transplantation because ventilator-dependency is a significant predictor of adverse outcomes. In other centers, however, successful lung transplantation has been performed on ventilated patients. Patients who develop an acute, reversible process and who are already on the waiting list for lung transplantation may be considered for short-term ventilation.

16. What are the most common causes of morbidity and mortality after pediatric lung transplantation?

One-year graft survival is reported at 75%. Pretransplant factors that affect survival include oxygen-dependence, the requirement for assisted ventilation, and the presence of aortopulmonary collateral vessels. Prolonged ischemic time and non-Caucasian, female recipients are linked with poorer outcomes.

Anastomotic stenosis and bronchomalacia occur more frequently in pediatric lung transplant recipients because of the small, narrow and compliant cartilage. Infants and small children under 3 years of age are at increased risk for graft injury due to aspiration secondary to gastroesophageal reflux.

It has been hypothesized that pediatric lung transplant patients are at a greater risk for infection than adult recipients because of smaller airways, impaired mucocilliary clearance, and a suboptimal cough reflex below the anastomosis site as a result of airway denervation. The infectious risk for pediatric patients is further heightened because of the social behavior of children, which is aggravated by infectious agents found in densely populated school and day care settings. Respiratory syntial virus, adenovirus, and parainfluenza are problematic for young recipients. Infections caused by *Aspergillus* are associated with high morbidity and present clinically as pneumonia, tracheobronchitis, aspergilloma, and systemic infection. Patients with CF are particularly at risk for developing allograft infections as a result of endogenous gram-negative organisms found in their sinuses and trachea. Several pediatric transplant centers have reported serious clinical problems with CF patients infected with *Bukholderia cepacia*.

Children with CF have additional complications that affect morbidity posttransplantation. Malabsorption of fat-soluble medications, such as cyclosporine, is problematic for patients with pancreatic insufficiency, necessitating close monitoring and evaluation of therapeutic blood levels. Additional sequelae of pancreatic insufficiency such as diabetes mellitus and osteoporosis are aggravated by corticosteroid therapy.

Bronchiolitis obliterans syndrome (BOS), a form of chronic rejection, continues to pose a threat to the achievement of long-term success in pediatric lung transplantation. It is a gradual destructive process of the small airways evident by decreasing airflow lung volumes found on pulmonary function. BO is diagnosed by either transbronchial biopsy or open lung biopsy. Prognosis remains poor because the majority of patients succumb to respiratory failure and death.

17. Describe the clinical presentation of acute rejection in pediatric lung transplantation.

The majority of pediatric patients who undergo transplantation experience at least one episode of acute rejection in the first year after transplant. The clinical signs and symptoms of acute rejection in pediatric lung transplantation range on a continuum from the patient being asymptomatic to severe respiratory distress. The diagnosis is complicated by symptoms that may either be subtle or difficult to distinguish from a respiratory infection.

Like adults, children may present with fever, cough, dyspnea, and fatigue. Physical examination of the chest may reveal wheezes and crackles. A greater than 10% fall in oxygen saturation and forced expiratory volume in 1-second (FEV_1) raises the index of suspicion of rejection. Acute rejection often presents as new or increased pleural effusions and air-space disease on chest radiograph. The diagnosis of rejection is confirmed by tissue obtained during a transbronchial biopsy. Before the development of flexible bronchoscopes for small children, there was a high morbidity associated with hemorrhage and perforation in young patients.

LIVER TRANSPLANTATION

18. What are disease-specific indications for pediatric liver transplantation?

Liver transplantation is standard therapy for children with end-stage liver failure caused by acute or chronic disease. Acute liver failure includes fulminant hepatitis, metabolic liver disease, inborn errors of metabolism, and liver tumors. Of the chronic liver diseases, biliary atresia accounts for approximately 43–50% of all pediatric liver transplants. Other indications include cholestatic liver disease, inherited metabolic liver disease, chronic active hepatitis, and cirrhosis.

19. When is the optimal timing of transplantation for children with end-stage liver failure?

Many pediatric transplant centers recommend early referral of children for liver transplantation when one or more of the following criteria are present:
- Intractable cholestasis
- Portal hypertension with variceal bleeding
- Severe hypersplenism with thrombocytopenia
- Refractory ascending cholangitis
- Failure of liver synthetic function with coagulopathy and hypoalbuminemia
- Failure to thrive and malnutrition
- Intractable ascites
- Encephalopathy (hyperammonemia and selected metabolic defects)
- Unacceptable quality of life (intractable pruritis or cholesteatomas associated with cholestatic liver disease)

20. What are the contraindications to pediatric liver transplantation?

Absolute contraindications in pediatric liver transplantation are rare. Relative contraindications in children include life-threatening or severely disabling extrahepatic multiorgan system failure not alleviated by transplantation, uncontrolled systemic sepsis of extrahepatic origin, and extrahepatic malignancy.

21. Which innovative surgical techniques are performed to expand donor availability and reduce waiting list deaths in pediatric liver transplantation?

Reduction of liver allografts is performed by surgically reducing an adult-sized or large cadaveric organ to fit into the child's smaller abdominal cavity. The left lateral segment of the liver is transplanted, whereas the right side of the donor organ is discarded. The disadvantage is that only one child benefits because suitable liver tissue remains unused. This intolerable waste led to the development of split liver transplantation.

The surgical creation of splitting a liver allograft was developed to enable one cadaveric donor allograft to be transplanted into two recipients, the smaller left lateral segment for a small child and the right lobe for an adult or larger child. Split liver transplantation increases the donor pool by allowing two recipients to benefit from one liver.

Living-related liver transplantation has been performed by removing the left lobe or left lateral segment of a parent or relative. The success rate for the recipient is similar to that reported for cadaveric transplantation, with donor morbidity and mortality reported as low. The primary benefit of living donor transplantation is that it allows for optimal timing of the transplant before the development of complications from end-stage liver disease. Because the graft is obtained from a healthy donor, there is minimal, if any, ischemic injury in the graft, and the total ischemic time is greatly reduced.

22. What are the most common causes of morbidity and mortality after pediatric liver transplantation?

According to the United Network for Organ Sharing [UNOS], 1-year graft survival is 71–87%. Patient survival is reported to be 81–94%. Factors that influence morbidity and mortality are the severity of liver failure, malnutrition, renal dysfunction, coagulopathy, and sepsis experienced preoperatively; allograft function; surgical complications; sepsis; and the side effect profile of immunosuppressants. In some situations, as in the case of hepatitis B virus, autoimmune hepatitis and giant-cell hepatitis are known to recur in the liver allograft.

The most important surgical complications in the pediatric patient are hepatic artery thrombosis (HAT), biliary leaks, bleeding, and bowel perforation. HAT occurs most often in infants and small children and is the most common cause of pediatric graft loss. HAT may present clinically as fulminant hepatic failure, biliary leaks, and late biliary stricture. The biliary complications occur because the biliary system is dependent on the hepatic artery. Bleeding is a function of the coagulopathy associated with poor graft function. Bowel perforation is most common in infants and children with biliary atresia who have had previous abdominal surgery.

23. Describe the clinical presentation of acute rejection in the pediatric liver transplant patient.

In the majority of situations, patients are asymptomatic, with elevated transaminases noted on routine monitoring. Clinically, patients may present with fever, fatigue, abdominal tenderness, irritability, and transaminitis with increasing bilirubin levels. Progressive symptoms may include ascites, jaundice, acholic stools, bile-stained urine, and renal impairment. A percutaneous liver biopsy confirms a diagnosis of rejection.

INTESTINAL TRANSPLANTATION

24. What are the primary indications for pediatric intestinal transplantation?

Intestinal transplantation is an accepted therapy for infants and children with irreversible intestinal failure who develop life-threatening complications related to total parenteral nutrition (TPN). Irreversible intestinal failure refers to a reduction in the functional gut mass required to satisfy body, nutrient, and fluid requirements. Short bowel syndrome, defective intestinal motility disorders including intestinal pseudo-obstruction, and congenital enterocyte abnormalities such as microvillus inclusion disease are the most common disorders referred for pediatric intestinal transplantation.

25. Which life-threatening complications of parenteral nutrition require consideration for intestinal transplantation?

TPN extends the life of children with intestinal failure and affords them the opportunity for quality of life when previously they would have died. However, TPN is associated with several life-threatening complications including irreversible TPN-induced liver disease, recurring life-threatening catheter-associated sepsis, loss of indwelling venous catheters due to recurring thromboses, and pulmonary embolism

26. Which unique factors are considered in the donor selection for pediatric intestinal transplant recipients?

Grafts for pediatric intestinal transplantation must be from an ABO-identical, age-, size-, CMV-matched donor. Donors with prolonged low cardiac output syndrome or those with a history of prolonged cardiopulmonary arrest are rarely accepted because of the likelihood of bowel ischemia.

27. What are the contraindications to intestinal transplantation?

The following clinical criteria exclude candidacy for pediatric intestinal transplantation:
- Profound neurologic disabilities
- Life-threatening diseases unrelated to the gastrointestinal system
- Severe immune deficiencies
- Nonresectable malignancies
- Multisystem autoimmune disease
- Insufficient vascular patency predicted to be less than 6 months

28. What are the most common causes of morbidity and mortality after pediatric intestinal transplantation?

Graft survival is estimated at 70–80% at 1 year and 50% at 5 years after transplantation. In the early postoperative period, patients with intestinal transplants may require extended intensive care because of graft malfunction and preoperative liver failure. Technical complications include biliary or intestinal anastomotic leaks, intestinal perforation, and hepatic artery thrombosis. In situations of a donor/recipient size mismatch, a delay in closing the abdominal wall may cause the patient to experience a respiratory distress syndrome related to an increase in intra-abdominal volume. The high levels of steroids and tacrolimus posttransplant often exacerbate pretransplant renal dysfunction.

There is a higher incidence of rejection (80–100%) in pediatric intestinal transplant recipients compared with other solid organ transplant groups. Consequently, a higher level of maintenance immunosuppression is required, which often leads to increased susceptibility to bacterial, fungal, and viral infections. Preoperative liver failure and sepsis also contribute to infectious complications. Patients are usually maintained on multiple antibiotic and antifungal regimens for several weeks after transplantation because infection is the primary cause of intestinal graft loss.

The presence of the Epstein-Barr virus (EBV) is associated with a higher incidence of posttransplant lymphoproliferative disease in intestinal transplant recipients because of the high prevalence of B-lymphocytes lining the gastrointestinal tract. Cytomegalovirus (CMV) is prevalent and often involves the allograft intestine. Clinical management includes the administration of ganciclovir alone or in combination with CMV high-titer immunoglobulin. Immunosuppression is rarely withdrawn because of the high incidence of rejection.

Patients continue on TPN initially and then are gradually weaned as oral or enteral nutrition is advanced. Because many of these children have not experienced the milestones for chewing, swallowing, and normal feeding behavior, they require a multidisciplinary approach of support to teach them to eat voluntarily. A small percentage of children require ongoing nocturnal enteral supplementation to ensure optimal nutrition to meet caloric and fluid requirements.

29. Describe the clinical presentation of acute rejection in the pediatric intestinal transplant patient.

Patients with intestinal transplants may present initially with nonspecific symptoms such as fever, abdominal tenderness, nausea, and vomiting. The stoma may become edematous, reddened, and friable with increasing drainage. With severe rejection, the patient likely experiences gastrointestinal bleeding, ulceration, and soughing of the intestinal mucosa.

There are no distinct clinical or predictive biochemical markers to identify rejection. Patients must undergo regular surveillance intestinal biopsy via endoscopy, which may demonstrate findings that are also consistent with infectious enteritis, making the diagnosis more difficult.

UNIQUE PEDIATRIC ISSUES

30. Why are viral infections problematic to the pediatric transplant patient?

Viral infections account for 25–30% of all posttransplant infections. Pediatric transplant recipients are five times more likely than adult recipients to develop primary viral syndromes. Infants and children are less likely to have preexisting immunity to community-acquired pathogens such as CMV and EBV and are therefore more likely to be seronegative at the time they receive a seropositive allograft. Such viruses are problematic because they are ubiquitous in the environment, and seroprevalence may exceed 90% in donor organs. Because the viruses are dormant in the donor organ tissue, they have the potential to become troublesome when the seronegative recipient receives immunosuppression.

31. Which two donor-associated viruses are particularly problematic in the first 6 months posttransplant?

Epstein-Barr virus (EBV) infection leads to a range of clinical illnesses including asymptomatic viremia, mononucleosis-type syndromes, proliferative tumors, and lymphomas. Following initial exposure, the EBV remains dormant for life. The pathogenesis of the exact events that trigger EBV proliferation are not known. However, we do know that EBV has the oncogenic potential to transform and immortalize B-lymphocytes, resulting in uncontrolled proliferation in patients taking immunosuppressive therapy.

The surveillance of EBV disease begins with the determination of the patient's seronegativity or seropositivity pretransplant to determine the risk once the EBV status of the allograft is known. Seronegative patients who receive a seropositive allograft should receive regular testing of the EBV antibody. Early detection of EBV polymerase chain reaction (PCR) is required following EBV seroconversion. Seroconverted patients with rising PCRs should be followed closely to identify early clinical symptomatology. Following an index of suspicion, patients require diagnostic imaging to determine the presence of EBV. EBV–posttransplantation lymphoproliferative disorder (PTLD) is confirmed by tissue sampling, preferably by excisional biopsy.

Treatment of EBV disease remains controversial, and there is no standardized treatment protocol among pediatric transplant centers. Goals of treatment may include the withdrawal of immunosuppression, the utilization of antiviral immunoglobulin therapy, and chemotherapy. Rituximab, an anti-CD-20 antibody has also been used successfully.

Cytomegalovirus (CMV) in pediatric transplant patients may be asymptomatic or may be exhibited by various symptoms ranging from fever, leukopenia, thrombocytopenia, pneumonitis, hepatitis, enteric ulceration, chorioretinitis, and allograft dysfunction.

There is no standardized protocol for the treatment of CMV among pediatric transplant centers. As with the treatment of EBV, treatment of CMV may include the withdrawal of immunosuppression and the use of antiviral therapy such as ganciclovir and immunoglobulin. Controversy remains related to the appropriate duration of therapy and the relevance of diagnostic markers in guiding clinical decision making.

32. Why is it so important for children to receive childhood immunizations before transplantation?

Vaccine-preventable diseases constitute a significant threat to pediatric solid organ transplant patients. It is highly recommended that these children be immunized before transplantation when the immunologic response is better. Live or live-attenuated vaccines are not recommended following transplantation, and immunization following transplantation may precipitate or potentiate rejection.

33. Is it safe for siblings to receive the measles-mumps-rubella vaccine?

Yes, despite the fact that measles-mumps-rubella (MMR) is a live-vaccine, there is no evidence of household transmission.

34. Is the immunosuppressed, varicella-zoster virus–seronegative patient at risk for contracting chicken pox?

The risk of varicella-zoster virus (VZV) relates to lifelong immunosuppressive therapy. High morbidity is associated with VZV that includes bacterial superinfection, pneumonitis, encephalitis, hepatitis, pancreatitis, and disseminated intravascular coagulation. Mortality rates as high as 25% have been reported in the transplant population.

35. What is the recommendation when a posttransplant patient is exposed to varicella-zoster virus?

The varicella-zoster vaccine is a live-attenuated vaccine currently contraindicated for children receiving immunosuppression. Patients who are VZV-seronegative posttransplant require passive immunization prophylaxis with varicella-zoster immunoglobulin [VZIG] 72–96 hours following exposure. VZIG is not indicated in patients who are VZV-seropositive. A diagnosis of varicella infection is based on the presence of a known exposure and the characteristic clinical appearance of the lesions; it is confirmed by the scraping of vesicular lesions for a positive identification of VZV through electron microscopy.

36. What is the treatment for an immunosuppressed patient who develops varicella-zoster virus?

The general principles of treatment for VZV include the administration of intravenous acyclovir, reduction or withdrawal of immunosuppression, and the monitoring of rejection. Transplant patients are usually switched to oral acyclovir providing that all existing lesions are dry and no new lesions appear. Patients who are concomitantly receiving acetylsalicylic acid (ASA) therapy should stop therapy because of the risk of Reye syndrome.

37. Is it safe for siblings to receive the chicken pox vaccine?

The benefit of vaccinating siblings outweighs the risk to the recipient and is therefore recommended. There are no patient precautions once the vaccine is administered to a sibling.

38. Describe the factors influencing the growth of pediatric transplant patients.

The majority of pediatric patients have preoperative stunted linear growth and malnutrition related to effects of their respective primary diseases in addition to end-stage organ failure. The severity of growth retardation is directly related to the age at onset of organ failure with the youngest infants experiencing the most severe limitations. Before transplantation, children with ESRD have had success in growth velocity with the use of recombinant human growth hormone (rhGH).

Achieving linear growth and maintaining optimal weight is of paramount importance to the pediatric transplant recipient's sense of well-being and ability to integrate into normal childhood and adolescent activities. The growth suppressant effect of corticosteroids, even in small doses, is well documented. Additional factors affecting growth velocity are allograft function, behavioral feeding problems, and the child's genetic growth potential. Caucasian recipients have improved growth potential in height compared with African-Americans or Hispanics.

All pediatric solid organ transplant recipients demonstrate the greatest catch-up growth in the youngest recipients, less than 6 years of age. Renal transplant patients demonstrate the greatest magnitude of growth retardation when compared with liver and heart recipients. One of the reasons suggested for this discrepancy is the younger age at transplant of liver and heart recipients and the shorter pretreatment course related to chronic and end-stage life-threatening disease.

39. Describe the unique features of pediatric noncompliance.

Noncompliance is an important focus for pediatric practitioners because it accounts for graft loss in 10–15% of all pediatric solid organ transplant patients. Noncompliance is viewed as the extent to which a patient's behavior coincides with the prescribed medical plan of care. It is a complex and multifaceted phenomenon, occurring on a continuum of adherence, partial adherence, and nonadherence.

The chronicity of organ failure and end-stage disease often leads to psychosocial and emotional problems in children and adolescents. Transplantation creates additional stressors for pediatric and adolescent patients who already struggle with low self-esteem and difficulty meeting the social, cognitive, educational, and vocational milestones of their healthy peers.

The cosmetic changes caused by immunosuppression, the strict medication regimen, diet and fluid restrictions, and the complexity and intensity of transplant follow-up commonly are manifested as noncompliance with the plan of care. Patients who suddenly or unexpectedly present with less cushinghoid features, subtherapeutic drug levels, decreased organ function, and late acute rejection should be assessed for nonadherence. A multidisciplinary, developmental, and educational approach is necessary to identify patients at risk and to implement initiatives to support patients and their families to plan for long-term graft survival.

BIBLIOGRAPHY

1. Al-Akash SI, Ettenger RB: Kidney transplantation in children. In GM Danovitch (ed): Handbook of Kidney Transplantation, 3rd ed. New York, Lippincott Williams & Wilkins, 2001, pp 332–364.
2. Atkinson P, Chatzipetrou M, Tsaroucha A, et al: Small bowel transplantation in children. Pediatr Transplant 1:11–118, 1997.

 3. Breinig MK, Zitelli B, Starzl TE, Ho M: Epstein-Barr virus, cytomegalovirus and other viral infections in children after transplant. J Infect Dis 156:273–279, 1999.
 4. Burroughs M, Moscona A: Immunization of pediatric solid organ transplant candidates and recipients. Clin Infect Dis 30: 857–869, 2000.
 5. Emre S: Living-donor liver transplantation in children. Pediatr Transplant 6:43–46, 2002.
 6. Fine RN: Growth following solid-organ transplantation. Pediatr Transplant 6:47–52, 2002.
 7. Fricker FJ, Addonizio L, Bernstein D, et al.: Heart transplantation in children: Indications. Pediatr Transplant 3:333–342, 1999.
 8. Huddleston CB: Lung transplantation: Recipient and donor outcomes in living donations. Rome, Italy, Programs and abstracts of the XVIII International Congress of the Transplantation Society, August 27–September 1, 2000.
 9. Kaufman SS, Atkinson JB, Bianchi A, et al: Indications for pediatric intestinal transplantation: A position paper for the American Society of Transplantation. Pediatr Transplant 5:80–87, 2001.
10. Kosmach B, Webber SA, Reyes J: Care of the solid organ transplant recipient. Pediatr Clin North Am 45:1395–1418, 1998.
11. Martin S: Posttransplant lymphoproliferative disease in a pediatric multivisceral transplant recipient. Crit Care Nurs 18:74–80, 1998.
12. Mazariegos GV, Reyes J: An update of current clinical practices in pediatric organ transplantation. Pediatr Rev 20:363–375, 1999.
13. Noyes BE, Kurland G, Orenstein DM: Lung and heart-lung transplantation in children. Pediatr Pulmonol 23:39–48, 1997.
14. Pandya A, Wasfy S, Hebert D, Allen UD: Varicella-zoster infection in the pediatric solid-organ transplant recipients: A hospital-based study in the prevaricella vaccine era. Pediatr Transplant 5:153–159, 2001.
15. Papalois VE, Majarian JS: Pediatric kidney transplantation: Historic hallmarks and a personal perspective. Pediatr Transplant 5:239–245, 2001.
16. Pirenne J, Koshiba T, Coosemans W, et al: Recent advances and future prospects in intestinal and multivisceral transplantation. Pediatr Transplant 5:452–456, 2001.
17. Stillwell PC, Mallory GB: Pediatric lung transplantation. Clin Chest Med 18:405–414, 1997.
18. Webber SA: 15 years of pediatric heart transplantation at the University of Pittsburgh: Lessons learned and future prospects. Pediatr Transplant 1:8–21, 1997.
19. West LJ, Pollock-Barsiv SM, Dipchand AI, et al: ABO-incompatible heart transplantation in infants. N Engl J Med 344:793–800, 2001.

20. INFECTIOUS DISEASE

Sandra A. Cupples, DNSc, RN

1. Why is infection in transplant candidates and recipients an important issue?

Infection is an important consideration for both transplant candidates and recipients. Many candidates may have a suboptimal response to vaccinations secondary to end-stage disease. Transplant candidates may also have preexisting infections associated with invasive catheters and devices (e.g., hemodialysis access devices, mechanical circulatory assist devices). Virtually all transplant recipients must take immunosuppressive agents to prevent rejection of the allograft, thereby increasing their risk of infection. This chapter discusses infection with respect to candidates, donors, and recipients. Information that applies to all adult solid organ transplant recipients is presented, as well as data specific to certain types of solid organ transplant procedures. Typical treatment options for the major posttransplant infections are presented. Recommendations regarding vaccinations for transplant candidates and recipients are summarized.

2. Name the types of infections that transplant candidates may harbor.

Transplant candidates may harbor preexisting active infections that, if undetected, may be especially problematic after transplantation. Major pretransplant infections among specific organ transplant candidates include the following[5]:

TYPE OF TRANSPLANT CANDIDATE	TYPE OF INFECTION
Kidney	Infection in native kidneys Occult abscesses Infections related to dialysis access devices or catheters Urinary tract infections
Pancreas	Urinary tract infections, particularly in women
Liver	Intra-abdominal infections (e.g., bacterial peritonitis) Aspiration pneumonia Catheter-related infections
Heart	Catheter-related infections Infections related to ventricular assist devices Pneumonia
Lung	Pneumonia Pulmonary bacterial or fungal colonization

3. Given that infections can be transmitted from the donor to the recipient, what does donor screening typically involve?

The donor's medical history is carefully reviewed, particularly with respect to vaccinations, prior infections, and unusual exposures to infection (e.g., residence in or travel to endemic areas, drug abuse, risky sexual behavior, or incarceration). In addition to the identification of current infection or colonization with organisms such as methicillin-resistant *Staphylococcus aureus* or vancomycin-resistant enterococci, donors are typically screened for the following agents[38]:

- Cytomegalovirus
- Human immunodeficiency virus
- Human T cell lymphotropic virus
- *Toxoplasma gondii*
- Epstein-Barr virus
- Hepatitis B virus
- Hepatitis C virus
- Syphilis
- History of tuberculosis or positive purified protein derivative (PPD) or other tuberculin test

4. Ideally, when should donor serologic testing be done?

Serum serologic testing ideally should be done before the administration of mass transfusions. If serologic testing is done after transfusion of the donor, the number of transfusions should be recorded. Often serologic testing is done both pre- and posttransfusion.

5. Is infection a significant problem after transplantation?

Infection is the leading cause of death in solid organ transplant recipients. Over two-thirds of recipients will have at least one episode of infection during the first posttransplant year.[34]

6. How are infection and rejection related?

The two major problems after solid organ transplantation are infection and rejection. Interventions designed to decrease the risk of rejection may increase the risk of infection. Conversely, interventions designed to decrease the risk of infection may increase the risk of rejection.

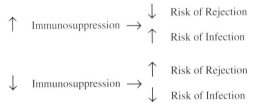

7. What are the two major sources of posttransplant infection?

Transplant recipients can develop infections from exogenous and endogenous sources:

EXOGENOUS SOURCES	ENDOGENOUS SOURCES
Allograft itself	Reactivation of latent infection
Blood transfusions	
Environment (hospital and community)	

8. When are transplant recipients at greatest risk for infection?

Transplant recipients are at increased risk for infection in the early postoperative period when immunosuppression doses are highest and any time immunosuppressive therapy is increased to treat rejection.

9. Which three factors determine the transplant recipient's risk for infection?

The three factors that determine the risk of infection are
1. Epidemiological exposure (hospital and community)
2. The patient's current preventive antimicrobial therapy (if any)
3. The patient's net state of immunosuppression

10. Discuss the two major types of exposure within the hospital environment.

Hospital exposures can be domiciliary or nondomiciliary. Domiciliary exposure occurs on the patient's unit, typically as a result of contamination of air or water with pathogens such as *Pseudomonas aeruginosa*. Other sources of domiciliary infection include vancomycin-resistant *Enterococcus faecium*, methicillin-resistant *Staphylococcus aureus*, and *Clostridium difficile* that are spread through person-to-person contact or through contaminated equipment.

Nondomiciliary exposure occurs when patients are exposed to contaminated air outside of the domiciliary unit, for example, during transport to other areas of the hospital such as radiology or surgery.[13]

11. Name the three major sources of community exposure.

The three major sources of community exposure include exposure to respiratory viruses, food-borne pathogens (e.g., salmonella), and the geographically restricted mycoses.

12. What is the patient's net state of immunosuppression?
The patient's net state of immunosuppression is the combined effect of the factors that influence the patient's susceptibility to infection. These factors include
- The current immunotherapy regimen
- Any concurrent infection caused by immune-modulating viruses: cytomegalovirus (CMV), Epstein-Barr virus (EBV), hepatitis B virus (HBV), hepatitis C virus (HCV), or human immunodeficiency virus (HIV)
- Any concurrent metabolic disorders such as malnutrition, uremia, diabetes mellitus
- Any concurrent neutropenia or lymphopenia
- Any disruption of normal endothelial and epithelial barriers such as indwelling catheters
- Any sequelae of the transplant surgery such as undrained fluid collections[13]

13. How are microorganisms that cause infection in transplant recipients classified?
The following are classifications of microorganisms[47]:

TYPE OF PATHOGEN	PATHOGENICITY	EXAMPLE
True pathogens	Cause classic infections	Influenza virus, typhoid, cholera
Sometime pathogens	Organisms that are benign under most circumstances but can cause lethal infections in transplant recipients if mucocutaneous barrier is disrupted	Normal gut flora *Staphylococcus aureus*
Nonpathogens	Organisms that rarely cause symptomatic disease in immunocompetent individuals but cause significant morbidity and mortality in transplant recipients	Opportunistic organisms such as *Aspergillus fumigatus*, *Cryptococcus neoformans*

14. What pharmacologic measures are taken to prevent infection?
Measures to prevent infection in transplant recipients may include the following:
- Administration of prophylactic antimicrobial therapy during the first few months posttransplant when immunosuppressant doses are highest
- Administration of antibiotic prophylaxis against infective endocarditis according to American Heart Association guidelines
- Periodic vaccinations per Centers for Disease Control and Prevention guidelines regarding administration of vaccines in immunosuppressed persons

15. What nonpharmacologic measures are recommended to prevent infection?
Nonpharmacologic measures to prevent infection vary among transplant centers and with the type of organ transplanted. Recommended measures for healthcare providers and patients/families may include the following:

HEALTHCARE PROVIDERS	PATIENTS AND FAMILIES
Wash hands frequently and thoroughly with antimicrobial soap.	Wash hands frequently and thoroughly with antimicrobial soap.
Use sterile technique per posttransplant protocols (e.g., central line dressing changes).	Avoid people with obvious signs of illness.
	Avoid raw or partially cooked foods of animal origin.
Follow reverse isolation procedures per posttransplant protocol.	Avoid cross-contamination between raw and cooked foods.
	Avoid unpasteurized products.
Conduct housekeeping per posttransplant hospital protocol.	Wash raw fruits and vegetables thoroughly before eating.

(Cont'd. on next page.)

HEALTHCARE PROVIDERS	PATIENTS AND FAMILIES
Use leucocyte-depleted or CMV-negative blood products for CMV-seronegative recipients.	Avoid potential animal sources of infection (e.g., cleaning cat litter boxes, bird cages, fish aquaria).
Use high-efficiency leucocyte blood filters.	Avoid close contact with infants and others who have recently received live virus vaccines (e.g., oral polio, varicella, or measles-mumps-rubella vaccines).
Discontinue indwelling lines and catheters as soon as possible.	
Obtain posttransplant infection surveillance tests per protocols.	
Avoid cross-contamination by staff members caring for patients with contagious infections.	Avoid potential sources of fungal infections during first posttransplant year (e.g., live plants, fresh flowers).
Use special masks to transport recipients through high-risk areas of hospital (e.g., construction sites that might contain *Aspergillus* spores).	Obtain yearly influenza vaccine (patients and household contacts) unless otherwise contraindicated.
Institution:	Use boiled (for at least 1 full minute) water or distilled water if safety of drinking water is questionable.
Monitor showers, toilet facilities, and air-conditioning systems for *Legionella*.	Avoid intravenous drug use.
Use high-efficiency particulate air-filtered air-handling systems if air supply is potentially contaminated, especially from construction.	Follow safe sex guidelines.
	Consult with transplant physician about travel to areas requiring malaria prophylaxis and/or vaccines.

CMV = cytomegalovirus.

16. Are certain infections more common at a particular time after transplantation?

Regardless of the type of organ transplant procedure, certain infections are more common at certain posttransplant periods. The following table is useful in making a differential diagnosis.[4,47,49]

TIME PERIOD	TYPE OF INFECTION	EXAMPLE
First month	Continuation of pretransplant infection	*Pseudomonas aeruginosa* infections in lung transplant candidates with cystic fibrosis
	Infections related to the surgical procedure, other iatrogenic procedures, and indwelling lines and catheters	Heart transplant: mediastinitis
	Transmission of infection by the donor allograft	Heart transplant: Transmission of *Toxoplasma gondii* via donor heart Lung transplant: transmission of *Candida* spp. from donor trachea
	Early reactivation of latent viruses	Reactivation of herpes simplex virus and human herpesvirus 6 infections
Months 2–6	Infections caused by opportunistic organisms or immunomodulating viruses	Reactivation of latent herpesvirus infections (cytomegalovirus, Epstein Barr virus), *Pneumocystis carinii*, *Listeria monocytogenes*
After 6 months	Community-acquired infections similar to those in immunocompetent individuals	Upper respiratory tract infections caused by sources such as influenza virus, adenoviruses.

17. Why do opportunistic infections develop after the first posttransplant month?

Calcineurin inhibitors (cyclosporine-based formulations and tacrolimus) prevent the synthesis of interleukin-2 and other lymphokines, thereby inhibiting both lymphocyte function and proliferation, effecting global cellular immune dysfunction, and predisposing the recipient to opportunistic infections. Development of these infections, however, is a function not only of the type of immuno-suppressive agents used but also the duration of immunosuppressive therapy. Therefore, these transplant-unique infections typically do not develop until 1 or more months after transplantation.[49]

18. In addition to time interval since transplantation, are there any other factors to consider in diagnosing infection?

FACTOR[4,24]	EXAMPLE
Pretransplant host factors	Age, nutritional status, comorbidities (e.g., diabetes mellitus), medications (e.g., steroid use), infection history (particularly infections that further suppress the immune system, such as CMV, EBV, HBV, HCV)
Preoperative factors	Invasive devices (e.g., intraaortic balloon pump, assist devices, mechanical ventilation)
Type of organ transplanted	Risk of infection greater for lung transplant recipients
Perioperative factors	Ischemic time, blood loss, transfusions
Donor factors	Donor CMV-seropositive, recipient CMV-seronegative
Immunosuppression regimen	Maintenance therapy (medications, doses, frequency); use of antilymphocyte therapy
Rejection history	Severity, treatment, and response to treatment
Current antimicrobial regimen (if any)	Use of prophylactic antiviral therapy to prevent CMV infection
Posttransplant exposure to nosocomial, community, or geographic sources of infection	Any recent hospitalizations; any community outbreaks of infection; any exposure to endemic fungi
Onset of symptoms	Bacterial infections usually manifest over a 24–48 hour period, but they can evolve over several (3–5) days

CMV = cytomegalovirus, EBV = Epstein-Barr virus, HBV = hepatitis B virus, HCV = hepatitis C virus,.

19. Why is the diagnosis of infection in transplant recipients often difficult?
The diagnosis of infection may be difficult for the following reasons:
- Immunosuppressive agents, particularly steroids, may diminish the inflammatory response to infection. As a result, signs such as fevers and elevated white blood cell count may be masked, and diagnostic tests such as skin testing and serologies may be less sensitive.
- Certain infections may not be associated with fever: undisseminated herpes simplex and herpes zoster infections, cryptococcal infections, and candidal infections.[11]
- Postoperative fevers may be caused by other factors such as rejection, adverse drug reactions, pulmonary embolism, deep vein thrombosis, malignancy, and allograft ischemia.[49]

20. How is infection in transplant recipients diagnosed?
Because traditional diagnostic tests may lack sensitivity, more sensitive diagnostic tests must be used early on, even for seemingly benign and often vague symptoms. Such tests may include the following:
- DNA probes
- Polymerase chain reaction
- Monoclonal antibodies for antigen detection
- Computed tomography
- Magnetic resonance imaging
- Biopsies

21. Name the important clinical manifestations of infection in organ transplant recipients.
Important clinical presentations include fever without any localizing findings, fever with headache, changes in level of consciousness or other central nervous system findings, unexplained skin lesions, and febrile pneumonitis.[22]

22. What does an infection workup typically include?

Patient evaluation includes a thorough history and physical examination as well as comprehensive diagnostic testing. More aggressive diagnostic procedures such as bronchoscopy, computed tomography scans, and biopsies are frequently required, as are pulmonary and infectious disease consultations.

23. What are the guidelines for assessment of infection in the transplant recipient?

The assessment of the transplant recipient is guided by the following:
- Careful examination of the sinuses, pharynx, lymph nodes, lungs, heart, abdomen, and skin is required.[4]
- Metastatic skin lesions, although seemingly benign, may be the first indication of a systemic infection caused by opportunistic organisms; biopsies of unexplained skin lesions are essential.
- Changes in level of consciousness may be subtle.
- Viral infections may have a subacute presentation.

24. What are the guidelines regarding various diagnostic tests?

TEST[10]	GUIDELINES
Conventional radiography or computed tomography (CT)	Essential in diagnosing infection of the chest and central nervous system, the two most important and common causes of life-threatening infection.
	Single-lung transplant recipients: Radiographic abnormalities in the native lung may make the diagnosis of infection in this lung more difficult.
	The presence of new infiltrates mandates an early, definitive diagnosis.[32]
	The depressed inflammatory response may significantly modify or delay the appearance of pulmonary lesions on the chest radiograph.[13]
Sinus films	Patients taking cyclosporine may be at increased risk for sinus infections. Acute sinusitis may be associated with minimal pain or tenderness; therefore, sinus films are key to diagnosing sinusitis.
CT	Often provides more accurate information than conventional radiography in determining the extent of infection and following the patient's response to therapy, especially in certain types of infection such as pulmonary infections due to fungi or *Nocardia*.
	Useful in determining which, if any, invasive diagnostic procedure would be indicated to arrive at a microbiologic diagnosis.
	For patients with concurrent or sequential respiratory infections, CT is useful in identifying the second causative agent.
	CT scan of brain is indicated for CNS infections caused by *Aspergillus* species, *Cryptococcus neoformans*, and *Listeria*.
	Abdominal CT is useful for suspected abscesses or adenopathy.[4]
	Use of contrast material depends on patient's current renal function.
Bronchoscopy	Early bronchoscopy is indicated for unexplained dyspnea or hypoxemia (regardless of chest radiography findings), severe pulmonary disease, or any radiographic findings that are suggestive of opportunistic infection.[4,11,32]
Ultrasonography (US)	Renal US is useful for diagnosing obstructions or fluid collections such as infected lymphoceles.
	Liver transplant recipients: Right upper quadrant US is useful in determining patency of vessels.[4]
Skin tests or serological response tests	May be of limited use for the following reasons:
	Immunotherapy may cause false-negative skin tests and circulating antibody tests.
	False-positive tests may be obtained in the absence of true infection because many pathogens such as *Candida* are common in the environment.

(Cont'd. on next page.)

TEST	GUIDELINES
Skin tests or serological response tests (cont'd.)	Antigen detection tests provide a semiquantitative assessment of microbial burden that may be used to guide therapy. Polymerase chain reaction assays provide important information about herpes group viruses in terms of viral load, prognosis, and therapeutic response.[47]
Histology	Extremely important because it facilitates a rapid, specific diagnosis and prompt initiation of pathogen-specific therapy, thereby avoiding multidrug therapy.
Endoscopy, colonoscopy	May be especially useful in diagnosing cytomegalovirus (CMV) infection, posttransplant lymphoproliferative disease, and *Clostridium difficile* and *Helicobacter pylori* infections.
Blood tests	Serologic testing may be less sensitive because of immunotherapy-mediated blunting of inflammatory response to infection.[34] Leukopenia may be due to CMV infection or medications such as ganciclovir, azathioprine, or mycophenolate mofetil. Liver enzymes may be elevated because of CMV infection, rejection, hepatitis (A, B, or C) infections, or medications.[4]
Urinalysis	Key in diagnosing urinary tract infections (UTIs) in renal transplant recipients, because many UTIs are asymptomatic in these patients; comprehensive urine cytodiagnostic tests are often indicated.

25. What are the most common causes of occult fever in transplant recipients?

The most common causes of occult fever for each posttransplant time period are listed below[10,22]:

First month	Technical complications related to the surgery, indwelling catheters, etc. Allograft rejection Antilymphocyte therapy (especially first few and last doses of a 10–14 day course) *Note:* Conventional drug fevers are uncommon.
Months 2–6	Viral infections (especially cytomegalovirus) Antilymphocyte therapy
After 6 months	Occult opportunistic infections Antilymphocyte therapy

26. What are the major bacterial, viral, fungal and protozoal pathogens that cause infection in transplant recipients?

The major pathogens that cause infection in transplant recipients listed are below[34,40,49]:

BACTERIAL	VIRAL	FUNGAL	PROTOZOAL
Enteric gram-negative bacteria	Cytomegalovirus	*Aspergillus* species	*Toxoplasma gondii*
Pseudomonas aeruginosa	Epstein-Barr virus	*Pneumocystis carinii*	*Cryptosporidium*
Legionella species	Herpes simplex virus	*Histoplasma capsulatum*	*Strongyloides stercoralis*
Nocardia asteroides	Varicella-zoster virus	*Coccidioides immitis*	
Listeria monocytogenes	Hepatitis B virus	*Blastomyces dermatitidis*	
Salmonella species	Hepatitis C virus	*Cryptococcus neoformans*	
Mycobacterium tuberculosis	Human herpesvirus-6	*Candida* species	
Nontuberculous mycobacteria	Papillomavirus		
	Adenoviruses		
	Respiratory syncytial virus		
	Influenza virus		
	Enterovirus		
	Papovavirus		

27. What are potential causes of fever of unknown origin?

A fever of unknown origin may be due to infectious or noninfectious causes[11,34,49]:

INFECTIOUS AGENTS	NONINFECTIOUS CAUSES
Systemic viral syndromes due to cytomegalovirus or Epstein-Barr virus	Rejection (especially in liver, kidney, and lung transplant recipients)
Disseminated tuberculosis	Organ ischemia secondary to infarction or decreased perfusion
Histoplasmosis	Pulmonary emboli
Cryptococcosis	Deep vein thrombosis
Systemic toxoplasmosis	Drug reactions to antilymphocyte therapy or antibiotics
Early *pneumocystis carinii* infection	Malignancy
	Organ ischemia secondary to infarction or poor perfusion

28. Are there any guidelines regarding hospitalization of transplant recipients with suspected infections?

Given the diagnostic challenges associated with infection in transplant recipients, it is generally recommended that patients be hospitalized for more aggressive testing if
- Chest infiltrates are present on chest radiography or computed tomography.
- Fevers of 38.5°C or higher persist.
- The patient appears toxic.
- The patient cannot perform routine activities of daily living.[10,11]

29. What are the unique characteristics of central nervous system infections in transplant recipients?
- Immunosuppressants may mask the signs of meningeal irritation.
- Changes in level of consciousness are often subtle.
- The simultaneous presence of unexplained fever and headache is the most reliable indication of a central nervous system (CNS) infection and warrants an immediate and complete neurological evaluation, including computed tomographic scan or magnetic resonance imaging of the brain and lumbar puncture (unless contraindicated).[10,13,34]

30. Name the four clinical central nervous system syndromes and associated pathogens that are typically observed in transplant recipients.

The four major central nervous system syndromes and their associated pathogens follow below.[10,13,22]

SYNDROME	ASSOCIATED PATHOGEN(S)
Acute meningitis	*Listeria monocytogenes*
Chronic or subacute meningitis	*Cryptococcus neoformans, Mycobacterium tuberculosis, Coccidioides immitis, L. monocytogenes, Histoplasma capsulatum, Nocardia asteroides, Strongyloides stercoralis*
Focal brain syndromes	Metastatic *Aspergillus* infection; occasionally *L. monocytogenes, Toxoplasma gondii, N. asteroides*
Progressive dementia	Polyomavirus, JC virus, herpes simplex virus, cytomegalovirus, Epstein-Barr virus

31. What three pathogens account for the majority of central nervous system infections in transplant recipients?

The majority of central nervous system infections in transplant recipients are caused by *Listeria monocytogenes, Cryptococcus neoformans*, and *Aspergillus fumigatus*.[49]

32. Which pathogens cause the greatest morbidity and mortality among transplant recipients?

Viruses cause the greatest morbidity and mortality among transplant recipients. The major posttransplant viral infections are caused by the herpes viruses (cytomegalovirus, Epstein-Barr virus, herpes simplex 1 and 2, and varicella zoster) and the hepatitis viruses. Compared with other populations, these viruses are more virulent, progress faster, and have a broader range of clinical sequelae in transplant recipients.

33. What are the clinical sequelae of viral infections?

Viral infections have both direct and indirect effects. Direct effects are the clinical syndromes associated with each pathogen (e.g., pneumonia, hepatitis). Indirect effects include the following:
- Alteration in the recipient's net state of immunosuppression such that the recipient is more susceptible to opportunistic infections such as aspergillosis or listeriosis
- Potential effect on the pathogenesis of allograft injury
- Potential role in oncogenesis[35]

34. What is the difference between infection with a herpes virus and disease caused by a herpes virus?

All herpes viruses are characterized by latency, which means that once a herpes virus is present, the patient harbors the viral genome for life. Immunosuppression can trigger the replication of latent herpes viruses. The term *infection* indicates viral replication as evidenced by culture or serologic testing. The term *disease* indicates that the recipient has specific symptoms that can be attributed to a herpes virus. Disease is diagnosed by demonstrating viremia or tissue invasion.[10,13]

35. Why is cytomegalovirus the most important pathogen that can affect transplant recipients?

Cytomegalovirus (CMV) is the single most common and most important pathogen that is encountered. CMV infection occurs in 30–70% of all solid organ transplant recipients; approximately 50 percent of these patients develop symptomatic disease.[40] CMV is particularly noteworthy because of its direct and indirect effects. Direct effects of CMV infection include tissue injury and clinical disease. The transplanted organ typically is more susceptible than native organs to the direct effects of CMV. Indirect effects include opportunistic superinfections, allograft injury, and rejection. There appears to be a bidirectional relationship between CMV and rejection because CMV can precipitate rejection and rejection-mediated inflammation (coupled with antirejection therapy) can increase CMV viral replication. Allograft-specific effects are as follows:

Hepatic allografts: Vanishing bile duct syndrome
Cardiac allografts: Accelerated cardiac vasculopathy
Lung allografts: Bronchiolitis obliterans
Kidney allografts: Glomerulopathy[13]

Some evidence suggests that CMV also has a possible role in oncogenesis.[37]

36. How is cytomegalovirus infection acquired?

There are three epidemiological patterns of CMV infection.

Primary (de novo) infection is acquired when a CMV-seronegative recipient receives either a CMV-seropositive allograft or blood products. Rarely, a CMV-seronegative recipient may acquire a primary infection through contact with an individual with an active CMV infection. Compared with the other two types of CMV infections, primary CMV infection has been associated with
- Higher rates of CMV infection and symptomatic disease
- Earlier onset of CMV posttransplant
- Higher rates of recurrent CMV episodes
- Increased risk of disseminated CMV disease
- Higher mortality rates[41]

Reactivation infection occurs when an endogenous, latent virus in a CMV-seropositive recipient is reactivated. Any inflammatory process or stress can promote reactivation (e.g., sepsis, rejection, antilymphocyte therapy).[47]

Superinfection occurs when a CMV-seropositive patient is infected with a new exogenous CMV strain from the allograft. It is important to note that the risk of a patient developing symptomatic CMV disease may be greater when the virus that is activated is of donor origin as opposed to recipient origin.[33,41,46]

37. Which transplant recipients are most likely to develop cytomegalovirus infection and disease?

In descending order, CMV disease occurs most frequently in the following types of transplant recipients[27]:

1. Heart-lung and lung
2. Small bowel
3. Kidney-pancreas
4. Heart
5. Liver
6. Kidney

The transplanted organ is more likely to be affected by CMV than a native organ. Thus, for example, CMV hepatitis primarily tends to occur in liver transplant recipients, intestinal CMV infection occurs primarily in small bowel transplant recipients.

Two groups of transplant recipients are at increased risk for symptomatic CMV disease:

• CMV-seropositive recipients who receive antithymocyte globulin or muromonab-CD3 for rejection therapy
• CMV-seronegative recipients who receive allografts from CMV-seropositive donors[37]

38. How costly is cytomegalovirus infection in terms of hospital resources?

The Transplant Infection Cost Analysis program recently examined hospital resource utilization associated with readmission for CMV infection in adult heart and renal recipients who were at least 2 years posttransplant. Data were obtained from two heart and three kidney transplant centers. Costs in dollars were standardized according to 1998 U.S. values. These data are summarized below.[19]

PARAMETER	HEART	RENAL
Range of days of inpatient care	2–95 days	1–56 days
Average number of inpatient days per recipient	10.9 days	10.5 days
Range of hospital charges	$2,323–$698,447	$1,947–$109,812
Average hospital charge per patient per readmission	$42,111	$22,598
Average hospital charge per day	$3863	$2152

It is important to note that these data do not reflect the total economic and social burden associated with CMV infection. Costs related to physician services, home health care, medications, lost productivity, decreased graft function, and retransplantation were not included in the analysis.

39. How common is Epstein Barr virus infection among transplant recipients?

Active Epstein Barr virus (EBV) replication occurs in 20–30% of transplant recipients who are on maintenance immunotherapy. However, the incidence increases to 80% of patients receiving antilymphocyte-antibody therapy.[13]

40. What are the consequences of Epstein Barr virus infection in transplant recipients?

The consequences of EBV infection range from a mononucleosis-like syndrome to posttransplant lymphoproliferative disease (PTLD).

41. What is posttransplant lymphoproliferative disease?

PTLD is a group of syndromes that range from a benign, self-limited form of polyclonal proliferation to aggressive, monoclonal malignant lymphomas that are highly resistant to therapy and result in significant morbidity and mortality. Among transplant recipients, primary infection with EBV is a significant risk factor for the development of PTLD.

PTLD typically develops between 8 and 18 months posttransplantation. It occurs most frequently within the abdomen. Diffuse involvement of nodal and extranodal tissue is common. The overall incidence of PTLD among solid organ transplant recipients is approximately 3%.[49]

42. What are the risk factors for posttransplant lymphoproliferative disease?

The risk factors for PTLD infection include
- Primary EBV infection
- Preceding CMV infection
- Antilymphocyte antibody therapy; cyclosporine or tacrolimus, which can cause reactivation of latent EBV infection and loss of surveillance against EBV-immortalized B-cells[13]
- Age of recipient: very young recipients who are predisposed to primary EBV and CMV infections; older recipients, owing to the possible relationship between the senescence of the immune system and the late development of PTLD[9]
- Type of allograft

43. Which type of transplant recipients have the highest incidence of posttransplant lymphoproliferative disease?

The incidence of PTLD is correlated with the type of allograft. In general, intestinal transplant recipients have the highest incidence of PTLD (reported incidence approximately 28%), followed in decreasing order by heart–lung (9.4%), lung (7.9%), heart (3.5%), liver (2.2%), and kidney (1%) transplant recipients.[31]

44. What are the clinical manifestations, diagnostic tests, and treatment options for posttransplant lymphoproliferative disease?

The clinical manifestations, diagnostic tests, and treatment options for PTLD include the following[27,34]:

CLINICAL MANIFESTATIONS	DIAGNOSTIC TESTS	TREATMENT OPTIONS
Fever of unknown origin	Computed tomographic scan	Treatment options are controversial.
Mononucleosis-like syndrome of fever, malaise and lymphadenopathy (with or without tonsillitis or pharyngitis)	Tissue biopsy	Benign polyclonal polymorphic B-cell lymphoma: Antiviral agents (acyclovir, ganciclovir) Decrease immunosuppression
Gastrointestinal symptoms: bleeding, abdominal pain, diarrhea, obstruction, perforation		Early malignant polyclonal polymorphic B-cell lymphoma: Antiviral agents (acyclovir, ganciclovir) Decrease immunosuppression Interferon-α
Weight loss		Gamma globulin
Night sweats		Anti-B-cell antibodies
Upper respiratory infection		Monoclonal polymorphic B-cell lymphoma:
Hepatocellular dysfunction		Decrease immunosuppression
CNS dysfunction: seizures, focal neurologic disease, change in state of consciousness		Chemotherapy Radiation Surgical resection

Data from Cupples SA, Lucey DL: Infectious diseases in transplantation. In Cupples SA, Ohler L (eds): Solid Organ Transplantation: A Handbook for Primary Health Care Providers. New York, Springer, 2002, pp 16–63.

45. What precautions should be taken for transplant recipients who are exposed to or acquire varicella-zoster virus ?

- Varicella-zoster virus (VZV)-seronegative recipients must report any exposure to VZV so that zoster immunoglobulin may be promptly administered.

- Chicken pox in transplant recipients is a medical emergency that requires hospitalization for intravenous therapy.[34]

46. What are the clinical implications of posttransplant hepatitis infections?

At 10 years posttransplant, approximately 10–20% percent of recipients with HCV infection and approximately 50% of recipients with HBV infection will have end-stage liver disease and/or hepatocellular carcinoma. Currently, the combination of interferon and ribavirin is the most effective therapy for HCV infections. However, many patients cannot tolerate this regimen.[47]

47. Discuss fungal infections in transplant recipients.

Although the incidence of fungal infections among transplant recipients is lower than the incidence of bacterial or viral infections, fungal infections have the highest mortality rates.

Fungal infection may be classified as infection with an opportunistic pathogen that rarely causes invasive disease in immunocompetent individuals and infection with one of the geographically restricted mycoses (histoplasmosis, coccidioidomycosis, or blastomycosis).Typical endemic areas include Central or South America, Southeast Asia, or the midwestern or southwestern areas of the United States.[34]

In transplant recipients, the three most common opportunistic fungal pathogens are *Candida*, *Cryptococci*, and *Aspergillus* species. Reported mortality rates range as follows: candidiasis, 23–71%; cryptococcosis, 0–60%; and aspergillosis, 20–100%.[48]

Originally classified as a protozoan, *Pneumocystis carinii* is now considered to be a fungal pathogen. Prophylaxis with trimethoprim-sulfamethoxazole has been highly effective in reducing the incidence of *Pneumocystis* pneumonia among transplant recipients.[48]

Antimicrobial agents that have been used to prevent or treat fungal infections include fluconazole, amphotericin B, and the newer, less nephrotoxic amphotericin B lipid complex. Nystatin suspension and clotrimazole troches are effective antifungal agents with activity against oral candidal infections.

48. Oral itraconazole is often prescribed for certain fungal infections. How can its absorption be increased?

Gastric acidity enhances the absorption of itraconazole. Gastric acidity is diminished by antacid therapy. Therefore, patients who take gastric antacid therapy may need to take itraconazole with a cola drink that lowers gastric pH temporarily.[6]

49. What are the major posttransplant parasitic pathogens?

The major parasitic pathogens are *Cryptosporidium* species, *Strongyloides stercoralis* and *Toxoplasma gondii*.

Cryptosporidium is a protozoan parasite that may cause severe, persistent, watery diarrhea. The organism is transmitted by fecal–oral or animal–person contamination and waterborne transmission.

Treatment options include fluid, electrolyte, and nutritional support. Spiramycin may be effective for some patients; however, this drug is poorly absorbed with food. High-dose intravenous spiramycin has been associated with increased stool output and volume loss.[12] Nonpharmacologic preventive measures include

- Boiling water for 5 minutes
- Using distilled water
- Avoiding use of ice cubes that have not been made with boiled or distilled water (e.g., in restaurants)
- Avoiding soda fountain drinks that have been reconstituted with tap water

Strongyloides stercoralis is an endemic intestinal nematode that can exist in the gastrointestinal tract for decades after the initial infection. An intact cell-mediated immune system prevents tissue invasion in the immunocompetent individual. However, after transplantation, disseminated strongyloidiasis can develop, precipitating a severe hemorrhagic enterocolitis and/or hemorrhagic pneumonia. Therapeutic agents include albendazole, ivermectin, and systemic antibacterial therapy for concomitant bacteremia or meningitis.

50. Discuss the risk of toxoplasmosis among heart and heart-lung transplant recipients.

Toxoplasmosis, a protozoal infection, occurs most frequently in heart and heart-lung transplant recipients because the *Toxoplasma gondii* pathogen encysts in the heart muscle. In heart transplant recipients, the overall incidence of toxoplasmosis ranges between 4 and 12%. However, the incidence is much higher in *T. gondii*-seronegative recipients who receive allografts from *T. gondii*-seropositive donors (approximately 50%). Primary toxoplasmosis typically occurs early in the postoperative period (6 weeks to 3 months). A reactivation infection (reinfection by latent organisms in a *T. gondii*-seropositive recipient) may be asymptomatic, less acute, and less life-threatening. Because toxoplasmosis can mimic rejection, a definitive diagnosis is made from the results of an endomyocardial biopsy.[11,40,46,49] Treatment options include pyrimethamine with folinic acid and sulfadiazine or clindamycin and pyrimethamine with folinic acid.[27]

51. Why are heart and heart-lung transplant recipients at increased risk for pneumonia?

Heart and heart-lung transplant recipients are at increased risk for pneumonia because of
- Disruption of the phrenic nerve
- Decreased protective pulmonary mechanisms
- Increased risk of aspiration and atelectasis
- Prolonged intubation[49]

52. Why are lung transplant recipients at increased risk for infection?

Lung transplant recipients are at increased risk for infection for the following reasons:
- The allograft is constantly exposed to the external environment.
- The allograft is denervated; this denervation results in a blunted cough reflex, decreased mucociliary clearance, and reactive hyperresponsiveness.
- Lymphatic drainage is interrupted.
- The anastomosis site may be associated with enhanced colonization, airway dehiscence, mediastinitis, bronchial stenosis, and postobstructive infection.
- Infections may be transmitted from the donor lung secondary to prolonged intubation and previous inactive infections.
- In single-lung transplantation, the native lung may harbor occult pretransplant infections or posttransplant infections.[2,44]

53. Where do most infections occur in lung transplant recipients?

Eighty percent of infections in lung transplant recipients occur in the lung, mediastinum, or pleural space.[2]

54. Which kidney transplant recipients are at increased risk for urinary tract infections?

Bacterial urinary tract infections (UTIs) are the most common complication following kidney transplantation. Recipients at increased risk for UTIs include those with
- Prolonged hemodialysis before transplantation
- Diabetes mellitus
- Postoperative bladder catheterization
- Allograft trauma
- Surgical complications associated with ureteral anastomosis

The incidence of UTIs in female recipients is twice that in male recipients.[25]

55. When do urinary tract infections typically occur?

Most UTIs occur within the first few months after kidney transplantation. However, UTIs may occur 6 months after transplantation or later. Recipients who are more likely to continue to have UTIs include those with
- Serum creatinine levels > 2 mg/dl
- Prednisone doses that exceed 20 mg/day
- Multiple treated rejection episodes
- Chronic viral infections[25]

56. In a kidney transplant recipient, what is the clinical significance of unilateral leg edema?

Unilateral leg edema on the side of the kidney transplant may be a sign of secondary infection of a wound-related lymphocele.

57. Why are urinary tract infections common among pancreas transplant recipients?

UTIs are common among pancreas transplant recipients for the following reasons:

- Diabetes is often associated with altered bladder function secondary to neurogenic changes and increased residual volume, both of which promote bacterial infection.
- Surgical trauma to the bladder may result in functional alterations.
- Duodenal contamination may be a nidus for bacterial infection.
- Alkaline and protein pancreatic secretions may promote bacterial growth.[20]

58. Why are urinalysis results in bladder-drained pancreas transplant recipients sometimes misleading?

Urinalysis results may be misleading because bladder-drained pancreas recipients tend to have an increased number of white and red blood cells in the urine. In addition, because the bladder mucosa is irritated by pancreatic enzymes, the urine often is positive for leukoesterase. Urine cultures and sensitivities should be obtained when a UTI is suspected.[45]

59. Tacrolimus is one of the major immunosuppressants used in liver and other types of transplantation. Given that tacrolimus is more than a hundredfold more potent than cyclosporine, why are infection rates not higher in recipients receiving tacrolimus?

It is thought that infection rates are not higher in recipients receiving tacrolimus because such recipients have fewer rejection episodes and therefore require less adjunctive immunosuppression therapy (e.g., antilymphocyte therapy).

60. Why do liver transplant recipients with a roux-en-Y choledochojejunostomy have a higher incidence of intrahepatic and biliary infections than recipients with a duct-to-duct anastomosis (choledochocholedochostomy)?

A roux-en-Y anastomosis is often performed in recipients with biliary strictures (e.g., recipients with primary biliary cirrhosis or previous bile duct surgery). This procedure may be associated with the reflux of enteric bacteria into the hepatobiliary system secondary to disruption of bowel integrity and sacrifice of the sphincter of Oddi.[41]

61. What factors predispose intestinal transplant recipients to infection?

Factors that predispose intestinal transplant recipients to infection include the following:

- The lengthy and involved transplant procedure
- Additional surgery (e.g., reexploration for complications such as perforation or dehiscence)
- The potential for rejection, ischemia, and posttransplant lymphoproliferative disease that can precipitate breakdown of the mucosal barrier and the subsequent migration of organisms from the intestinal lumen to other tissues and organs[53]

62. Summarize key points about bacterial, viral, and fungal infections in the various types of solid organ transplant recipients.

Key Points about Bacterial Infections in Solid Organ Transplant Recipients

Bacteria: General
- Bacteria are the most common causes of infection. The transplant site is the most common site of bacterial infection, and bacterial pneumonias are common among all types of transplant recipients.[11]

Lung transplant
- Bacteria are the etiologic agents in approximately 50% of infectious complications.[44]
- Bacterial pneumonias are the most frequent infectious complication.[44]

(Cont'd. on next page)

Key Points about Bacterial Infections in Solid Organ Transplant Recipients (Continued)

Lung transplant (*cont'd.*)
- Infections caused by *Pseudomonas* pathogens are particularly common in recipients who undergo lung transplantation for cystic fibrosis.[15]
- The most frequent bacterial pathogens are gram-negative rods.[2]

Liver transplant
- Bacterial infections are the most common type of infection among liver transplant recipients.[41]
- Of recipients, 35–70% have at least one bacterial infection; overall incidence: 0.8–1.46 episodes per recipient.[41]
- Infections that involve the liver, biliary tract, peritoneal cavity, surgical site, and bloodstream are most common.[42]
- Bacteremia is more common among liver transplant recipients than any other type of transplant recipient.[11]

Kidney transplant
- Bacterial infections occur in approximately 47% of recipients.[42]
- Urinary tract infections are the most common bacterial infections.[34]
- Recipients have a high incidence of asymptomatic urinary tract infections; therefore, surveillance cultures are often required.[42]

Heart transplant
- Bacterial infections occur in 21–30% of recipients.[42]
- Pneumonia is the most common bacterial infection.[42]
- Mediastinitis generally is caused by gram-positive bacteria (*Staphylococcus aureus*, coagulase-negative *S. aureus*), but gram-negative bacteria have also been identified as etiologic agents.[49]

Pancreas/kidney-pancreas transplant
- Bacterial infections occur in 35% of recipients.[42]
- The most common bacterial infections are wound and intra-abdominal infections. The most common pathogens are enteric bacteria.[42]

Key Points about Viral Infections in Solid Organ Transplant Recipients

Cytomegalovirus (CMV): General
- The single most important pathogen; common in all types of solid organ transplant recipients.[11]
- During the first posttransplant year, over 50% of recipients have evidence of viral replication.[37]

Lung transplant
- CMV is the most important and most frequent viral pathogen.
- The rate of CMV infection and disease is higher among lung transplant recipients than any other solid organ recipients.[44]
- The reported incidence of CMV disease is 50–80% in lung and heart-lung recipients.[50]
- The lung is the most common site of invasive CMV disease.

Liver transplant
- CMV infection occurs in 30–50% of recipients; symptomatic disease develops in approximately half of these recipients.[41]

Kidney transplant
- CMV is the most important pathogen in renal transplant recipients.[35]
- The reported incidence of CMV disease is 8–25%.[50]

Heart transplant
- The gastrointestinal tract is the most common site of CMV infection.
- The risk of CMV disease is 50–75% in CMV-seronegative recipients who receive an allograft from a CMV-seropositive donor.[36]
- The reported incidence of CMV disease is 8–25%.[50]

(Cont'd. on next page.)

Cytomegalovirus (CMV): General *(cont'd.)*

Pancreas/kidney-pancreas transplant
- The reported incidence of CMV disease is 50% in pancreas and kidney-pancreas recipients.[50]
- Some studies indicate that kidney-pancreas recipients have a higher prevalence of CMV disease than isolated kidney recipients.[11]

Hepatotropic viruses, hepatitis B virus (HBV), and hepatitis C virus (HCV): General
- HBV and HCV are common causes of liver disease among transplant recipients.[7]
- HCV may be transmitted by the allograft itself or by transfusion of blood products. After parenteral exposure, HCV seroconversion typically occurs within 3 months, but may not occur for 12 months.[7]

Lung transplant
- Minimal information is available about viral hepatitis in lung transplant recipients.[7]

Liver transplant
- Without adequate prophylaxis, HBV graft reinfection occurs in 80–100% of hepatitis B surface antigen-positive recipients. This rate is significantly reduced with the use of long-term, high-dose hepatitis B immunoglobulin with or without lamivudine.[14]
- Chronic HCV infection is the most common cause of end-stage liver disease that necessitates transplantation. After transplant, HCV reinfection occurs in virtually all patients.[21]

Kidney transplant
- Renal transplant recipients have the second highest prevalence of hepatitis infections.[11]
- In patients with HBV infection, the clinical manifestations of chronic liver disease are typically not apparent in the first 1–2 years after transplant. After 2 years, recipients develop progressive chronic liver disease and/or hepatocellular carcinoma.[35]

Heart transplant
- Little is known about the clinical course of HCV infection in heart transplant recipients, although there have been anecdotal reports of cholestatic liver disease and liver failure in this population.[7]

Pancreas/kidney-pancreas transplant
- Minimal information is available about viral hepatitis in pancreas transplant recipients.[7]

Herpes simplex virus (HSV-1, HSV-2): General
- Oral lesions often extend beyond the lip and involve the oral cavity and esophagus.[11]
- At least 50% of recipients are HSV-seropositive at the time of transplant; 40% will later develop HSV disease.[16]

Lung transplant
- Reported incidence: up to 18%
- Most infections are clinically significant.[44]
- Lung allografts are particularly susceptible to HSV infection; pulmonary involvement may occur from viremia, aspiration, or contiguous spread from the oropharynx via the trachea.[16]

Liver transplant
- Most HSV infections are reactivation of latent infections in HSV-seropositive recipients. Visceral infections are rare.[41]

Kidney transplant
- The most common manifestation is herpes labialis.[23]
- Most infections are reactivated; disseminated disease is rare.[35]

Heart transplant
- Most HSV infections are reactivated from the latent state. Reactivation is typically seen as herpes labialis.[49]

Pancreas/kidney-pancreas transplant
- There are anecdotal reports of possible transmission of HSV-2 from seropositive donors to seronegative transplant recipients.[17]

Key Points about Fungal Infections in Solid Organ Transplant Recipients

Fungal: General
• Fungal infections have been reported in all types of transplant recipients and are associated with higher mortality rates than any other type of infection.[18]

Lung transplant
  • Reported prevalence of invasive infection: 14–36%
  • Reported mortality: *Candida* spp: 27%
                     Aspergillus spp: 21–100%[18]
  • Infections frequently involve the abdominal cavity and may be associated with fungemia. Invasive infection is most commonly caused by *Candida* spp.[18]

Liver transplant
  • Reported prevalence of invasive infection: 7.5–42%
  • Reported mortality: *Candida* spp: 10%-59%
                     Aspergillus spp: 50–100%[18]
  • Recipients have the highest incidence of invasive fungal infections of all solid organ transplant recipients.[40] The reported incidence is 4–42%.[48]

Kidney transplant
  • Reported prevalence of invasive infection: 5–6%
  • Reported mortality: *Candida* spp: 23–71%
                     Aspergillus spp: 20–100%[18]
  • The most common infections include candidiasis, aspergillosis, cryptococcosis, and zygomycosis.[1]
  • The urinary tract is the most common site of fungal infection.[29]

Heart transplant
  • Reported prevalence of invasive infection: 4–20%
  • Reported mortality: *Aspergillus* spp: 32–64%[18]
  • The preponderance of aspergillosis infection in the lungs is unique to heart transplant recipients.[18]
  • Fungal agents that have been implicated in mediastinitis include *A. fumigatus* and *Candida* spp.[49]

Pancreas/kidney-pancreas transplant
  • Reported prevalence of invasive infection: 19–35%
  • Reported mortality: unknown[18]
  • The risk of invasive fungal infection is associated with the surgical method whereby pancreatic exocrine secretions are drained (e.g., duodenocystostomy drainage may facilitate candidal colonization of the bladder).[18]

Aspergillus species: General
  • Aspergillosis is acquired mainly by inhalation of spores.[29]
  • Primary site of infection is the lung; secondary sites often include the brain, gastrointestinal tract, heart, kidney, liver or spleen. Disseminated disease has a poor prognosis.[11]

Lung transplant
  • Colonization occurs in 22–85% of recipients at some time posttransplant.[44]
  • Invasive aspergillosis occurs in 13–26% of colonized recipients.[44]
  • Lung transplant recipients have the highest incidence of invasive aspergillosis.[41]

Liver transplant
  • Infection with *Aspergillus* species is relatively uncommon; however the mortality rate is high, especially for infections caused by *A. fumigatus*.[30]
  • Liver transplant recipients have the second highest incidence of invasive aspergillosis.[41]

Kidney transplant
  • Although *A. fumigatus* and *A. flavus* have been associated with life-threatening infections,[39] renal transplant recipients are generally at lower risk for invasive aspergillosis.[28]

(Cont'd. on next page.)

***Aspergillus* species: General** *(cont'd.)*

Heart transplant
- The prevalence of invasive aspergillosis is approximately 6%; the overall mortality is 78%.[28]

Pancreas/kidney-pancreas transplant
- *Aspergillus* infections are similar to those in kidney transplant recipients.[48]

***Candida:* General**
- Candidiasis is the most common fungal infection.[52]
- Most cases of candidiasis arise from endogenous sources.[29]
- Mucosal infections are most common; liver and lung transplant recipients are at highest risk for visceral or disseminated candidiasis.[11]

Lung transplant
- Colonization may interfere with healing of the bronchial anastomosis, thereby precipitating tracheobronchitis and leakage, which may prove fatal.[48]

Liver transplant
- Over 50% of fungal infections are due to *Candida* spp.[30]
- Liver transplant recipients have the highest incidence of invasive candidiasis.[41]
- Extensive abdominal surgery is a risk factor for invasion of the gastrointestinal tract.[48]

Kidney transplant
- Asymptomatic candiduria can be serious due to risk of obstructing candidal fungal balls, ascending pyelonephritis, and sepsis (particularly in diabetic patients with bladder dysfunction).[34]

Heart transplant
- Candidal infection may cause rupture of the aortic anastomosis secondary to mycotic aneurysm.[29]

Pancreas/kidney-pancreas transplant
- Risk factors for candidiasis include indwelling bladder catheters, diabetes mellitus, and draining of exocrine secretions into the bladder. These secretions create a nonacidic environment that promotes *Candida* colonization.[40]

63. Summarize the treatment options for common posttransplant viral, bacterial, and fungal infections.

Treatment options for common posttransplant infections include the following[10]:

TYPE OF INFECTION	TREATMENT OPTIONS
Cytomegalovirus (CMV) infection	Intravenous ganciclovir followed by oral ganciclovir CMV hyperimmune globulin (for tissue-invasive disease) Foscarnet (for ganciclovir-resistant organisms or patients who cannot tolerate ganciclovir)

Epstein-Barr virus (EBV) infection	Acyclovir
	Posttransplant lymphoproliferative disease (PTLD)—benign polyclonal polymorphic B cell hyperplasia:
	    Acyclovir
	    Ganciclovir
	    Decreased immunosuppression (possibly)
	
	PTLD—early malignant polyclonal polymorphic B cell lymphoma:
	    Acyclovir Gamma globulin
	    Ganciclovir Anti-B cell antibodies (anti-CD 20)
	    Interferon-α Decreased immunosuppression (possibly)
	
	Monoclonal polymorphic B cell lymphoma:
	    Chemotherapy Resection
	    Radiation Decreased immunosuppression

(Cont'd. on next page.)

TYPE OF INFECTION	TREATMENT OPTIONS	
Herpes simplex 1 and 2	Acyclovir Ganciclovir Famciclovir	Valacyclovir Foscarnet
Hepatitis	Hepatitis B: hepatitis B immunoglobulin Hepatitis C: interferon and ribavirin	
Listeriosis	Meningeal doses of penicillin or ampicillin Gentamicin Trimethoprim-sulfamethoxazole (for patients allergic to penicillin)	
Norcardiosis	Sulfasoxazole Trimethoprim-sulfamethoxazole Amikacin	Imipenem Third generation cephalosporins Minocycline
Legionellosis	Quinolones (levofloxacin, ciprofloxacin) Rifampin	Doxycyline Macrolide antibiotics Trimethoprim-sulfamethoxazole
Mycobacterial infection	Isoniazid Rifampin	Pyrazinamide Ethambutol
Aspergillosis	Amphotericin B Itraconazole	
Candidiasis	Clortrimazole Mycostatin Fluconazole	Amphotericin B followed by fluconazole (for critically ill or unstable patients)
Cryptococcosis	Amphotericin B Amphotericin B and 5 flucytosine Fluconazole	
Pneumocystis	TMP-SMZ Pentamidine Dapsone-trimethoprim	Atovaquone Clindamycin primaquine
Coccidioidomycosis	Amphotericin B Fluconazole (maintenance therapy) Itraconazole (maintenance therapy)	
Histoplasmosis	Amphotericin B Itraconazole (maintenance therapy)	
Cryptosporidosis	Fluid and electrolyte replacement Nutritional support Spiramycin (effective for some patients)	
Toxoplasmosis	Pyrimethamine with folinic acid and sulfadiazine Clindamycin and pyrimethamine with folinic acid	
Strongyloidiasis	Albendazole Ivermectin	

64. List the general guidelines for treatment of infection in transplant recipients.
In the immunosuppressed patient, it is important to remember that[10]
- The most important determinants of survival are often how quickly a diagnosis is made and how soon microbe-specific therapy is started.
- Antimicrobial therapy is guided by the results of the history and physical, gram stains, and other diagnostic tests.
- In general, broad-spectrum, empiric antibiotics are avoided. More specific therapy that is based on diagnostic tests is preferred.[24]

• Antimicrobial therapy typically is not prescribed for fixed courses; instead, therapy is based on microbial burden. The greater the microbial burden, the longer and more intense the antimicrobial therapy. Therapy is continued until laboratory results and clinical evidence demonstrate that active infection has been eradicated.
• It is better to prevent than treat infection; therefore, prophylactic or preemptive antimicrobial agents are frequently administered.

65. What are the three ways in which antimicrobial therapy is used for transplant recipients?

Antimicrobial therapy can be used for
• Therapeutic use: treatment of an established infection
• Prophylactic use: administration of antimicrobial therapy to an entire population of patients to prevent common infections
• Preemptive use: administration of antimicrobial therapy to a subgroup of patients who are at high risk for clinically significant infection based on established clinical, epidemiologic, or laboratory data

66. What are the goals of antimicrobial therapy?

The three goals of antimicrobial therapy are eradication of active infection, limitation of any pathologic effect, and prevention of recurrence.[36]

67. Are there any special precautions regarding antimicobial therapy?

Antimicrobial agents can cause both pharmacokinetic and idiosyncratic interactions with the patient's immunosuppressive agents. Pharmacokinetic interactions occur because cyclosporine and tacrolimus are metabolized by way of the cytochrome P450 hepatic enzyme system. Antimicrobial agents that downregulate the cytochrome P450 system cause serum cyclosporine and tacrolimus levels to increase and place the patient at greater risk for nephotoxocity, overimmunosuppression, and infection. Other antimicrobials upregulate the cytochrome P450 system and can result in inadequate immunosuppression and increased risk of graft rejection. Idiosyncratic nephrotoxicity can occur in recipients who have normal renal function.[4,10,43,47,49,51]

↑ CYCLOSPORINE OR TACROLIMUS LEVELS	↓ CYCLOSPORINE OR TACROLIMUS LEVELS	POTENTIAL TO CAUSE ADDITIVE NEPHROTOXICITY
Azithromycin	Imipenem	Acyclovir
Clarithromycin	Isoniazid	Aminoglycosides
Erythromycin	Rifabutin	Amphotericin B
Fluconazole	Rifampin	Ciprofloxacin (high dose)
Itraconazole	Sulfamethoxazole	Erythromycin
Josamycin	Nafcillin	Foscarnet
Ketoconazole		Ketoconazole
		Pentamidine
		Trimethoprim-sulfamethoxazole (high doses)
		Quinolones (high doses)
		Vancomycin

Data from Cupples SA, Lucey DL: Infectious diseases in transplantation. In Cupples SA, Ohler L (eds): Solid Organ Transplantation: A Handbook for Primary Health Care Providers. New York, Springer, 2002, pp 16–62.

68. Why is it important to update transplant candidates' immunizations?

Immunosuppressed patients typically have a suboptimal response to vaccinations. Therefore, it is important to update transplant candidates' immunizations before transplantation. Preferably, vaccines should be administered as early as possible in the disease course because vaccines often are less effective in patients with severe end-organ dysfunction.[5]

69. What vaccines are commonly recommended for adult transplant candidates?

VACCINE[5]	CONSIDERATIONS[5]
Hepatitis A virus	Recommended especially for liver transplant candidates, preferably early in the disease process, before the onset of end-stage cirrhosis.
Hepatitis B virus (HBV)	HBV vaccine series is recommended for HBV-seronegative candidates. Consider enhanced-potency regimen and/or additional doses for certain subsets of patients (e.g., patients on hemodialysis, alcoholic patients, diabetic patients, vaccine nonresponders).
	Consider accelerated-schedule vaccine series for patients who may undergo transplantation within a short time period. Pretransplant HBV immunity is especially important for nonhepatic candidates who may receive an allograft from a hepatitis B surface antigen-negative, hepatitis B core antibody-positive donor.
Influenza virus	Recommended yearly (in appropriate season) to prevent severe influenza infection or secondary bacterial pneumonia. Especially important for candidates with heart or lung disease. Household contacts of candidates should also receive vaccine (unless otherwise contraindicated).
Varicella virus	Consider vaccine for all nonimmune transplant candidates.
Tetanus-diphtheria toxoid	Update booster before transplantation if candidate has not received it in the preceding 5 years. For candidates who have not received primary series, administer series before transplantation.
Measles-mumps-rubella	Administer series according to standard recommendations before transplantation.
Poliovirus	Administer inactivated poliovirus vaccine (IPV) before transplantation. Use IPV (rather than live oral poliovirus vaccine) for household contact of transplant patients.
Haemophilus influenzae type B (HIB) conjugate vaccine	Adult candidates may have previously developed protective titers. Asplenic, hypogammaglobulinemic, or other immunocompromised candidates: measure HIB titers and revaccinate accordingly.
Meningococcal	Consider administration for transplant candidates who will be entering college within 1–2 years.

70. Are there any standard vaccine protocols for transplant recipients?

Standard vaccine protocols have not been developed. There is some concern that vaccines may stimulate the immune system and trigger a rejection episode. Immune response to vaccines may be variable. However, two vaccines that are commonly recommended are

1. Pneumococcal vaccine approximately every 6 years

2. Tetanus booster every 10 years, although some transplant centers prefer to treat tetanus-related wounds with tetanus immunoglobulin alone[3]

71. Should transplant recipients receive an annual influenza vaccine?

The effectiveness of influenza vaccines is controversial, and transplant centers differ in terms of flu vaccine policies. Factors that may influence whether any given transplant recipient should receive the influenza vaccine include time since transplant, most recent biopsy results, current level of immunosuppressants, and current clinical status. However, household contacts of the transplant recipient should receive an annual influenza vaccine, unless otherwise contraindicated.

72. Should transplant recipients receive live attenuated vaccines?

Because there is a risk that viral replication may be facilitated in immunocompromised patients, it is generally recommended that transplant recipients avoid the following live attenuated vaccines[8]:

- Oral polio vaccine
- Measles-mumps-rubella vaccine
- Bacilli Calmette-Guerin
- Small pox vaccine
- TY21a typhoid vaccine
- Yellow fever vaccine (if severely immunocompromised)

73. Should the oral polio vaccine be given to any of the transplant recipient's household or intimate contacts?

The oral polio vaccine (OPV) should not be administered to any household or intimate contact. If this vaccine is inadvertently administered to a household or intimate contact, the transplant patient must avoid close contact with the recipient of the OPV for approximately 1 month (the period of maximum secretion of the virus).[8]

74. Thus far, you have focused on infection prevention for transplant recipients. How can nurses and other clinicians protect themselves against infections that transplant recipients may have?

Nurses and other healthcare workers should take several precautions to prevent transmission of infection from the transplant recipient to the clinician, including the following[6]:

- Pregnant, CMV-seronegative clinicians should avoid direct care of recipients with active CMV.
- VZV-seronegative clinicians should avoid direct care of recipients with chickenpox or herpes zoster. VZV-seronegative clinicians should consider vaccination.
- Standard precautions should be followed with all patients, but particularly those with Hepatitis B or C. Hepatitis B vaccination is recommended for clinicians.
- Pregnant, parvovirus-seronegative clinicians should avoid direct care of recipients with known or suspected parvovirus infections.
- Isolation precautions (identical to those followed for nontransplant patients) are recommended during initial therapy for tuberculosis.
- Standard precautions should be followed for recipients with multiresistant bacterial infections.
- Immunosuppressed clinicians should consult with their physicians for more specific guidelines.

BIBLIOGRAPHY

1. Abbott KC, Hypolite I, Poropatich RK, et al: Hospitalizations for fungal infections after renal transplantation in the United States. Transpl Infect Dis 3:203–211, 2001.
2. Alexander BD, Tapson VF: Infectious complications of lung transplantation. Transpl Infect Dis 3:128–137, 2001.
3. Avery RK: Infections and immunizations in organ transplant recipients: A preventive approach. Cleve Clin J Med 61:386–392, 1994.
4. Avery RK: Infectious disease and transplantation: Messages for the generalist. Cleve Clin J Med 61:305–314, 1998.
5. Avery RK, Ljungman P: Prophylactic measures in the solid-organ recipient before transplantation. Clin Infect Dis 33(Suppl 1):S15–S21, 2001.
6. Avery RK, Mossad SB: Solid organ transplant-related infectious disease for the home care clinician. Home Health Care Consultant 6(8):29–39, 1999.
7. Bzowej NH, Wright TL: Viral hepatitis in the transplant patient. In Bowden RA, Ljungman P, Paya CV (eds): Transplant Infections. Philadelphia, Lippincott-Raven, 1998, pp 309–324.
8. Centers for Disease Control and Prevention. Recommendations of the Advisory Committee on Immunization Practices (ACIP): Use of vaccines and immune globulins in persons with altered immunocompetence. MMWR Morb Mortal Wkly Rep 43(RR-4): 1–18, 1993.
9. Cockfield SM: Identifying the patient at risk for post-transplant lymphoproliferative disorder. Transpl Infect Dis 3:70–78, 2001.

10. Cupples SA, Lucey DL: Infectious diseases in transplantation. In Cupples SA, Ohler L (eds): Solid Organ Transplantation: A Handbook for Primary Health Care Providers. New York, Springer, 2002, pp 16–63.
11. Dummer S: Infections in transplantation. In Makowa L, Sher L (eds): Handbook of Solid Organ Transplantation. Austin, TX, Landes Bioscience, 1995, pp 305–335.
12. Fishman JA: Pneumocystis carinii and parasitic infections in the immunocompromised host. In Rubin RH, Young LS (eds): Clinical Approach to Infection in the Compromised Host, 3rd ed. New York, Plenum, 1994, pp 275–334.
13. Fishman JA, Rubin RH: Infection in organ transplant recipients. N Engl J Med 338(24):1741–1751, 1998.
14. Fontana RJ, Hann HL, Wright T, et al: A multicenter study of lamivudine treatment in 33 patients with hepatitis B after liver transplantation. Liver Transplant 7:504–510, 2001.
15. Frost AE: Role of infections, pathogenesis, and management in lung transplantation. Transplant Proc 31:175–177, 1999.
16. Gnann JH: Other herpesviruses: Herpes simplex virus, varicella-zoster virus, human herpesvirus types 6, 7 and 8. In Bowden RA, Ljungman P, Paya CV (eds): Transplant Infections. Philadelphia, Lippincott-Raven, 1998, pp 265–285.
17. Goodman JL: Possible transmission of herpes simplex virus by organ transplantation. Transplantation 47:609–613, 1989.
18. Hadley S, Karchmer AW: Fungal infections in solid organ transplant recipients. Infect Dis Clin North Am 9:1045–1074, 1995.
19. Henderson R, Carlin D, Kohlhase K, et al: Multicenter US study of hospital resource utilization associated with cytomegalovirus-related readmission of renal and heart transplant patients. Tranpl Infect Dis 3(Suppl 2):57–59, 2001.
20. Henry ML: Pancreatic transplantation. In Makowka L, Sher L (eds): Handbook of Organ Transplantation. Austin, TX, Landes, 1995, pp 289–303.
21. Keeffe EB: Liver transplantation at the millennium: Past, present, and future. Clin Liver Dis 4:241–255, 2000.
22. Kontoyiannis DP, Rubin RH: Infection in the organ transplant recipient. Infect Dis Clin North Am 9:811–822, 1995.
23. Kubak BM, Holt CD: Infectious complications of kidney transplantation and their management. In Danovitch GM (Ed): Handbook of Kidney Transplantation, 2nd ed. Boston, Little Brown, 1996, pp 187–213.
24. Miller LW: Long-term complications of cardiac transplantation. Prog Cardiovasc Dis 33:229–282, 1991.
25. Munoz P: Management of urinary tract infections and lymphocele in renal transplant recipients. Clin Infect Dis 33(Suppl 1):S53–S57, 2001.
26. Patel R, Paya CV: Cytomegalovirus infection and disease in solid organ transplant recipients. In Bowden RA, Ljungman P, Paya CV (eds): Transplant Infections. Philadelphia, Lippincott-Raven, 1998, pp 229–244.
27. Patel R, Paya CV: Infections in solid organ transplant recipients. Clin Microbiol Rev 10:86–124, 1997.
28. Patterson DL, Singh N: Invasive aspergillosis in transplant recipients. Medicine 78:123–138, 1999.
29. Paya CV: Fungal infections in solid organ transplantation. Clin Infect Dis 16:677–688, 1993.
30. Paya CV: Prevention of fungal and hepatitis virus infections in liver transplantation. Clin Infect Dis 33(Suppl 1):S47–S52, 2001.
31. Preiksaitis JK, Cockfield SM: Epstein-Barr virus and lymphoproliferative disorders after transplantation. In Bowden RA, Ljungman P, Paya CV (eds): Transplant Infections. Philadelphia, Lippincott-Raven, 1998, pp 245–263.
32. Rizk NW, Faul JL: Diagnosis and natural history of pulmonary infections in transplant recipients. Chest 117:303–305, 2000.
33. Rubin RH: Cytomegalovirus in solid organ transplantation. Transpl Infect Dis 3(Suppl 2):1–5, 2001.
34. Rubin RH: Infection in the organ transplant recipient. In Rubin RH, Young LS (eds): Clinical Approach to Infection in the Compromised Host, 3rd ed. New York, Plenum Medical Book, 1994, pp 629–705.
35. Rubin RH: Infectious disease complications of renal transplantation. Kidney Int 44:221–236, 1993.
36. Rubin RH: Prevention and treatment of cytomegalovirus disease in heart transplant patients. J Heart Lung Transplant 19:731–735, 2000.
37. Rubin RH, Kemmerly SA, Conti D, et al: Prevention of primary cytomegalovirus disease in organ transplant recipients with oral ganciclovir or oral Acyclovir prophylaxis. Transpl Infect Dis 2:112–117, 2000.
38. Schaffner A: Pretransplant evaluation for infections in donors and recipients of solid organs. Clin Infect Dis 33(Suppl 1):S9–S14, 2001.
39. Sia IG, Paya CV: Infectious complications following renal transplantation. Surg Clin North Am 78:95–122, 1998.
40. Singh N: Infections in solid organ transplant recipients. Am J Infect Control 25:409–417, 1997.
41. Singh N: Infectious diseases in the liver transplant recipient. Semin Gastroint Dis 9(3):136–146, 1998.

42. Soave R: Prophylaxis strategies for solid-organ transplantation. Clin Infect Dis 33 (Suppl 1):S26–S31, 2001.
43. Sollinger H, Pirsch J: Transplantation Drug Pocket Reference Guide, 2nd ed. Austin, TX, Landes Bioscience, 1996.
44. Speich R, van der Bij W: Epidemiology and management of infections after lung transplantation. Clin Infect Dis 33(Suppl 1):S58–S65, 2001.
45. Steen DC: The current state of pancreas transplantation. AACN Clin Issues 10:164–175, 1999.
46. Thaler SJ, Rubin RH. Opportunistic infections in the cardiac transplant patient. Curr Opin Cardiol 11:191–203, 1996.
47. Tolkoff-Rubin NE, Rubin RH: Recent advances in the diagnosis and management of infection in the organ transplant recipient. Semin Nephrol 20:148–163, 2000.
48. Tollemar JG: Fungal infections in solid organ transplant recipients. In Bowden RA, Ljungman P, Paya CV (eds): Transplant Infections, Philadelphia, Lippincott-Raven, 1998, pp 339–350.
49. Tucker PC: Infectious complications. In Baumgartner WA, Reitz B, Kasper E (eds): Heart and Lung Transplantation, 2nd ed. Philadelphia, Saunders, 2002, pp 355–371.
50. van der Bij W, Speich R: Management of cytomegalovirus infection and disease after solid-organ transplantation. Clin Infect Dis 33(Suppl 1):S33–S37, 2001.
51. Wagoner LE: Management of the cardiac transplant recipient: Roles of the transplant cardiologist and primary care physician. Am J Med Sci 314:173–184, 1997.
52. Wheat LJ: Fungal infections in the immunocompromised host. In Rubin RH, Young LS (eds): Clinical Approach to Infection in the Compromised Host, 3rd ed. New York, Plenum Medical Book, 1994, pp 211–237.
53. Williams L, Horslen SP, Langnas AN: Intestinal transplantation. In Cupples S, Ohler L (eds): Solid Organ Transplantation: A Handbook for Primary Health Care Providers. New York, Springer, 2002, pp 292–333.

21. LONG-TERM COMPLICATIONS OF SOLID ORGAN TRANSPLANTATION

Sharon M. Augustine, RN, CRNP, and
Maureen P. Flattery, RN, MSN, C-ANP

1. What are the most common complications following solid organ transplantation?

Many long-term complications are associated with solid organ transplantation, the most frequent of which include the following:

- Acute and chronic rejection
- Infection
- Osteoporosis
- Renal insufficiency
- Malignancy
- Hyperlipidemia
- Hypertension
- Diabetes mellitus
- Gastrointestinal dysfunction
- Cognitive impairment
- Sexual dysfunction

2. Explain the difference between acute and chronic rejection.

Despite common misperceptions, the difference between acute and chronic rejection has little to do with how long after transplantation the rejection episode occurs. Transplanted organs are at risk of rejection because of the ability of the immune system to recognize and respond to donor antigens as non-self. This response may occur through the activation of lymphocytes (cellular rejection) and antibodies (humoral rejection).

Acute rejection may occur as early as 7–10 days after transplantation when antigens on the surface of the grafted organ are recognized as foreign or non-self. As a result of the recognition process, lymphocytes travel to the area, with resultant interstitial or perivascular infiltration. On the other hand, acute rejection may occur years after transplantation. When acute rejection is accompanied by cellular necrosis, it is generally considered to be a serious rejection episode that requires augmentation of immunosuppression.

Chronic rejection generally refers to an antibody response (humoral rejection) that causes vasculopathy. The vasculopathy is manifested in similar ways across different types of organ transplantation—for example, accelerated graft atherosclerosis (AGA) in heart transplantation, bronchiolitis obliterans in lung transplantation, renal artery stenosis in kidney transplantation, and ductopenia in liver transplantation.

3. How is acute rejection best diagnosed?

As in many areas in medicine, diagnosis is usually accomplished using a set of diagnostic methods. Two basic approaches to assessment are routine surveillance tests to diagnose the problem promptly, even before patients are symptomatic, and clinical assessment based on history and symptoms. Tissue biopsy remains the definitive diagnostic tool for either routine surveillance or suspected rejection. Adjunctive diagnostic tests are organ-specific. For example, an echocardiogram is helpful in determining cardiac function in heart transplant recipients. In liver transplant recipients, baseline and current liver function tests are compared. In addition, organ-specific symptoms of organ failure are clues to the possibility of rejection and should prompt further physical assessment as well as laboratory and other diagnostic testing.

4. When is rejection treated?

The severity of acute rejection determines whether clinicians decide to treat. Each organ has its own scale with descriptive criteria for the severity of rejection. It is rare that upon pathologic examination of donor tissue some lymphocytes are not seen. Treatment becomes necessary when lymphocytic infiltrates are associated with necrosis. Clinical correlates are specific to failure of the organ transplanted.

5. Why do infections remain a significant source of morbidity after transplantation?

Infection risk is greatest immediately following transplantation, and, although it decreases over time, it continues to be a cause of significant morbidity in this population. Immediately following surgery, the recipient is generally debilitated, may be in an intensive care setting, has invasive lines, and is taking high-dose immunosuppressant medications. Bacterial infections, especially nosocomial infections, occur most frequently. Viral infections, specifically cytomegalovirus (CMV) and Epstein-Barr virus (EBV), have been implicated in both acute illnesses and the development of long-term sequelae. Fungal infections, particularly candidiasis and aspergillosis, and protozoal infections, such as *Pneumocystis carinii* (PCP), are also of concern. Additionally, transplant recipients in certain geographic areas are at risk for developing infections endemic to their particular areas, e.g., coccidioidomycosis in the southwestern United States and blastomycosis in the southern United States.

6. What measures are taken to minimize the risk of infection?

Prevention is the best method of minimizing the risk of infection. Careful hand washing and attention to the appropriate aseptic or sterile procedures during hospitalization are vital. Each institution has its own organ-specific protocol for infection prophylaxis. A typical protocol might include the following:
- Antifungal medications (clotrimazole, ketoconazole)
- Sulfamethoxazole-trimethoprim for PCP prophylaxis
- Ganciclovir or valganciclovir for CMV prophylaxis (particularly for CMV-seronegative recipients of CMV-seropositive allografts)

Patients are also encouraged to assume an active role in preventing infection and are typically instructed to
- Monitor body temperature daily and immediately report any temperature elevations or other signs and symptoms of infection to the transplant team.
- Avoid obvious risks of infection such as tattooing.
- To the extent possible, avoid individuals with communicable illnesses.
- Obtain routine vaccinations, with the exception of vaccines that contain live viruses.

It is important to remember that immunosuppressed patients are at risk for developing uncommon infections. Therefore, any unusual presentation or illness should be investigated thoroughly. (See chapter 20).

7. Why is osteoporosis such a significant problem in transplant recipients?

Pretransplant factors often predispose patients to low bone density. Chronic problems such as renal failure, loop diuretics, prerenal azotemia, passive or active liver congestion, history of tobacco use, hypogonadism, and insufficient dietary calcium and weight-bearing exercise may all contribute to bone loss. Immunosuppressive medications including steroids, cyclosporine, tacrolimus, azathioprine, mycophenolate mofetil, and rapamycin have direct and indirect effects on bone and mineral metabolism.

Steroids are the most challenging immunosuppressive medications to manage because they remain the cornerstone of the prevention and treatment of rejection in most types of solid organ transplantation. Corticosteroid therapy affects bone density by
- Increasing urinary calcium excretion while reducing intestinal absorption.
- Increasing levels of parathyroid hormone.
- Decreasing skeletal growth factors including androgen and estrogen synthesis.
- Increasing bone resorption.
- Decreasing bone formation by osteoblasts.[18]

8. Clinically, how is osteoporosis defined?

By definition, osteoporosis is the loss of bone mass to the extent that patients are at risk for fractures with only minimal trauma. Therefore, any degree of osteoporosis is cause for concern and warrants preventive management. Operationally, the World Health Organization (WHO) defines osteopenia as a bone mineral density (BMD) between 1 standard deviation (SD) and 2.5 SD below the mean of young normal controls. Osteoporosis is defined as a BMD > 2.5 SD below the mean of young normals.

9. When should clinicians begin to monitor patients for osteoporosis?

Many transplant centers obtain baseline bone density scans for all transplant candidates. Information from the baseline scan can be compared with posttransplant bone density scans.

Early screening and prevention are important because the most significant period of bone loss is the first 6 months after transplantation, with the most dramatic loss often seen during the first 3 months. The practical and clinical consequences of bone loss during this period are important because 36% of patients experience fractures during the first year after transplantation.

10. What tests are included in the routine screening for osteoporosis?

A guideline for osteoporosis evaluation should include the following:
- Measurement of BMD by dual-energy x-ray absorptiometry (DEXA) scan of the spine and hips. Some centers use other tests to measure BMD, such as quantitative computed tomography (CT)
- Laboratory tests
  - Calcium
  - 25-OH vitamin D
  - Osteocalcin
  - Intact parathyroid hormone
  - Alkaline phosphatase
  - Chemistry levels
  - Assessment of urinary calcium and markers of resorption (urinary pyridinoline cross-links or N-telopeptides)

These tests are important for baseline benchmarks.

11. What supplements and medications should patients take to help prevent osteoporosis?

It is generally recommended that all patients on steroid or calcineurin inhibitor therapy take dietary supplements totaling 1500 mg of calcium and 800–1000 mg of vitamin D. Patients diagnosed with osteoporosis by DEXA scan and patients with fractures should also take an inhibitor of bone resorption, such as one of the bisphosphonates (alendronate, etidronate), calcitonin (which can be administered by subcutaneous injections or nasal spray), or estrogen (unless otherwise contraindicated). Some evidence suggests that bisphosphonate therapy may be helpful in preventing transplant-related osteoporosis.

It is recommended that patients take bisphosphonates immediately upon rising in the morning with a full glass of water at least 30 minutes before ingesting any other food or liquids (to optimize absorption) and remain upright for at least 30 minutes after swallowing the medication (to prevent esophagitis and esophageal erosion, which frequently occur with bisphosphonate therapy).

12. What is the cause of renal dysfunction in the transplant recipient?

Although renal dysfunction is most commonly seen as a side effect of the immunosuppressive regimen, other causes of nephrotoxicity should be investigated. In the renal transplant recipient, renal dysfunction can be caused by acute or chronic rejection, as well as by the effects of the disease process, such as hypertension or diabetes, that led to the need for transplantation.

13. How is renal insufficiency treated?

Renal sufficiency may be treated by reducing the patient's dose of calcineurin inhibitor (cyclosporine or tacrolimus). However, this dose reduction must be weighed against the risk of precipitating rejection. Although high trough blood levels of these drugs are more likely to lead to nephrotoxicity, renal insufficiency can also occur at low trough levels. The patient's volume status should be evaluated to determine if dehydration is a contributing factor. In addition, the patient's medication profile should be reviewed to identify other nephrotoxic medications (such as nonsteroidal anti-inflammatory drugs, diuretics, certain antibiotics, and antihypertensive medications) that could be the cause of synergistic or additive nephrotoxicity.

14. What are some potential consequences of renal insufficiency?

Renal insufficiency can lead to volume overload. Because many medications are cleared through the kidneys, renal insufficiency can result in inadequate clearance of medications and toxic side effects. Calcineurin inhibitors are nephrotoxic; therefore, renal insufficiency can limit immunosuppression options. In some patients, renal insufficiency progresses to end-stage renal disease, dialysis, and renal transplantation.

15. How often does cancer occur in the transplant recipient? What are the most common manifestations?

The prevalence of cancer in the solid organ transplant population has been estimated to range from 4–18% with an average of 6%.[15] The risk increases over the life of the transplanted organ. Transplant recipients tend to develop tumors that are uncommon in the general population. The most common malignancies are carcinoma of the skin and lips, lymphomas, and Kaposi's sarcoma. Of interest, malignancies that typically occur in the general population, carcinomas of the breast, lung, prostate, and colon, do not occur more frequently among transplant recipients and may even occur less frequently.[16]

16. How is cancer in transplant recipients treated?

The key to successful treatment is early diagnosis. Cancer screening should include regular assessment of the skin, face, and scalp for lesions and investigation of any constitutional complaints including evaluation for lymphadenopathy, as well as routine, age-appropriate cancer screening as recommended by the American Cancer Society.

Skin cancer treatment includes surgical excision, cryosurgery, and chemotherapy. Acyclovir and ganciclovir as well as radiation therapy or surgical excision of a single infected lymph node have been used to treat lymphomas, including posttransplant lymphoproliferative disease (PTLD). Reduction or cessation of immunosuppressive therapy may also be attempted. In some cases, it may be necessary to completely withdraw therapy. In these cases, a choice must be made between the viability of the graft and the life of the patient. Unfortunately, extrarenal transplant recipients have no alternative therapy should their graft fail.

17. What can transplant recipients do to help prevent cancer?

Transplant recipients should be alerted to their increased risk of developing cancer and encouraged to incorporate the following practices into their lifestyles:
- Stop smoking.
- Perform routine self-examination of skin.
- Undergo routine cancer screening according to American Cancer Society guidelines.
  - Schedule annual check-up with dermatologist.
    - Obtain prompt treatment of any premalignant or malignant skin lesions.
  - Schedule pelvic examination with Papanicolaou test for women.
  - Schedule mammogram/self breast examination for women.
  - Schedule prostate examination and prostate-specific antigen test for men.
  - Schedule sigmoidoscopy/colonoscopy in patients > 50 years of age.
- Observe sun precautions:
  - Avoid undue exposure to sunlight.
  - Avoid tanning beds.
  - Wear wide-brimmed hats, sun visors, sunglasses, and protective clothing.
  - Use a sunscreen lotion that filters out ultraviolet-B rays.

18. What is the cause of posttransplant hyperlipidemia?

There are several causes for hyperlipidemia following solid organ transplantation. The most common cause is preexisting hyperlipidemia. The immunosuppressive regimen has also been implicated. Cyclosporine has been associated with increased serum cholesterol and triglyceride levels.[14] Although tacrolimus also can cause hyperlipidemia, tacrolimus-induced hyperlipidemia is generally not as significant as that which occurs with cyclosporine-based regimens.[21] Steroid therapy has long been associated with elevated cholesterol levels. Rapamycin use has also resulted in hyperlipidemia.

19. How should hyperlipidemia be treated?

Hyperlipidemia is a known risk factor for the development of coronary artery disease. Therefore, solid organ transplant recipients should be encouraged to incorporate healthy dietary habits into their lifestyle. However, a low-fat, low-cholesterol diet alone may not be sufficient to control serum lipid levels. The class of drugs called *statins* (3 hydroxy-3 methylglutaryl coenzyme A [HMG-CoA] reductase inhibitors) has been shown to not only reduce serum cholesterol in the general population, but also in solid organ transplant recipients. A secondary benefit of this class of drugs is an improvement in endothelin function and perhaps inhibition of allograft inflammatory activity.

Several studies have examined the efficacy of different statins (pravastatin and atorvastatin). All have been found to be beneficial. Formulary requirements or prescriptive preference may influence the choice of drug.

Caution must be used when prescribing these medications for patients who also take a calcineurin inhibitor. This combination of medications can lead to rhabdomyolysis, a potentially life-threatening complication. Patients should be encouraged to report any muscle pain or weakness following the initiation of lipid therapy. Hepatic function and serum creatinine phosphokinase (CPK) should be evaluated on a regular basis.

20. List some causes of posttransplant hypertension.

Hypertension, like many other posttransplant complications, has many causes.

1. In the kidney transplant recipient, hypertension in the donor as well as uncontrolled renin secretion from the remaining native kidney or renal artery stenosis can lead to hypertension.

2. Preexisting hypertension in any type of solid organ transplant recipient contributes to the development of posttransplant hypertension.

3. Cyclosporine has been associated with a decrease in endogenous nitric oxide and the loss of the diurnal variation in blood pressure, which result in renal vascular constriction, a hyperrenin state, and an increase in total peripheral resistance.

4. Corticosteroid therapy contributes to the development of hypertension by increasing intravascular volume.

21. What are the treatment options for hypertension?

Posttransplant hypertension should be treated as strictly in this population as in any other group of patients with cardiovascular risk factors, including those with essential hypertension and diabetes mellitus. Recipients should be encouraged to incorporate health-promoting activities into their daily lives, including weight loss, cessation of smoking, and regular exercise. These methods alone, however, probably will not control calcineurin inhibitor-induced hypertension. Calcium channel blockers are effective in achieving blood-pressure control and exhibit a synergistic effect on the calcineurin inhibitor. (The patient may be able to take less of the calcineurin inhibitor to maintain a comparable therapeutic blood level.) In addition, evidence suggests that tacrolimus induces less hypertension than cyclosporine. Therefore, tailoring of the immunosuppressant regimen may be indicated. It may be necessary to use more than one antihypertensive agent to reduce the morbidity associated with this complication—for example, angiotensin-converting enzyme inhibitors, angiotensin II receptor blockers, alpha agonists, or vasodilators.

22. Why do so many recipients require insulin therapy after transplantation?

Immunosuppressant medications, particularly steroids but also calcineurin inhibitors, are diabetogenic. Steroids influence insulin resistance, glucose uptake, insulin receptor sensitivity, and insulin production. Cyclosporine and tacrolimus may contribute to insulin resistance and decreased insulin secretion and may have a toxic effect on pancreatic beta cells.

23. Is the treatment for posttransplant diabetes mellitus similar to the treatment of diabetes in the general population?

Yes, the Diabetes Control and Complications Trial (DCCT) recommends tight control of blood glucose levels for all patients. Results from this trial indicated that a 2% decrease in average HbA_{1c} was associated with a 60% reduction in risk of diabetic retinopathy, nephropathy, and neuropathy. Therefore, it is important to follow DCCT guidelines that recommend intervention for blood glucose levels of > 126 mg/dl on two consecutive tests in order to reduce the risks of end-organ damage.[5]

24. Do all recipients experience cognitive impairment following transplantation?

No, they do not. However, there are contradictory findings in the literature regarding such issues as

- Pre- to posttransplant improvement in neurocognitive function
- Declining neurocognitive functioning in the posttransplant period
- The reversibility of posttransplant neurocognitive deficits

Unfortunately, there is no question that a significant percentage of recipients experience some degree of neurocognitive deficit following transplantation.

25. What is the cause of posttransplant neurocognitive deficits?

A number of physiologic factors may affect neurocognitive functioning before and after transplantation. These include

- Organ-specific causes such as low perfusion states in end-stage heart failure, poor oxygenation in chronic lung diseases, and metabolic abnormalities in kidney and liver failure
- The effects of cardiopulmonary bypass
- Comorbidities such as other neurologic illnesses, cerebrovascular events, or infection
- Concomitant psychiatric disorders
- Concomitant substance abuse
- The effects of medications, particularly cyclosporine

26. How are transplant recipients assessed for neurocognitive deficits?

Unless a patient complains about poor memory or an inability to think clearly, neurocognitive deficits may go unnoticed. Patients may interact normally during a clinic visit, but still have difficulty in their everyday lives. Patients who appear noncompliant with the medication regime may actually have difficulty remembering when and how to take each drug. Other cues may include the following:

- Distractibility and inability to focus on tasks
- Inability to remember important information or keep appointments
- Failure to report important signs and symptoms
- Inability to understand complex information
- Inability to perform multistep tasks

Some transplant centers routinely have patients evaluated by a psychiatrist or neuropsychologist. If such evaluation is not the case, transplant clinicians should specifically ask patients (and, with the patient's consent, family members) about their cognitive function. Patients with cognitive deficits should be referred to a specialist as soon as possible. The consultant will do extensive neurocognitive testing and provide patients and family members with strategies that may be useful for minimizing the effects of these deficits.

27. What factors contribute to sexual dysfunction?

Many factors contribute to impotence following transplantation. For many men, impotence is a preexisting condition, related to both the chronic illness that led to the need for transplantation (e.g., hypertension, diabetes, or coronary artery disease) and the medications used to treat that illness (e.g., beta-blocker therapy for congestive heart failure). Following transplantation, the medications used to prevent rejection and to treat the side effects of the immunosuppressive regimen may contribute to changes in sexual function.

Women, too, can experience changes in sexual function. Such changes may be related to loss of libido and/or the onset of menopause. Psychological factors, such as fear of infection or rejection or a loss of intimacy with a significant other, can also contribute to sexual dysfunction.

28. Is there effective treatment for sexual dysfunction?

Unfortunately, many patients are disappointed after transplantation when they do not recover sexual function. Patients and their significant others may be too embarrassed to discuss problems, especially with a health care provider of the opposite sex. Therefore, it is important that health care providers try to put the patient at ease. One can validate the importance of the patient's problem with a simple statement: "Many patients have reported problems with sexual function following transplant. Please let me know if you notice any changes or have any concerns."

Assessment should include a careful history. It may be necessary to refer the patient to a urologist or gynecologist for further evaluation and treatment. The widespread publicity about and availability of sildenofil (Viagra) helped to destigmatize the problem. For certain patients, sildenofil is an effective treatment for sexual dysfunction. However, it may be contraindicated in patients with cardiovascular disease.

29. What are the most frequent gastrointestinal complications experienced by transplant recipients?

The most frequently occurring gastrointestinal (GI) complications are gastritis, peptic ulcer disease, perforated viscus, pancreatitis, and hepatitis. The latter two complications are more difficult to diagnose in patients with pancreatic and liver transplants, respectively. Given that glucocorticoid therapy is often associated with GI irritation and hemorrhage, antisecretory compounds and H_2-histamine receptor antagonists are frequently prescribed for the first 6–12 months posttransplant when steroid doses are high.

30. Why may gastrointestinal problems go undiagnosed?

Even though immunosuppressant medications, especially steroids, are contributing factors to GI complications, the masking effects of these drugs often prevent or delay recognition of the problem. One must remember that relatively mild and vague symptoms can lead to catastrophic consequences if left untreated. Hypercalcemia due to hyperparathyroidism can lead to bleeding after kidney transplantation. Infection or superinfection with opportunistic organisms can also cause inflammation and ulceration.

BIBLIOGRAPHY

1. Asberg A, Hartmann A, Fjeldsa,E, Holdaas H: Atorvastatin improves endothelial function in renal transplant recipients. Nephrol Dial Transplant 16:1920–1924, 2001.
2. Augustine SM, Yeo CJ, Buchman TG, et al: Gastrointestinal complications in heart and heart lung transplant patients. J Heart Transplant 10:547–556, 1991.
3. Baumgartner WA, Reitz B, Kasper E, Theodore J: Heart and Lung Transplantation, 2nd ed. Philadelphia, W.B. Saunders, 2002.
4. Cameron DE, Traill TA: Complications of immunosuppressive therapy. In Baumgartner, WA, Reitz BA, Achuff, SC (eds): Heart and Lung Transplantation, Philadelphia, W.B. Saunders, 1990, pp 237–248.
5. Costanzo MR, Cross AM, Haas GS: Posttransplant care/medical complications. In Norman DJ, Suki WN, Young TE (eds): Primer on Transplantation, 2nd ed. Thorofare, NJ, American Society of Transplant Physicians, 1998, pp 343–361.
6. Diabetes Control and Complications Trial Research Group: The effect of intensive treatment of diabetes on the development and progression of long-term complications in insulin-dependent diabetes mellitus. N Engl J Med 329:977–986, 1993.
7. Joseph JC: Corticosteroid-induced osteoporosis. Am J Hosp Pharm 51:188–197, 1994.
8. Fellstrom B: Risk factors for and management of post-transplantation cardiovascular disease. Bio Drugs 15:261–278, 2001
9. Flattery MP: Incidence and treatment of cancer in transplant recipients. J Transpl Coord 8:105–112, 1998.
10. Jindal RM: Posttransplant diabetes mellitus—A review. Transplantation 58:1289–1298, 1994.

11. Koomans HA, Lightenberg G: Mechanisms and consequences of arterial hypertension after renal transplantation. Transplantation 72:S9–S12, 2001.
12. Looker AC, Johnston CC, Wahner HW, et al: Prevalence of low femoral bone density in older US women from NHANES III. J Bone Miner Res 10:796–802, 1995.
13. Midtvedt K, Neumayer HH: Management strategies for posttransplant hypertension. Transplantation 70:SS64–SS69, 2000.
14. Nemunaitis J, Deeg, JH, Yee GC: High cyclosporine levels after bone marrow transplantation associated with hypertriglyceridemia. Lancet 2(8509):744–745, 1986.
15. Penn I: Depressed immunity and the development of cancer. Cancer Detect Prev 18:241–252, 1994.
16. Penn, I. Occurrence of cancers in immunosuppressed organ transplant recipients. In Terasaki PI (ed): Clinical Transplants. Los Angeles, CA, UCLA Tissue Typing Laboratory, 1990, pp 53–62.
17. Presti JC, Stoller ML, Carroll PR: Urology. In Tierney LM, McPhee SJ, Papadakis MA (eds): Current Medical Diagnosis and Treatment. Stamford, CT, Appleton & Lange, 1998, pp 896–898.
18. Rodino MA, Shane E: Osteoporosis after organ transplantation. Am J Med 104(5):459–469, 1998.
19. Rubin RR, Pryrot M: Implications of the DCCT: Looking beyond tight control. Diabetes Care 17:235–236, 1994.
20. Shane E, Rodino MA, McMahon DJ, et al: Prevention of bone loss after heart transplantation with antiresorptive therapy: A pilot study. J Heart Lung Transplant 17:1089–1096, 1998.
21. Taylor DO, Barr ML, Radovancevic B et al: A randomized, multicenter comparison of tacrolimus and cyclosporine immunosuppressive regimens in cardiac transplantation: Decreased hyperlipidemia and hypertension with tacrolimus. J Heart Lung Transplant, 18:336–345, 1999.

22. PREGNANCY AFTER TRANSPLANTATION

Jamie D. Blazek, RN, MPH, CCTC, FNP-C

1. Have there been successful pregnancies after solid organ transplantation?

Yes. The first reported successful pregnancy occurred in 1958. The mother, a renal transplant recipient, had received a kidney from her identical twin sister. The largest number of reported pregnancies has occurred in renal transplant recipients. Successful outcomes for both mother and child have also been reported in kidney–pancreas, liver, heart, heart–lung, liver–kidney, and lung transplant recipients.

2. What effect does end-stage organ disease have on female reproductive function?

When a major organ fails, there are both physiologic and psychological factors that can result in reproductive failure. Normal menstruation depends on a delicate balance of precise fluctuations in ovarian and pituitary hormone levels, the characteristics of the endometrium, the autonomic nervous system, vascular changes, prostaglandins, enzymes, nutrition, and psychological factors. Menstrual abnormalities from amenorrhea to metromenorrhagia can occur in women with end-stage organ disease as a result of gonadotropic dysfunction, hormonal imbalances, and anemia. Decreased libido, poor self-esteem, poor nutrition, and altered body image also alter reproductive function.

3. Do menstrual cycles resume after transplantation?

Yes. Many women with previous end-stage organ disease may think that they are postmenopausal only to find that regular menstruation resumes following successful transplantation.

4. Explain the physiology of the menstrual cycle.

The typical menstrual cycle begins with endocrine feedback between the hypothalamus and the anterior pituitary gland where follicle-stimulating hormone is released, resulting in the ripening of an ovarian follicle. The ripening follicle produces the estrogens, estrone, estradiol, and estriol, which thicken the lining of the uterus. Luteinizing hormone from the pituitary gland stimulates the follicle to rupture and release an ovum. Prolactin, also from the pituitary gland, turns the remaining follicle case into the corpus luteum, which secretes progesterone. Meanwhile, the ovum travels down the fallopian tube to the uterus. Progesterone ripens the uterus lining, preparing it for implantation of a fertilized ovum. If fertilization and implantation do not occur, estrogen and progesterone levels fall, and the uterus lining begins to slough.

5. Does transplantation or the use of immunosuppressant agents affect fertility?

No. Transplantation itself does not affect fertility. On the contrary, there typically is a significant improvement in quality of life after transplantation. Most women resume a relatively normal lifestyle. The sexual dysfunction and loss of libido associated with end-stage organ failure resolve, ovulations resumes, and fertility returns. No adverse affects on fertility have been associated with three of the major immunosuppressants: prednisone, cyclosporine, and azathioprine.

6. Where can I obtain additional information about pregnancy and transplantation?

The National Transplantation Pregnancy Registry (NTPR) is an excellent resource. This registry was established in 1991 at Thomas Jefferson University. Over the past 10 years, the registry has collected data on the outcomes of (1) 1,192 pregnancies in 774 female transplant recipients and (2) 896 pregnancies fathered by male transplant recipients. Registry data include information about the long-term outcomes of recipients and offspring. Additional information about the NTPR is found at the end of this chapter.

7. How safe is pregnancy following transplantation?

The safety of pregnancy in transplant recipients must include concern for three outcomes—the mother, the infant, and the allograft. Data from the NTPR indicate that "in the majority of female recipients studied, pregnancy does not appear to cause excessive or irreversible problems with graft function, if the function of the transplant organ is stable prior to pregnancy. However, a small percentage of recipients identified within each organ system may develop rejection, graft dysfunction, and/or graft loss that may be related to the pregnancy and may occur unpredictably. Outcomes are not entirely similar among all organ systems, and one must consider risks on an individual organ basis"[4] (p. 129). Some transplant programs strongly discourage posttransplant pregnancies, particularly for heart and lung transplant recipients. Given the fact that some women with end-stage organ disease may seek transplantation for the purpose of improving their ability to become pregnant, other centers, depending on the type of organ transplant, have adopted a more liberal attitude towards posttransplant pregnancy.

8. What is the transplant coordinator's role in reproductive counseling for transplant candidates?

Optimally, reproductive counseling for a female transplant candidate of childbearing age should begin before transplantation. During pretransplant interviews, the transplant coordinator should obtain a careful menstrual history (onset and pattern) and identify any previous and current birth control methods. The patient's desire for future children also should be determined. At this time, the potential for posttransplant pregnancy can be briefly discussed. This interview sets the stage for future discussions on this topic.

9. When should posttransplant reproductive counseling begin?

Normal menses can resume as early as 1 month following transplantation. Therefore, reproductive counseling should be provided in the first few weeks following transplantation, either during discharge teaching or at the first posttransplant clinic appointment. Appropriate birth control methods should be instituted as soon as sexual intercourse is resumed. Information regarding the advantages and disadvantages of various birth control methods should be provided, either by the transplant coordinator or by the patient's gynecologist.

10. Which birth control methods are safe for female transplant recipients?

Condoms, diaphragms, and spermicidal jellies have traditionally been the preferred methods of birth control for transplant recipients. Simultaneous use of more than one of these methods increases their overall effectiveness. Use of intrauterine devices (IUDs) such as coils has been discouraged because of the attendant risk of pelvic infections. Antirejection medications may also decrease the effectiveness of IUDs. Immunosuppressive agents increase the hazards associated with oral contraceptive methods and place the transplant recipient at greater risk of thromboembolism, hypertension, accelerated coronary artery disease, gastrointestinal disorders, and depression.

Some transplant centers have recently allowed their female transplant recipients to use low-dose oral contraceptive pills (OCPs). However, several case reports have indicated that concurrent use of cyclosporine and OCPs can result in higher cyclosporine concentrations. Androgens, estrogens, and progestins can increase cyclosporine concentration, most likely because of a reduction in hepatic cyclosporine metabolism. If cyclosporine and low-dose OCPs are administered concurrently, the patient's serum cyclosporine level and clinical response must be carefully monitored. OCPs are always contraindicated in patients with a history of deep vein thrombosis and clotting disorders such as Budd-Chiarri syndrome.

11. Are there any ethical issues associated with pregnancy in transplant recipients?

Several major ethical issues are associated with pregnancy following transplantation:
- Concerns about whether a woman with a limited lifespan or a potentially limited ability to care for a child should become pregnant.

- Concerns about the potential long-term effects of exposure to immunosuppressant agents in utero. It is unknown whether these offspring and future generations will be predisposed to infertility, malignancy, or congenital abnormalities.
- Concerns that women who have undergone heart transplantation for peripartum cardiomyopathy may have a recurrence of this disease in a subsequent posttransplant pregnancy.
- Concerns that familial cardiomyopathy may develop in the fetuses of women who have undergone heart transplantation for this disease.
- Concerns about the emotional well-being of the offspring of a transplant recipient who experiences graft rejection and the possible need for retransplantation.

Nurses, physicians, psychologists, social workers, ethicists, and clergy can provide information, guidance, and support to women and their partners as they cope with these difficult issues. The decision to become pregnant after transplantation should be made carefully so that immediate and long-term outcomes for all concerned may be optimized.

12. List some guidelines associated with optimal outcomes for both mother and child

In general, it is recommend that transplant recipients
- Postpone pregnancy for at least 1 year, and preferably 2 years, after transplantation when the risk of rejection is lower and immunosuppressant doses are lower and more stable.
- Have stable graft function (i.e., no evidence of rejection, graft dysfunction, or deterioration).
- Have good renal function (serum creatinine < 1.5 mg/dl; creatinine clearance > 75 ml/hr) at the time of conception.
- Be relatively normotensive or have hypertension that is well controlled.
- Be normoglycemic or have diabetes mellitus that is well controlled.
- Have overall good health.

13. Why is an interdisciplinary approach to pregnancy recommended?

An interdisciplinary approach is recommended to optimize outcomes for the mother and infant. In addition to an obstetrician with expertise in high-risk pregnancies, interdisciplinary team members typically include the transplant surgeon, transplant physician (e.g., cardiologist, hepatologist, nephrologist, pulmonologist), transplant coordinator, anesthesiologist, psychologist, social worker, pharmacist, dietician, and nurses who will provide prenatal, intrapartum, and postpartum care.

14. Describe the etiology of normal physiologic changes in pregnancy and their possible effects in transplant recipients.

PHYSIOLOGIC CHANGE	ETIOLOGY	POSSIBLE EFFECT IN TRANSPLANT RECIPIENT
↑ Blood volume	↓ Red blood cell mass ↓ Plasma expansion	Hemodilution may → ↓ in serum drug levels
↑ Cardiac output	↑ Stroke volume and heart rate	Heart transplant recipients: In denervated heart, cardiac output ↑ because of ↑ in circulating volume and circulating catecholamines
↑ Heart rate	↑ Circulating catecholamines ↓ Stroke volume	Exacerbation of ↑ heart rate due to cyclosporine
↑ Stroke volume	↑ Intravascular volume ↑ Venous return	Heart transplant recipients: Rejection may → systolic/diastolic dysfunction, thereby interfering with heart's ability to ↑ stroke volume
Right ventricular enlargement; tricuspid regurgitation	↑ Blood volume	Heart transplant recipients: Exacerbation of biopsy-induced tricuspid regurgitation

(Cont'd. on next page)

PHYSIOLOGIC CHANGE	ETIOLOGY	POSSIBLE EFFECT IN TRANSPLANT RECIPIENT
↑ Triglycerides ↑ Cholesterol	↑ Triglyceride synthesis stimulated by estrogen	Exacerbation of prepregnancy hyper-lipidemia and graft atherosclerosis
Weight gain	↑ Total body water because of intra-cellular expansion in growing organs (uterine, placental, fetal) and ↑ extracellular expansion (plasma volume, organs, amniotic fluid)	Weight gain may be aggravated by prednisone; ↑ blood volume may ↓ serum concentration of immuno-suppressants
Sodium retention	↑ Tubular absorption of sodium	↑ Edema; exacerbation of fluid retention caused by prednisone
↓ T-lymphocytes ↓ T-helper cells	Hormonal factors	↑ Risk of infection ↓ Risk of rejection
↓ Glucose tolerance	↓ Tissue sensitivity to insulin; effects of human placental lactogen that ↑ lipolysis, ↑ free fatty acid blood levels, ↓ sensitivity to insulin	↑ Risk of diabetogenesis for patients on prednisone, tacrolimus
Hyperemic, edema-tous gums	Chemical changes in connective tissue; ↑ in hydrophyilic mucopolysaccharides	Exacerbation of gum hyperplasia associated with immuno-suppressants
Stomach: ↓ motility, ↓ tone	Systemic relaxation of smooth muscles	Exacerbation of gastrointestinal symptoms associated with immunosuppressants
Gastroesophageal reflux; heartburn	Lower esophageal sphincter pressure ↓ because of smooth muscle relaxa-tion effects of progesterone; ↑ intra-abdominal pressure in 3rd trimester	Exacerbation of reflux due to ulcero-genic effects of chronic steroid use; gastrointestinal symptoms ↑ by azathioprine and prednisone
↑ Risk of urinary tract infection	↑ Glomerular filtration rate → ↓ glucose and amino acids in urine; ↑ urethral dilation → ↓ incidence of urinary tract infection	Risk of urinary tract infection ↑ because of immunosuppression
↑ Risk of chole-lithiasis	↓ Motility, ↑ volume in gallbladder; diluted bile; ↓ solubility of cholesterol → formation of crystals and stones	May exacerbate risk of colelithiasis associated with azathioprine

Adapted from Cupples SA: Cardiac transplantation in women. Crit Care Nurs Clin North Am 9:521–533, 1997, with permission.

15. What does routine prenatal monitoring involve?

ACTIVITY	RATIONALE
Monitor for infection (obtain leukocyte counts; screen for cytomegalovirus and other herpes virus infections).	Latent cytomegalovirus infections can be reactivated by allograft rejection and the hormonal changes associated with pregnancy.
Monitor for hypertension, edema and proteinuria. (Women are typically required to record blood pressure and weight daily).	Hypertension is a side effect of many immuno-suppressant medications.
Gestational diabetes screening: Monitor fasting blood glucose levels, and perform glucose tolerance tests as indicated.	Certain immunosuppressants (e.g., prednisone, tacrolimus) may induce diabetes.

16. What nutritional guidelines are recommended for pregnant transplant recipients?

To ensure maximal intrauterine fetal growth, a pregnant woman should eat approximately 2300 calories per day, with increases in protein, folic acid, calcium, iron, and vitamins A, B_6, B_{12}, and C. Prenatal vitamins are recommended.

17. What medications are typically administered during the intrapartum period?

Broad-spectrum antibiotics are usually initiated once the patient's membranes have ruptured; they are continued for a short time after delivery to prevent incisional infections related to either an episiotomy or cesarean section. Patients who are allergic to penicillin must take carefully selected alternative antibiotics to prevent toxic interactions with immunosuppressive agents. If the patient's creatinine clearance is decreased, the dose of renally excreted antibiotics may have to be lowered. Additional intravenous doses of steroids may be administered during labor.

18. What factors are associated with risks to the mother?

Maternal risks depend on the type of organ transplant, the stability of graft function, and the type and amount of immunosuppression that the woman is currently taking. In general, negative outcomes (e.g., maternal death, fetal loss, and graft loss) are more common in women with poor graft function, hypertension, and renal dysfunction and in women who are on higher doses of immunosuppression.

19. Is there one preferred immunosuppression regimen for pregnant transplant recipients?

There is no preferred immunosuppressive protocol for pregnant transplant recipients. It is recommended, however, that serum immunosuppression levels be monitored closely throughout the prenatal and postpartum periods to assure therapeutic levels. Changes in the mother's blood volume may result in the need to increase or decrease doses of immunosuppressive agents.

20. Why do calcineurin inhibitors predispose recipients to preeclampsia?

Calcineurin inhibitors such as cyclosporine and tacrolimus decrease the production of endogenous nitric oxide. Because nitric oxide is a mediator of smooth muscle relaxation, interference with the production of nitric oxide may increase sensitivity to vasoconstrictors and thereby predispose transplant recipients to preeclampsia.[6]

21. What are the major maternal risks associated with the various types of solid organ transplantation?

TYPE OF TRANSPLANT	MAJOR MATERNAL RISKS
Renal	Deterioration of renal function and ultimate loss of the allograft may occur when serum creatinine levels are elevated prior to conception.
	Further deterioration of renal function can result if blood pressure is not adequately controlled.
	Preeclampsia, characterized by hypertension and proteinuria during pregnancy, can lead to hypertensive crisis (eclampsia) if not adequately treated.
	Gestational diabetes can adversely affect renal graft function.
	NTPR data indicate the following:*
	• Incidence of hypertension is higher among recipients on cyclosporine-A-based regimens than those on tacrolimus.
	• Incidence of diabetes is lower among recipients on cyclosporine-A-based regimens than those on tacrolimus.
	• Recipients with a prepregnancy history of allograft rejection or elevated serum creatinine levels before or during pregnancy may be at increased risk for preeclampsia and warrant closer surveillance during pregnancy.
	• Successful pregnancy outcomes have been reported in recipients on cyclosporine-A-based regimens regardless of the length of the interval between transplant and conception; however, the incidence of pregnancy termination was highest in women with an interval ≤ 6 months.

(Cont'd. on next page)

TYPE OF TRANSPLANT	MAJOR MATERNAL RISKS
Liver	Hypertension, hyperbilirubinemia, preeclampsia, gestational diabetes, and graft rejection can occur.
	Preeclamptic patients are more likely to have low serum albumin levels because of loss of albumin in the urine.
	Complications associated with prenatal hypertension are more common if the woman has renal dysfunction at the time of conception.
	Graft loss and poor maternal outcomes have been associated with pregnancies occurring within 6 months of transplantation and recurrence of hepatitis B and C infections.
	NTPR data indicate the following:*
	• The incidence of hypertension during pregnancy and preeclampsia are lower in recipients on tacrolimus compared with recipients on cyclosporine-A-based regimens.
	• The incidence of diabetes during pregnancy is higher in recipients on tacrolimus compared with cyclosporine-A-based regimens.
	• Women with biopsy-proven acute rejection during pregnancy had poorer newborn outcomes and increased risk of recurrent rejection postpartum.
Pancreas	Hypertension, preeclampsia, graft rejection, and infections have been associated with pregnancy among pancreas transplant recipients.[†]
	Postpartum graft loss is more likely if rejection occurs during pregnancy.
Heart	Hypertension, preeclampsia, deteriorating renal function, and diabetes are associated with poorer pregnancy outcomes.
Lung	Hyperemesis gravidarum (frequent vomiting during pregnancy) may lead to inadequate levels of immunosuppression.
	Acute rejection and chronic rejection have been reported, as well as graft loss and death.[‡]
	Significant perinatal complications such as shortness of breath and infection place the pregnant recipient at particularly high risk.
	Although data from recent NTPR entries indicate more favorable outcomes than those of earlier entries, the overall risks for female lung transplant recipients appear greater than those for other organ recipients.*

* NTPR data from Armenti VT, Radomski JS, Moritz MJ, et al: Report from the National Transplantation Pregnancy Registry (NTPR): Outcomes of pregnancy after transplantation. In Cecka JM, Terasaki PI (eds) Clinical Transplants 2000. Los Angeles, UCLA Immunogenetics Center, 2001, pp 123–134.

† From Armenti VT, Moritz MJ, Jarrell BE, Davidson JM: Pregnancy after transplantation. Transplant Rev 14(3):145–157, 2000; Armenti VT, Radomski JS, Moritz MJ, et al: Report from the National Transplantation Pregnancy Registry (NTPR): Outcomes of pregnancy after transplantation. In Cecka JM, Terasaki PI (eds) Clinical Transplants 2000. Los Angeles, UCLA Immunogenetics Center, 2001, pp 123–134; Bumgardner GL, Matas AJ: Transplantation and pregnancy. Transplant Rev 6(3):139–162, 1992.

‡ From Donaldson S, Novotny D, Paradowski L, Aris R: Acute and chronic lung allograft rejection during pregnancy. Chest 110(1):293–296, 1996; Gertner G, Coscia L, McGrory C, et al: Pregnancy in lung transplant recipients. Prog Transplant 10(2):109–112, 2000.

22. Is the incidence of allograft rejection higher when a transplant recipient becomes pregnant?

With the exception of lung transplant recipients, there does not appear to be a higher rate of rejection provided that graft function is good at the time of conception and immunosuppression levels and graft function are monitored closely throughout pregnancy. If rejection is detected, it should be treated. Although the number of pregnancies among lung transplant recipients is small, higher rates of both chronic and acute rejection have been reported in this population.

23. How is acute rejection during pregnancy treated?

Acute rejection episodes during pregnancy are treated by increasing the amount of immunosuppression, usually with corticosteroids. This treatment option potentially increases the risk of both drug toxicity and infections. However, successful maternal and newborn pregnancy outcomes have been reported when rejection episodes have been treated with a variety of agents, including muromonab-CD3.

24. What are the pregnancy categories of the major immunosuppressants?

PREGNANCY CATEGORY B (NO FETAL RISK)	PREGNANCY CATEGORY C (FETAL RISK CANNOT BE RULED OUT)	PREGNANCY CATEGORY D (EVIDENCE OF FETAL RISK)
Corticosteroids (prednisone, methylprednisolone)	Cyclosporine A (Sandimmune, Neoral)	Azathioprine (Imuran)
Basiliximab (Simulect)	Tacrolimus (Prograf)	
	Antithymocyte globulin (Atgam, ATG)	
	Antithymocyte globulin (Thymoglobulin)	
	Orthoclone (OKT3)	
	Mycophenolate mofetil (CellCept)	
	Gengraf (cyclosporine capsules USP [modified])	
	Daclizumab (Zenapax)	
	Sirolimus (Rapamune)	

Adapted from Armenti VT, Radomski JS, Moritz, MJ, et al: Report from the National Transplantation Pregnancy Registry (NTPR): Outcomes of pregnancy after transplantation. In Cecka JM Terasaki PI (eds): Clinical Transplants 2000. Los Angeles, UCLA Tissue Typing Laboratory, 2001, pp 123–134, with permission.

25. Why are cyclosporine levels monitored closely during the early postpartum period?
Cyclosporine tends to concentrate in the placenta. After delivery, cyclosporine levels may increase suddenly. Therefore, it is important to monitor cyclosporine levels closely and adjust the dose accordingly.

26. What maternal and fetal risks are associated with the use of prednisone, cyclosporine, and azathioprine?

	PREDNISONE	CYCLOSPORINE	AZATHIOPRINE
Maternal	Infection	Infection	Infection
	Masking of signs of infection	Hypertension	Hepatotoxicity
	Impaired wound healing	Nephrotoxicity	Gastrointestinal disorders
	Peptic ulcer disease	Hepatotoxicity	Nausea, vomiting
	Ulcerative esophagitis		
	Steroid-induced diabetes		
	Hypertension		
	$\uparrow$ Potassium excretion		
	Emotional instability		
Fetal	Spontaneous abortion	Pregnancy category C	Pregnancy category D
	Premature membrane rupture	Crosses placenta	Crosses placenta
	Adrenal insufficiency	Prematurity	Leukopenia
	Placental insufficiency	Immunodeficiency	Thrombocytopenia
	Exopthalmos	Autoimmunity	
		Intrauterine growth retardation	

From Cupples SA: (1997) Cardiac transplantation in women. Crit Care Nurs Clin North Am 9:521–533, 1997, with permission.

27. What are the potential risks to the developing fetus and neonate?

The major risks to the fetus and neonate are spontaneous abortion, preterm delivery (< 37 weeks), intrauterine growth retardation, low birth weight, neonatal infection, neonatal mortality, and birth defects.

- The rate of fetal loss is dependent on graft function. In general, when graft function is good, the incidence of abortion approximates that of the general population (8–9%). When graft function is poor, rates of spontaneous abortion can exceed 50%.
- Higher rates of prematurity and intrauterine growth retardation are more common in mothers who have renal insufficiency, graft dysfunction, poorly controlled hypertension and/or diabetes, and who have been treated for rejection during pregnancy.
- Low levels of immunosuppressants have been measured in neonates during the first few days following birth; however, these concentrations usually drop to undetectable levels within a week.
- There are case reports of neonatal infections, although most are related to maternal infections with either the human immunodeficiency virus or cytomegalovirus. Neonatal infections such as pneumonia can also be related to prematurity.
- The reported rate of birth defects in children of transplanted women appears to be similar to that of the general population.

28. What types of birth defects have been reported in offspring of female transplant recipients?

Alcoholic embryopathies	Meningomyelocele
Anal atresia	Microcephaly
Anencephaly	Mitochrondrial cardiomyopathy
Cataracts	Patent ductus arteriosus
Cerebral palsy	Polycystic kidneys
Cleft palate	Premature closure of fontanelles
Congenital heart disease	Pulmonary artery stenosis
Diaphragmatic hernia	Pyloric stenosis
Ear defects	Strabismus
Limb deformities	Trisomy 21
Hydrocephalus	Tuberous sclerosis
Hypospadius	Umbilical hernias
Inguinal hernias	Ureteral abnormalities
Intra-articular hemangioma	Ventricular septal defect

29. Given that endomyocardial biopsy under fluoroscopic guidance may expose the fetus to radiation, name some alternative methods that can be used for rejection surveillance in pregnant heart transplant recipients.

Alternative methods include the following:
- Echocardiographically-guided endomyocardial biopsy
- Echocardiography (baseline and periodic calculation of ejection fraction)
- Cytoimmunologic monitoring
- Right heart catheterization in the presence of clinical signs and symptoms of rejection

30. Describe the preferred method of delivery and analgesia for heart transplant recipients.

Vaginal delivery is preferred. Labor may be induced to ensure that all necessary resources and personnel are available for the delivery. Epidural anesthesia is generally preferred for both vaginal delivery and cesarean section. With the controlled administration of epidural anesthesia, it is easier to achieve a balance between volume loading and peripheral vasodilatation.

31. Why is the number of pregnancies following heart transplantation expected to increase?

Since 1984, more than 2000 pediatric heart transplant procedures have been performed. As these recipients come into their childbearing years, it is anticipated that the number of posttransplant pregnancies will increase.

32. Is breastfeeding recommended for transplant recipients?
Many reports cite detectable levels of immunosuppressive drugs (azathioprine, prednisone, and cyclosporine) in breast milk. The levels vary from case to case and may be influenced by maternal serum levels. The significance of this finding is not well understood because the risk of the low concentrations to the infant has not been studied. Despite the fact that transplant physicians and obstetricians traditionally have discouraged transplant recipients from breastfeeding, there are documented individual cases of women who have breastfed their infants with no apparent untoward effect on the child. If the mother chooses to breastfeed her infant, it is important to monitor maternal serum immunosuppressant levels, immunosuppressant levels in the breast milk, infant serum immunosuppressant levels, and signs of immunosuppressant toxicity in the infant

33. Are there any problems with male transplant recipients fathering a pregnancy?
Pregnancies fathered by transplant recipients have not been as thoroughly studied as pregnancies among female transplant recipients. However, in general, the outcomes of such pregnancies have been favorable and appear to be similar to outcomes of pregnancies in the general population.

34. Where can I obtain more information on the care of the pregnant transplant recipient?
The National Transplantation Pregnancy Registry (NTPR)
1025 Walnut Street
605 College Building
Philadelphia, PA 19107
Phone: 215-955-2840
Fax: 215-923-1420
Toll free: 877-955-6877
e-mail: NTPR.registry@mail.tju.edu
The NTPR is a great resource for management of pregnant transplant patients. The NTPR collects data not only on pregnant female transplant recipients but also male recipients who have fathered offspring. Enrollment forms can be requested from the registry. Transplant coordinators provide these forms to prospective parents who agree to participate in the registry. The patient fills out the enrollment form at the end of the pregnancy, regardless of outcome. It is important to capture all outcomes: elective and spontaneous abortions, births (live and stillborn), as well as maternal and neonatal complications. The NTPR also conducts long-term follow-up on the offspring. Transplant coordinators receive a small honorarium for each pregnant transplant patient who enrolls.

BIBLIOGRAPHY

1. Armenti VT, Herrine KH, Radomski JS, Moritz MJ: Pregnancy after liver transplantation. Liver Transplant 6:671–685, 2000.
2. Armenti VT, Moritz MJ, Davidson JM: Drug safety issues following transplantation and immunosuppression: Effects and outcomes. Drug Safety 19:219–232, 1998.
3. Armenti VT, Moritz MJ, Jarrell BE, Davidson JM: Pregnancy after transplantation. Transplant Rev 14(3):145–157, 2000.
4. Armenti VT, Radomski JS, Moritz MJ, et al: Report from the National Transplantation Pregnancy Registry (NTPR): Outcomes of pregnancy after transplantation. In Cecka JM, Terasaki PI (eds) Clinical Transplants 2000. Los Angeles, UCLA Immunogenetics Center, 2001, pp 123–134.
5. Bumgardner GL, Matas AJ: Transplantation and pregnancy. Transplant Rev 6(3):139–162, 1992.
6. Casele HL, Laifer SA: Association of pregnancy complications and choice of immunosuppressant in liver transplant patients. Transplantation 65:581–582, 1998.
7. Cupples SA: Cardiac transplantation in women. Crit Care Nurs Clin N Am 9:521-533, 1997.
8. Donaldson S, Novotny D, Paradowski L, Aris R: Acute and chronic lung allograft rejection during pregnancy. Chest 110:293-296, 1996.
9. Gertner G, Coscia L, McGrory C, et al: Pregnancy in lung transplant recipients. Prog Transplant 10:109–112, 2000.
10. Jordan E, Pugh L: Pregnancy after cardiac transplantation: Principles of nursing care. J Obstet Gynecol Neonat Nurs 25:131–135, 1996.

11. Kainz A, Harabacz I, Cowlrick IS, et al: Analysis of 100 pregnancy outcomes in women treated systemically with tacrolimus. Transplant Int 13:S299–S300, 2000.
12. Kim K, Sukhani R, Slogoff S, Tomich P: Central hemodynamic changes associated with pregnancy in a long-term cardiac transplant recipient. Am J Obstet Gynecol 174:1651–1653, 1996.
13. Penn I: Pregnancy in solid organ allograft recipients: Literature scan. Transplantation 1997 First Quarter Review XII(2):1–24, 1997.
14. Poole JH: Liver transplant and pregnancy. J Perinatal Neonatal Nurs 11(4):25–35, 1998.
15. Scott JR, Wagoner LE, Olsen SL, et al: Pregnancy in heart transplant recipients: Management and outcomes. Obstet Gynecol 82:324–327, 1993.
16. Wilson GA, Coscia LA, McGrory CH, et al: National Transplantation Pregnancy Registry: Post-pregnancy graft loss among female pancreas-kidney recipients. Transplant Proc 33:1667–1669, 2001.

23. COPING WITH TRANSPLANTATION

Janet B. Mize, RN, BSN, CCTC, CCM

COPING WITH TRANSPLANTATION

1. How can transplant team members help patients to deal with the stressors associated with the transplant evaluation process?

The transplant evaluation process is inherently stressful. Patients must deal with numerous diagnostic tests, unexpected delays, and fears that abnormal test results might eliminate them from further consideration for transplantation. This can be a particularly difficult time for patients who are accustomed to exercising control over their affairs; often these patients attempt to control the disease and the transplant process as well. It is helpful if transplant team members

- Thoroughly explain the rationale for the various diagnostic tests
- Allow patients to participate in the scheduling of diagnostic tests, thereby providing them some control over the situation and affording them an opportunity to adjust to the reality of the need for an organ transplant.
- Understand the conflicting emotions that patients may experience at this time
- Permit patients to verbalize their feelings. (*Note:* It is often useful to schedule an interview with the transplant team social worker or other mental health provider early in the evaluation process. The appointment often provides both the time and the appropriate setting for patients to express their frustrations.)

2. How can transplant professionals help patients to work through their initial denial?

Patients often experience denial when they first learn of the need for an organ transplant. Often, patients do not believe they are as ill as they really are. Denial, coupled with a sense of loss of control, may lead to defiance and noncompliance with recommendations regarding such issues as substance-abuse cessation and dietary guidelines. It is important for healthcare providers to understand and acknowledge the patient's denial, provide periodic explanations of the patient's clinical status, offer gentle reminders about the rationale for any required behavioral modification, and suggest additional resources, as indicated (e.g., smoking cessation programs, nutritional counseling).

3. Why is the waiting period more difficult to cope with today than 10 years ago?

Ten years ago, the average waiting time for a solid organ transplant was considerably shorter than it is today. More often than not, candidates received their transplants before they became morbidly ill. However, as waiting times increased and medical management of the transplant candidate became more challenging, frustrations increased accordingly—not only for transplant candidates, but also for their families and transplant team members. Thus, it has become increasingly more important to incorporate adaptive coping mechanisms into the entire transplant process.

4. What can transplant professionals do to help candidates and family members to cope with long organ-waiting times?

Often patients mistakenly believe that once they are placed on the waiting list, an organ will become readily available. As the waiting period goes on, waiting for that phone call becomes more and more difficult. Transplant professionals can help patients and family members to cope by

- Providing a good explanation of the organ allocation system and anticipated waiting time
- Suggesting projects and tasks that can help patients and family members to remain involved in their transplant care, such as keeping journals, organizing a medication system,

keeping a calendar of appointments, and establishing a 24-hour care plan to be followed posttransplantation.
- Partnering the patient with a recipient mentor of a similar age and gender
- Encouraging attendance at support group meetings

5. Why are support groups helpful?

Waiting for an organ transplant is not easy. It brings with it difficult life changes and can arouse powerful emotions such as fear and guilt. These emotions always need to be addressed and are best handled with a positive attitude, a supportive network of family and friends, and a good relationship with the transplant team. Participation in a transplant support group is one way of coping with the emotional ups and downs of the waiting period. Learning that others share similar emotions helps candidates and family members to know that they are not alone. Support group members often share effective strategies for coping with the many stressors associated with the waiting period. Transplant recipients who participate in support group meetings offer tremendous hope for candidates and family members. These recipients are living proof that transplantation works!

6. Why does end-stage disease often interfere with effective coping?

Chronic disease eventually takes its toll on any individual. When patients are at the point of needing an organ transplant, they may feel as if they are at the end of their rope. Often they have dealt with the signs and symptoms of their disease for many years and quite frankly feel as if they cannot continue to do so. Patients who enter the transplant process at this stage may possess marginal or maladaptive coping skills and have little hope that they will ever see healthier days.

Along with despair, many end-stage diseases cause confusion, irritability, chronic fatigue and depression—all of which can interfere with effective coping. It is important that transplant team members try to understand the difficulty that patients may have with the physical and emotional demands of a rigorous evaluation testing schedule. Such understanding can go a long way toward strengthening the team's relationship with the patient and facilitating adaptive coping mechanisms.

7. Describe the stressors that candidates and family members face during the organ waiting period.

While each patient's situation is unique, typical stressors that are encountered during the waiting period include
- Fear that a donor organ will not become available in time
- Uncertainty about how long the waiting period will last
- Deteriorating health status
- Financial concerns, especially if the candidate is unable to work
- Changing roles and lifestyles (Caregivers often must become the primary breadwinner in the family. The role reversal and subsequent lifestyle changes may generate conflicting emotions within the family unit.)

8. How does "guilt" factor into the transplant process?

Guilt can rear its ugly head throughout the transplant process. Patients often feel guilty about earlier behaviors that may have precipitated their end-stage disease (e.g., previous alcohol or drug use). While waiting for the transplant, both patients and family members may feel guilty about "wishing" for a donor to become available, knowing that this means that someone "has to die." Following transplantation, recipients may experience "survivor's guilt" and conflicting emotions about knowing that "someone died" so that they could have a second chance at life. Throughout the transplant process, patients often feel guilty because they are a source of worry to their loved ones.

It is important that patients and family members know that such feelings are common and a natural part of dealing with an organ transplant. However, if these feelings continue for a long period of time, the transplant mental health professional should be consulted.

9. Why is the patient's caregiver at risk for "burn-out"?

More often than not, the transplant process is more difficult on the caregiver than the patient. For at least some portion of this process, the caregiver may have to become the primary bread-winner, assume responsibility for daily activities within the home, and function as a "single parent"—all while caring for the chronically ill patient. Often, this added workload creates additional stressors for both the caregiver and the patient. Before and after transplant, it is essential that the caregiver take breaks whenever possible. The transplant team should encourage caregivers to explore options for respite care so that burnout is minimized.

10. What can healthcare professionals do to help patients become more compliant?

Both pre- and posttransplant medical regimens can be quite complicated and overwhelming for patients. The following strategies are useful for giving patients responsibility for their care and enhancing compliance:

- Have the patient keep a journal to record weights, vital signs, medication changes, future medical appointments, and questions for the transplant team. Review this documentation at each clinic appointment.
- Enroll the patient in a transplant-specific pharmacy program. Such programs simplify the medication-ordering process. In addition, the pharmacists are excellent resources for patients and families.
- Take advantage of every "teachable moment." Use each encounter to assess patients' knowledge and review important material.
- Help the patient to devise a user-friendly medication system.

11. What type of medication system do you suggest?

Transplant candidates and recipients typically take many medications throughout the day. Patients may have problems remembering to take their medications exactly as prescribed. One of the following medication systems may help to simplify this process.

- Have the patient purchase a fishing tackle box or craft box with individual compartments. Label the *columns* with the days of the week and the *rows* with the time of day (e.g., morning, afternoon, evening, bedtime). (*Note:* the typical pill containers that are available in drugstores are usually not large enough to accommodate a weeks' worth of medications).
- Have the patient use a combination of small (snack-sized) and large zip-close plastic bags. Use the small plastic bags for specific doses throughout the day. Label the small bags with their respective dosing times (e.g., morning, afternoon, evening, bedtime). Put all of the individual dose bags into the larger bag. Label the larger bags with the days of the week.
- For patients who have a particularly difficult time remembering to take medications, suggest that the patient use a pill container with a built-in alarm system.

What works for one patient may not work for another. Occasionally, patients have to try one or more of the above medication systems to determine which one works best for them.

12. How can you be certain that patients are taking their medications correctly?

Once a particular system for medication is established with the patient, the nurse's job becomes easier. However, it is still important to review medications periodically with patients. Have the patient bring in the medication system and explain how it is used. Question the patient about both prescribed and over-the-counter medications. Many over-the-counter medications, herbal supplements, and teas can adversely interact with prescription medications. Encourage patients to call whenever they have questions about medications or whenever another healthcare provider prescribes a new medication.

13. What advice can you give to patients whose medication schedules "control" their lives?

Immediately after discharge, all of the patient's and family's activities tend to rotate around the medication schedule. They have been drilled about compliance, accuracy, and record-keeping. Some patients may even set an alarm clock to remind them of the time to take the next medication and then sit patiently next to the clock waiting for it to ring! Although this type of behavior is understandable in the early posttransplant period, long-term obsession over medications is not healthy. Even though medications are certainly an important part of posttransplant life, patients must learn to relax and realize that there may be occasions when a dose is taken late or even missed. Most transplant centers advise patients to either follow written instructions regarding such medication mistakes or to contact a member of the transplant team for further directions.

Medication schedules and trough immunosuppressant blood draws may become more complicated once the recipient returns to work or school. Often conflicts can be resolved by reviewing the recipient's daily activities and medication regimen. It may be possible to have trough levels drawn in the evening instead of the morning. Or these levels may be drawn at a local laboratory that is closer to the recipient's home, school, or job.

Regardless of the specific issue, it is usually possible to work out a medically sound but "livable" schedule that compliments, rather than dictates, the recipient's lifestyle.

14. Can transplant recipients tell when their immunosuppression levels are too high?

Certain transplant recipients may get a "feel" for their immunosuppression levels, similar to that which diabetic patients get when their blood glucose levels are too high or low. These recipients may have an exacerbation of the side effects normally associated with certain immunosuppressants (e.g., tremors or headaches). Some recipients are so attuned to side effects that they are able to predict their immunosuppressant levels with a surprising degree of accuracy. It is important to listen to these patients and draw immunosuppressant levels accordingly. However, recipients must be instructed not to adjust their doses themselves.

15. How can recipients minimize the unsightly side effects of immunosuppressant medications?

Unfortunately many immunosuppressants cause unsightly physical changes such as skin irritation and eruptions, excessive hair growth, gingival hyperplasia, facial fullness, and weight gain. Side effects are difficult for all transplant recipients; however, they may be particularly problematic for women and adolescents. During the pretransplant period, it is important for transplant professionals to discuss the potential side effects and identify strategies for dealing with them:
- Use of approved hair removal techniques
- Surgery for gingival hyperplasia
- Sensible diet and regular exercise for weight control
- Hairstyles that minimize facial fullness

16. How can transplant professionals help family members to cope with the recipient's steroid-induced mood changes?

Steroid therapy is often associated with mood swings. Although transplant professionals are accustomed to dealing with these side effects, family members are often taken by surprise. Life at home may get at little "touchy" at times when the recipient becomes quick-tempered or emotional. Family members may complain that recipients are not well enough to care for themselves yet are well enough to be irritable or demanding. Reassurance is the greatest gift one can give family members at this point. Assure them that, in most cases, mood swings and irritability decrease as steroid medications are weaned and possibly discontinued. Unless these symptoms are reflective of the recipient's underlying personality, this too shall pass.

It is also essential that family members take care of themselves by getting away from time to time. Even short breaks can effectively reduce stress levels. Friends and other relatives are generally quite willing to provide respite care. Family members may feel guilty about leaving the recipient, so it is important to let them know that it is "OK" to get away, even if only for a few hours.

17. What helps the patient, caregivers, and healthcare professionals deal with the confusion that some patients experience?

Patients with end-stage disease and transplant recipients may experience confusion from time to time. For example, liver transplant candidates may have encephalopathy; transplant recipients may have neurocognitive deficits secondary to immunosuppressant medications. Confusion, however, may have its greatest impact on caregivers and healthcare professionals. Consequently, these individuals may be tempted to take total control of the situation. Although this approach may be the easiest, it is not necessarily the best for the patient. Given that periods of confusion may wax and wane, it is important to allow patients to exercise as much autonomy and control as possible on days when they are less confused.

However, it is equally important to recognize times when the patient is confused. Clues that indicate confusion might include

- Asking the same question several times over a short period of time
- Overlooking activities of daily living (e.g., shaving, brushing teeth)
- Forgetting to take medications
- Experiencing difficulty in simple tasks such as dialing the telephone.

Lists of "to do" activities might be useful during periods of confusion. However, lists are effective only if the patient remembers to look at the list! Verbal and written reminders (e.g., notes pasted to the bathroom mirror or medicine cabinet) are helpful adjuncts.

18. What are some indications that a patient's driving might have to be restricted?

Chronic disease and certain medications can impair concentration, slow reflexes, and increase response time. Clinic visits are a good time to assess a patient's ability to drive safely. Question patients about the need to pull over and rest, any situations in which they forgot where they were going, or any occasions when they went through a red light or stop sign without realizing it. These are all subtle signs that a patient's driving might have to be restricted.

19. How can transplant professionals help recipients to cope with postdischarge "separation anxiety"?

Transplant recipients often experience "separation anxiety" when they are first discharged. This anxiety may be more intense for recipients who live far from the transplant center. Despite comprehensive discharge teaching, the complex dos and don'ts of the posttransplant regimen may be overwhelming once the recipient leaves the security of the hospital. Anxiety may manifest itself in numerous calls to the transplant office, calls that may seem to have little purpose. However, these "comfort calls" are the recipient's way of reaching out for reassurance that everything is all right. It behooves transplant professionals to understand the motive behind these calls and invest time in assessing the recipient's transition to home. Over time, the calls typically decrease in frequency as the recipient is reassured that all is well and begins to enjoy the comforts of home.

20. What causes impotence in certain transplant recipients?

Impotence in the early postoperative period may be associated with lack of energy, depression, or medications. Erectile dysfunction may resolve as the recipient's recovery progresses, energy returns, and steroid-induced depression decreases. If this condition persists, however, a urology consultation may be warranted. It is important for transplant clinicians to remind recipients to check with the transplant team before taking any medications prescribed by other healthcare providers.

21. When is it safe for a transplant recipient to travel?

The recipient's potential to travel depends on the recipient's age, degree of pretransplant morbidity, type of transplant procedure, and course of recovery. Other factors to consider include the mode of travel, destination, and availability of medical care should it be required at any time during the trip. Most transplant centers do not permit recipients to travel until their clinical status is stable, incisions are well-healed, and mobility has returned. Travel to foreign countries is usually restricted during the first posttransplant year.

22. Are there any tips for transplant recipients who are planning a trip?

Following transplantation, planning a trip requires a little more thought. It is generally recommended that recipients

- Keep their medications with them at all times. Medications should not be packed in a suitcase that will be checked.
- Take at least 3 days' worth of extra medications with them (in case their return is delayed).
- Obtain the name and telephone number of a transplant center close to their destination.
- Make arrangements for any special needs (such as a wheelchair or special diet).
- Take a letter (on hospital stationery) that lists the date of transplant, all current medications, and the name of a contact person at the transplant center of record.
- Carry a bottle of hand cleanser or disposable hand wipes for frequent hand-washing.
- Depending on the destination and mode of travel, carry or pack several small bottles of distilled water.

23. When can transplant recipients return to work?

Return to work typically depends on a number of factors such as the time interval since transplant, type of work, and potential for exposure to environmental hazards. Many recipients can return to their former occupations. However, some recipients may have to seek an alternative type of employment (e.g., those whose former occupations involved heavy physical labor or those who worked in an environment that exposed them to chemicals, infections, or other hazards). Many transplant centers recommend that recipients return to work gradually; for example, they could work part-time for several weeks. Many employers require written authorization from the transplant center regarding the number of hours a recipient may work and any limitations on the recipient's activities.

Ideally, discussions about posttransplant employment should begin in the pretransplant period so that the transplant center's expectations regarding return to work can be communicated to the patient and vocational training needs can be identified. Referral to a vocational rehabilitation counselor may be required. In some situations, it may be possible for the patient to begin vocational training during the pretransplant waiting period.

24. Why may some transplant recipients be tempted to engage in risky behavior?

Transplantation gives recipients a new lease on life. Occasionally, this *joie de vie* is accompanied by a sense of invincibility, particularly in younger recipients. After they have settled into a posttransplant routine, certain recipients may be tempted to engage in risky behaviors such as smoking, excessive drinking, drug abuse, or unsafe sexual practices. Or they may participate in activities such as skydiving or bungie-cord jumping that can result in blunt trauma to the transplanted organ. Transplant clinicians may have to remind recipients of the dangers inherent in these activities. Referral to a mental health professional or substance abuse counselor may be warranted.

25. Can transplant recipients have pets?

Pets can be therapeutic in many respects. They offer companionship, diversion, and opportunities for exercise. Some studies have indicated that pets also help to lower blood pressure and decrease stress. There are some precautions, however, that transplant recipients must observe. Some transplant centers restrict recipients from having birds or reptiles. Others recommend that recipients avoid changing litter boxes and cleaning fish aquariums. Before discharge, it is important to determine if the recipient has any pets and to discuss center-specific guidelines.

26. Are transplant recipients allowed to communicate with their donor families?

At one time, recipients were not permitted to contact their donor families. Some transplant programs still strongly discourage this practice. Today, however, many recipients want to personally thank their donor families for the gift of life they have received.

Written communication is typically anonymous and is initiated by the recipient. Recipients often share information about themselves (e.g., occupation, family situation, hobbies) and talk about their transplant experience and life after the surgery. In most instances, donor families welcome and appreciate this communication because the recipient's well-being is a great source of comfort and peace. Donor families frequently write back to the recipient. Sharing information about the donor often helps donor families through the grieving process. Occasionally, however, a donor family may choose not to respond to a recipient's letter.

Under certain circumstances, anonymous communication may progress to direct communication and even meetings between the recipient and donor family. For this to happen, both parties must agree to nonanonymous communication and sign a waiver releasing their right to confidentiality.

Communication between recipients and donor families may be mediated by the Donor Family Advocacy office of the local organ procurement organization.

27. Does life after transplant ever return to normal?

The term "normal" is relative. Some would argue that taking immunosuppressive medications twice a day for the rest of one's life and other aspects of the posttransplant regimen are not "normal." Others contend that transplantation involves trading one chronic disease for another. Nevertheless, many transplant recipients resume active lifestyles, return to work or school, travel extensively, and enjoy the good life. In short, they treasure their "second chance at life" and are deeply appreciative of the gift of life that has been given to them.

BIBLIOGRAPHY

1. Benning CR, Smith A: Psychological needs of family members of liver transplant patients. Clin Nurs Spec 8:280–288, 1994.
2. Bohachick P, Reeder S, Taylor MV, et al: Psychosocial impact of heart transplantation on spouses. Clin Nurs Res 10:6–25, discussion 26–28, 2001.
3. Collins EG, White-Williams C, Jalowiec A: Impact of the heart transplant waiting process on spouses. J Heart Lung Transplant 15:623–630, 1996.
4. Collins EG, White-Williams C, Jalowiec A: Spouse quality of life before and 1 year after heart transplantation. Crit Care Nurs Clin North Am 12:103–110, 2000.
5. Cupples SA, Nolan MT, Augustine SM, et al: Perceived stressors and coping strategies among heart transplant candidates. J Transpl Coord 8:179–187, 1998.
6. Fedewa MM, Oberst MT: Family caregiving in a pediatric renal transplant population. Pediatr Nurs 22:402–407, 417, 1996.
7. Hanton LB: Caring for children awaiting heart transplantation: Psychosocial implications. Pediatr Nurs 24:214–218, 1998.
8. Hirth AM, Stewart MH: Hope and social support as coping resources for adults waiting for cardiac transplantation. Can J Nurs Res 26:31–48, 1994.
9. Hwang HF: Patient and family adjustment to heart transplantation. Prog Cardiovasc Nurs 11:16–18, 39, 1996.
10. Kaba E, Thompson DR, Burnard P: Coping after heart transplantation: A descriptive study of heart transplant recipients' methods of coping. J Adv Nurs 32:930–936, 2000.
11. Kurz JM: Desire for control, coping, and quality of life in heart and lung transplant candidates, recipients, and spouses: A pilot study. Prog Transplant 11:224–230, 2001.
12. Lindqvist R, Carlsson, Sjoden PO: Coping strategies and health-related quality of life among spouses of continuous ambulatory peritoneal dialysis, haemodialysis, and transplant patients. J Adv Nurs 31:1398–1408, 2000.
13. Nickel R, Wunsch A, Egle UT, et al: The relevance of anxiety, depression, and coping in patients after liver transplantation. Liver Transpl 8:63–71, 2002.
14. Olbrisch ME, Benedict SM, Ashe K, et al: Psychosocial assessment and care of organ transplant patients. J Consult Clin Psychol 70:771–783, 2002.
15. Parr E, Mize J: Coping with an Organ Transplant. New York, Avery, 2001.
16. Pelletier-Hibbert M, Sohi P: Sources of uncertainty and coping strategies used by family members of individuals living with end-stage renal disease. Nephrol Nurs J 28:411–417, 419; discussion 418–419, 2001.
17. Rodrigue JR, Davis GL, Howard RJ: Psychological adjustment of liver transplant candidates. Clin Transplant 7:228–229, 1993.
18. Singer HK, Ruchinskas RA, Riley KC, et al: The psychological impact of end-stage lung disease. Chest 120:1246–1252, 2001.
19. Stubblefield C, Murray RL: Making the transition: Pediatric lung transplantation. J Pediatr Health Care 14:280–287, 2000.
20. Suddaby EC, Flattery MP, Luna M: Stress and coping among parents of children awaiting cardiac transplantation J Transpl Coord 7:36–40, 1997.
21. Thomas DJ: Returning to work after liver transplantation: Experiencing the roadblocks. J Transpl Coord 6:134–138, 1996.

24. RISK MANAGEMENT FOR TRANSPLANT COORDINATORS*

Linda Ohler, MSN, RN, CCTC, FAAN

1. What areas in the current practice of a transplant coordinator can be considered risky?

Several areas in the practice of a transplant coordinator can become risky. Although many of the daily interactions seem routine, the coordinator's handling of telephone communications, e-mail, faxes, and documentation carries many potential risks. This chapter addresses potential problems for nurses who are working in outpatient settings and providing advice to patients across state lines. Because most of the nurse's educational background focused on the care of hospitalized or acutely ill patients, practice in an outpatient setting must be carefully evaluated to ensure that interventions are within the scope of state nurse practice acts.

2. Describe potential problems associated with providing advice to patients across state lines.

Telephone communications are part of everyday practice for transplant coordinators. In talking with patients on the telephone, providing them with consultations, advice, and information, the coordinator must consider potential risks with regard to practice issues outside of the state nurse practice acts. Many transplant patients do not live in the state where they underwent transplantation. Therefore, nurses communicate with patients across state lines and may not be licensed to practice in the state where the patient lives. It is important to be familiar with the nurse practice acts in each state where the nurse gives advice or instruction. The National Council of State Boards of Nursing (NCSBN) has been addressing such concerns as the practice of nursing across state lines. The NCSBN is working with various states to implement a mutual recognition for practice as well as interstate agreements. Information about how laws for interstate nursing practice may affect the coordinator may be accessed at www.ncsbn.org or at each state board of nursing.

3. Are there any risks in communicating with patients by phone?

Two areas of concern with telephone communication include misunderstandings about information given to patients or family members and about messages left on voice mail or recorders. It is easy to misunderstand verbal phone messages. The number 15 can sound like 50 over the phone. Add to this patients for whom English is a second language and you have many opportunities for complex phone interactions that may result in errors. Leaving messages on voicemail or on a recorder carries much potential for breach of confidentiality. One may leave the message on the wrong phone, or a family member may forget to tell the patient about the message. If the message is left at a patient's place of employment, one may breach confidentiality if someone else listens to the message. It is a nurse's responsibility to talk with the patient directly rather than leave a message with instruction. The nurse may leave a message for the patient to call back, but it remains the his or her responsibility to contact the patient with information.

Patients may minimize symptoms when calling to report a problem. Most patients want the problem fixed through a telephone consultation and do not want to return to the clinic or be admitted to the hospital. As a result, experienced coordinators with excellent communication skills know the importance of triaging patient calls. The message that the coordinator receives may state, "I have this painful pimple behind my ear," but the coordinator must respond with great care, beginning with questions to further determine whether the patient's complaint really is a pimple or the beginning of a more serious disorder such as shingles from a herpes infection.

---

* The information contained in this chapter is not meant to take the place of legal advice. It is recommended that each nurse contact the risk management or legal department of his or her institution to determine areas of potential practice risks.

With the busy schedules that transplant coordinators keep, long hours and patient complaints can put coordinators at risk for communication failures. Trying to second-guess what a patient or family is reporting can contribute to miscommunication. This danger is especially true with patients or families who call several times a day or week. A coordinator may not triage as thoroughly and may collect incomplete information when patients or families call repeatedly. In the process of stereotyping callers, the coordinator may make the mistake of collecting incomplete information or jumping to conclusions. Not talking with the patient directly is another area that may contribute to miscommunication. Communication skills are a key component of the expert clinical transplant coordinator's role. Having standard-of-care protocols for triaging in place may also help to prevent miscommunication during patient and family phone calls.

When triage of patient problems is done by phone, communication is complicated by the fact there are no written instructions for the patient or family to refer to once the instructions have been given. Because of the complexities of posttransplant care and medication regimens, patients and families are often overwhelmed by the instructions they receive. Without written instructions for future reference, the patient and family may make inaccurate interpretations from memory that cause a failure in the actual implementation of instructions. Phone instructions, or any verbal instructions, have the potential to create misunderstandings. Coordinators should ask patients to repeat the instructions and suggest that the instructions be written in the patient's transplant diary. Because most patients are discharged with a diary-type booklet for keeping track of their medications and recording daily vital signs, it is a good idea to educate patients on maintaining written instructions based on phone conversations with transplant professionals.

4. Some transplant patients and their families call frequently. Does the transplant coordinator have to document every conversation?

Documentation of phone calls can be a challenge if the coordinator is following hundreds of outpatients. Documentation of communication with patients is crucial. Whether refilling a prescription or giving a patient advice while on call, the coordinator must document all interactions, directions, and changes in patient status. The date and time should be documented with each entry along with the purpose of the call. Documentation should also include a statement about the advice given to the patient or caller, any discussions or consultations with physician regarding the call, and the patient's response to the advice. If patients are given a warning about the risk of not complying with the advice, that information must be documented as well. Although documentation is one of the first skills covered in nursing education, it is also one area that most practicing nurses can improve. Documentation is not only a legal responsibility, but also a method for team members to communicate events and any changes in medications or patient status.

5. Patients want to communicate by e-mail. What safeguards should the transplant coordinator take with this form of communication?

Electronic communication has become a way of life for many of us. In healthcare many concerns have been raised over communicating with patients via e-mail. For patients who are connected to e-mail servers, communication with doctors and nurses is much easier by e-mail than trying to contact them by phone. But several concerns for healthcare professionals should be addressed before entering into communications with patients via e-mail. The American Medical Informatics Association in Bethesda, Maryland, has recommended guidelines for electronic communication with patients. Before starting electronic communication, it is highly recommended that written informed consent be obtained from the patient for this form of communication. It is important to point out that although the medical institution's firewalls may be secure, the patient's home computer probably does not have the same protection of confidential information.

6. What guidelines should be established with patients for e-mail communications?

In establishing guidelines with patients for electronic mail communications, nurses and physicians should discuss key issues for the content of information to be shared by e-mail. For instance, patients should always have their full name on each e-mail communication for proper

identification. Many people use a screen name that may be impossible to associate with a particular patient. Patients should know when to expect a response to their e-mail communication. It is
best to have an automatic reply stating that the e-mail communication is not intended for emergencies and that patients should call a specified number for any emergency. The automatic reply
may also state when patients may expect a response or whom to contact if the office is closed.
Breaches in confidentiality can occur in sending an e-mail to the wrong person. The table below
outlines considerations for establishing e-mail communication with patients.

Establishing e-mail Communication with Patients

1. Obtain written consent from each patient for e-mail communication.
   a. Explain that all e-mail correspondence becomes part of the patient's medical record.
   b. Establish with whom e-mail communication will be shared.
   c. Explain potential security risks; describe how breaches in confidentiality may occur.
2. Establish guidelines with each patient for appropriate use of e-mail communication.
   a. Not for use in emergency
   b. Whom to contact if no personnel are in the office
   c. Refilling prescriptions
   d. Requests for referrals
   e. Laboratory/test results
   f. Making appointments
3. Ask patients to include their full name in each message.
4. Establish the expected turn-around time for a reply.

7. Are there any other concerns about e-mail communication?

Writing style in e-mail communication is often quite casual; however, e-mail communication
with patients should not be casual. Long-term relationships with patients can potentially result in
a loss of professional boundaries. It is natural for patients to want to be special. They have gone
through a lot with their illnesses and subsequent transplants. Coordinators often are seen as a life-
line to patients and families. Patients may use e-mail communication as an avenue for friendly
communication. Avoiding casual conversational styles often helps patients to realize that this
form of communication is for medical information and communication of instructions.

8. How does the coordinator document e-mail communications?

Copies of all e-mail correspondence must be kept in a patient's medical record. This record
keeping includes the physician's communication with a patient as well as that from all other team
members. Copies of the patient's e-mail as well as the provider's response should be maintained
as part of the medical record.

9. What are the major concerns in faxing patient documents?

Several concerns related to breaches in confidentiality arise with the use of faxes to communicate patient information. First, the medical provider needs written consent to share a patient's
medical records with another physician's office or laboratory. The written consent should be
maintained in the patient's medical record. In addition, fax machines must be kept in a secure
area to prevent other patients or visitors from reading information left on the fax machine. Being
certain that one has the correct fax number is important to ensure that medical information is not
sent to an unintended receiver. Each of these instances carries a potential for breaches in the confidentiality of a patient's private medical information.

10. Are there risks in patient evaluations?

During the evaluation process for transplantation, patients and families are often highly anxious. They want to pass the tests and be listed for transplantation. Most believe their quality of
life will greatly improve with a new organ. Thus, there is much at stake for them to convince the
transplant team that the patient is a good candidate and that the family support is steadfast and

dedicated. While team members evaluate the patient physically and psychosocially, coordinators often have the greatest role in educating and guiding patients and families through the process.

Coordinators and team members must provide consistent messaging to patients and families. From the initial phone conversation between the coordinator and patient, information is being conveyed. It is recommended that the initial visit for transplant evaluation consist of education for the patient and family. Understandably, some patients such as heart or liver patients are often acutely ill and unable to participate in the education process. In such cases, the family needs extra support and clear information. Information may need to be repeated on several occasions when anxieties are high.

The key to managing risks is in the messaging. Patients and families need to understand the evaluation and listing process, the allocation of organs, and the complexities of long-term follow-up after transplantation. Establishing good relationships and trust is very important.

11. What are the risks involved when listing a patient for transplantation?

Once a patient has completed the evaluation process to determine if transplantation is necessary and whether it is the best option, the listing process begins. Forms are completed, and information is sent by secure computer systems or by fax to the United Network of Organ Sharing (UNOS) (see chapter 1). It is a good idea for the listing nurse to confirm with another team member that the information being transmitted is correct. Serious errors have been made in listing patients, such as including an incorrect blood type. Failure to list a patient has also been reported. Such errors can occur when roles or messages are unclear. Inaccurate communication about which lung to transplant can result in serious morbidities or mortality. Verification of the information being transmitted is the best practice.

Not listing a patient can be an issue for nurses as well. If the transplant team has determined that a patient is not a candidate for transplantation, the patient must be notified. Who will communicate this decision to the patient and family must be resolved in advance, perhaps in a team meeting. Documentation of the team decision, the rationale for the decision, and all communication with the patient is very important. It is highly recommended that a letter be sent to the patient with a copy to the referring physician that states why the patient was not listed for transplantation. Being denied a transplant can produce a very emotional response from the patient and family. Documentation is important.

12. What does one need to document when the patient is contacted for the transplant?

Notifying a patient at home that a potential donor organ may be available requires documentation. Many patients remain at home waiting for a transplant and may carry a pager for notification. When the on-call coordinator is contacted about a potential donor organ, the patient is contacted either by phone or by pager. There have been instances when the patient has forgotten the pager or cannot be reached. The coordinator needs to document the date and times of the calls, including the phone numbers used in each attempt.

Once contacted, the patient and family must receive clear instructions. They will, undoubtedly, be very emotional and may not remember all instructions. Ask them to repeat the instructions and to write them down. On rare occasions, a patient reached at home has second thoughts and tells the coordinator the transplant is too risky or not wanted. It is very important for the coordinator to document this conversation and to document the communication with the transplant surgeon as well. It is a good practice to notify the patient's referring physician of this event.

13. Are there risks in preparing patients for discharge?

Posttransplant care is often complex with dosages of antirejection medications being changed and individualized regularly to meet each patient's needs. Postoperative complications, patient education needs, home care arrangements, and prescription orders add to the complexity of care. The fact that patients are discharged earlier adds stress for the nurses who must ensure that all education and discharge preparations are completed and documented. More importantly, nurses must ensure that the patient understands information that has been presented. Most transplant coordinators have on-call responsibilities and are available to respond to patient questions or concerns. There must be good communication channels among staff nurses, inpatient coordinators, clinical nurse specialists, and the on-call coordinator to facilitate a patient's transition to home and self-care.

Communication strategies are important for all team members responsible for this complex patient population. Many transplant programs have residents and fellows who follow transplant patients. Often their rotation is for 4–8 weeks. This short period certainly does not provide them with the opportunity to become experts in transplantation. Staff physicians usually oversee daily or twice-daily rounds on transplant patients. Although some transplant coordinators maintain a single role as inpatient coordinator, others rotate weekly or monthly in the role of inpatient coordinator. The rotation almost always occurs on the same day as the rotation of staff physicians, residents, and interns. Thus patients may have an entirely new transplant team at the beginning of each month. Communication, both verbal and written, is crucial to optimizing continuity of care. One idea for enhancing that communication is to have one member of the transplant team rotate on the 15th of the month rather than on the first, which allows one person to be the continuity force for communication.

Some transplant centers are hiring nurse practitioners to fulfill the role of transplant coordinator to cover the discharge needs and outpatient follow-up care. Although this is an excellent role for nurse practitioners, most nurses must continue to practice within state guidelines for registered nurses. Writing physician orders, writing discharge prescriptions, and dictating discharge summaries are a few of the tasks being asked of nurse-coordinators in various hospital settings, especially if there is no resident or fellow following transplant patients. If the physician orders are cosigned, the task is not harmful. Writing discharge prescriptions on presigned prescriptions, however, is very risky. While physician assistants are accustomed to dictating discharge summaries, most nurses have neither the educational background nor the legal right to fulfill this practice.

14. Does a nurse who is on call for patients with problems face any risks?

Nurses face several potential problems when they are on call after hours and on weekends. The potential problems arise when the nurse steps outside of the realm of nursing practice or fails to document any interactions or discussions with patients or family members. Weekend or evening calls may entail simple questions about patient care issues, such as wound management or what to do about a skipped dose of medication. It is very easy for an experienced transplant nurse to answer most patient questions. However, only written standard protocols protect nurses who triage calls from patients and families. Many common problems prompt a call from a transplant patient, and nurses who take the responsibility for being on call should ascertain that their licenses are protected with written standard protocols. Such protocols should be developed with team physicians.

15. How does the nurse-coordinator know what standard protocols are needed to ensure safe practice?

Transplant patients have many common complications such as infections and rejections after transplantation. Written protocols that direct nurses in the care of the patient with fevers, rashes, rigors, shortness of breath, abdominal pain, or other common symptoms not only protect the nurse on call who is caring for patients but also ensure that the team is working within a common framework. For instance, if a patient calls with a temperature of 39°C, the response from each coordinator or physician will be the same if all team members are using the same written protocols.

Although rejection symptoms vary with each organ system, transplant teams can easily develop standard protocols that reflect and identify criteria for detecting rejection. Liver teams have different criteria for determining a potential rejection than lung teams or heart teams. Developing standard protocols for teams to follow when triaging calls from patients saves time and frustration, and may even save a graft.

16. How does the team develop written standard protocols?

Team meetings are usually held weekly in most transplant centers. The weekly meeting provides staff with the opportunity to discuss issues such as standardized protocols. Reaching team consensus may take a few meetings, but the results are worth the time. The group may decide to start by determining which problems are most common in their particular patient population. Lung patients have different problems from renal recipients, but there are common issues related to infections. Symptoms of rejection vary.

Starting with a list of common problems in a particular patient population is the first step in developing standard protocols. Developing a list of questions to ask the patient is of great value in standardizing triage for nurses on call. Team consensus on interventions for each patient problem identified helps to shape the standard protocol. Each nurse should have these standardized protocols available for reference when on call as well as in the transplant clinic office when triaging patient problems. Using standard care protocols protects a nurse from stepping out of the boundaries for the scope of nursing practice.

17. How can the transplant coordinator document information when he or she is on call?

Most transplant coordinators are on call for coordinating a transplant, whereas others carry that responsibility plus being the first call source for patients with questions and emergencies. Documentation of events while on call ensures accurate communication of any changes in patient medications, health status, or instructions given to the patient or family. How can a nurse document these events when not in the hospital or at home? Although carrying a pager, cell phone, and notebooks filled with candidate information is certainly a familiar scenario for all transplant coordinators, tools for documentation are not always readily available or convenient. In addition, while personal digital assistants are an excellent resource, not all coordinators have that luxury. Thus, developing a system for documenting patient information while on call is important for each center.

Carrying blank progress notes is one possibility. Documenting information on progress notes can be helpful so long as the notes are maintained in a safe and secure place where they are not accessible for others to read. The use of a dictation system is another method for managing on-call events. Keeping a small dictaphone available for on-call coordinators is a tool that may improve documentation of information. In a large multiorgan transplant center where several nurses are on call covering pediatrics, adult, abdominal and thoracic transplantation, the use of a central dictation line may be more cost effective. Nurses may dictate into a service from their cell phone or home phone. The information is typed and sent to the coordinator for signature and placed into the patient's medical record. The nurse must be certain to record the date and time of the interaction.

Some transplant centers provide the on-call nurse with a computer that permits access to patient information using security codes to enter the hospital's system. Nurses can access candidate records for the transplant or posttransplant records of medication dosages and history summaries through the use of a computer and coded system. Documentation can be updated through this system and downloaded into the patient's medical record. Thus, a weekend for the on-call transplant coordinator may be quite an electronic experience with cell phones, pagers, dictaphones, and lap-top computers.

18. What are key points to document when on call?

All communication with a patient or family member must be documented. Any instructions given to the patient and the patient's response to the instructions should be documented along with any changes in dosages of medications. Consultation with a physician should be documented along with any verbal orders. The physician giving the verbal orders must sign the orders in the patient's chart, unless the transplant coordinator is a licensed nurse practitioner with prescribing privileges.

Key Documentation Points

• Date, time of call	• Instructions given	• Patient/family response
• Problem reported	• Name of consultant or physician	to instructions
• Identity of caller: patient	with whom the nurse spoke	• Any changes in medications
or family member	• Instructions from consultant	• Plan of care
• Assessment of the problem	or physician	• Written verbal orders

19. Why does the coordinator need to write a plan of care in the documentation?

The plan of care is one of the greatest communication tools for team members who follow the coordinator in the care of each patient. Excellent documentation of a patient call is very helpful to the next coordinator or physician caring for the patient, but a plan of care communicates and guides the nurse or physician to better continuity of care. For instance, if the dose of medication is changed for a patient, the plan of care may include a follow-up trough level of a calcineurin inhibitor or a check with the patient on a reduction of symptomatic side effects. The documentation should explain why was the dosage changed and include any modifications to the plan of care following that change Documenting the plan of care is a form of effective communication with team members.

20. What are the coordinator's responsibilities with patient test results in the posttransplant follow-up phases of care?

Most patients follow a protocol of tests during the follow-up phases of posttransplant care. The frequency of biopsies, laboratory tests, and diagnostic tests is usually written for transplant coordinators to follow. Most centers have flow sheets in which data is entered from the standard test results. It is not uncommon, however, for additional tests to be ordered. In most transplant centers, coordinators are responsible for gathering test results and documenting them in the chart or on the flow sheets.

All tests that are ordered should be written on the patient's flow sheet to ensure that the test results are gathered. The coordinator should have a reminder system for following up on unscheduled tests. A note placed on a calendar or on a "to-do" list is a clear reminder to check results of the tests. All test results should be reviewed with the physician and documented in the progress notes. Having a method for following up on unscheduled tests is very important in patient care and risk management. The development of a method would be a good process-improvement project for a transplant clinic to ensure patient safety and decrease risks to nursing practice.

21. What is the role of a transplant coordinator with regard to informed consent?

Physicians explain risks and benefits to patients before diagnostic tests and surgical procedures. The transplant coordinator is often the educator for patients and their families and the conveyor of information. Team members depend on one another in patient care issues. Even though the physician has explained the risks and benefits of transplantation, medications, and diagnostic tests, the coordinator should always follow up with basic information. Asking the patient what the physician discussed is a good place to start with patient education.

Applebaum conducted a study on a group of patients to determine their understanding of informed consent.[2] Five days after signing an informed consent document, patients were asked to describe the studies in which they were participating. Few could adequately describe the study in which they were enrolled. Applebaum described this phenomenon as "therapeutic misconceptions." Patients may interpret risks and benefits very differently from what is presented to them. Coordinators should ask what the patients know about the medications or the procedure and should correct any misconceptions. The coordinator's role in informed consent is educating patients and families and ensuring the accuracy of their understanding.

22. Does the coordinator have to document every medication refilled?

Yes, all refills must be documented with the name of the physician authorizing the refills, the date, and the name of the pharmacy. Many patients require written prescriptions for refills because of insurance requirements. With the number of medications that transplant patients take, writing prescriptions can be a time consuming process for any transplant center. Documenting prescription refills helps to determine the appropriate use of medications. Some transplant centers ask for a 5-day notice for written refills. Such notice provides coordinators with adequate time for preparing prescriptions and having them signed appropriately by physicians or nurse practitioners.

23. What should the coordinator do to prevent breaches in patient confidentiality?

Patient confidentiality has become a major concern for healthcare providers in recent years. Advances in communication technology have brought added risks for patient confidentiality. Outpatient charts should be contained in a secure area when the clinic is unattended. Fax machines should be kept in a secure area away from visitors and patients. Telephone communications with patients should be conducted away from waiting rooms and visitors. Computers should be shut down when physicians and nurses are away from their desks, or their offices should be locked when the computer is unattended.

For presentations of case reports at meetings or in journals, patient initials, names, or identifying characteristics should be avoided. The International Council of Medical Journal Editors (www.icmje.com) recommends written informed consent from patients or families when publication of case reports is a possibility. Patient confidentiality has become a very important part of nursing practice.

BIBLIOGRAPHY

1. Anastasia PJ, Blevins MC: Outpatient chemotherapy: Telephone triage for symptom management. Oncol Nurs Forum 24(Suppl):13–22, 1997.
2. Applebaum PS, Roth LH, Lidz CW, et al: False hopes and best data: Consent to research and the therapeutic misconception. Hastings Center Rep 17(2):20–24, 1987.
3. Frank-Stromborg M, Christensen A: Nurse documentation: Not done or worse, done the wrong way—Part 1. Oncol Nurs Forum 28:697–702, 2001.
4. Kane B, Sands D: Guidelines for the clinical use of electronic mail with patients. JAMIA 5:104–111, 1998.
5. Lloyd MG: Practical risk management considerations for clinical email in ambulatory care. J Healthcare Risk Manage 21(3):11–17, 2001.
6. McLean P: Telephone advice: Is it safe? Can Nurse 94(8):53–54, 1998.
7. National Council of State Boards of Nursing. www.ncsbn.org. Accessed May 10, 2002.
8. Ohler L, Daine V: Telecommunication: Cautions and risks for nurses. Prog Cardiovasc Nurs 16(4):172–175, 2001.
9. Spielberg AR: On call and on line: Sociohistorical, legal and ethical implications of email for the patient-physician relationship. JAMA 280:1353–1359, 1998.

25. PATIENT EDUCATION

Linda Ohler, MSN, RN, CCTC, FAAN

1. Why is patient education in transplantation important?

The current successes in transplantation have been attributed to various interventions such as surgical techniques, newer immunosuppressive agents, and biological markers for rejection. Transplant patient education, however, is seldom recognized as a contributing factor to improved outcomes. Although outcomes of educational interventions have been studied in other areas of healthcare, few studies have reported the benefits of patient education in transplant populations. Studies that have covered education primarily address discharge teaching and compliance issues rather than the effectiveness of patient education on outcomes.

Education of transplant patients should not be viewed as a luxury. Building structured educational programs takes time initially but may save time ultimately in terms of long-term patient follow-up. Comprehensive patient and family education programs may decrease the volume of calls after discharge, increase compliance through understanding, and improve outcomes in graft survival. Patients learn when to call the transplant coordinator, what symptoms to report, how to properly take medications, and many other self-care techniques that may improve outcomes.

2. Who provides patient education for transplantation?

Transplant coordinators are responsible for educating potential candidates and their families about the process of transplantation from the evaluation phase through the listing and waiting phases. The primary focus in discharge teaching is preparation of patients for self-care after leaving the hospital setting. Although staff nurses in critical care and step-down units often provide the majority of discharge teaching, such education is usually accomplished in concert with transplant coordinators and many of the transplant team members.

Some transplant centers have developed multidisciplinary teaching programs in which the pharmacist provides education about medications, the dietitian provides information about nutritional aspects of care, and physical therapists or exercise physiologists consult with patients on individualized fitness programs. Educational maps may be used to help with the continuity of teaching and to communicate the progress with patient education. Programs may be individualized for a patient and family, or they may provide group education sessions on specified topics.

3. How can one educate a critically ill patient in need of a transplant?

Although the approaches outlined in this chapter address ideal educational programs for transplant candidates and recipients, some patients may be too ill to participate in the programs. In such cases, families often benefit from the education. Understanding the goals of transplantation and the complexity of the process to attain those goals is usually beneficial to families. Patients who become acutely and critically ill may not be aware that a transplant is being considered. This group of patients requires more time to recover emotionally, psychologically, and physically before they are ready to learn.

4. What key factors should be considered when planning educational programs for patients?

Several important factors to consider when planning educational interventions with patients are emotional status, physical health, readiness to learn, and learning style. Because individuals process information in different ways, a multisensory approach to teaching is recommended. Information takes a different pathway to the brain when we use our eyes and other pathways when we use our hands or our ears. It has been said that learners retain 10% of what they read, 20% of what they hear, 30% of what they see, 50% of what they see and hear, 70% of what they say, and 90% of what they say and do. Thus, the more senses that are included in educational programs, the greater the likelihood of a successful experience. Multisensory instruction applies several approaches. For example, by using slides during didactic presentations, encouraging participatory discussions, providing examples of concepts, and encouraging patients to take notes, the educator stimulates multiple senses during the teaching–learning process. Listening to the presentation evokes the auditory sense; viewing the slides calls upon the visual sense; and taking notes provides tactile stimulation. Return demonstrations in which a patient or family member actually performs an injection or a dressing change are remembered better than if the demonstration alone serves as the education.

5. There is so much for patients and families to learn. How should educational programs be structured ?

Setley developed a theory called the *Four Stages of Learning*. The stages are identified as exposure, guided learning, independence, and mastery. This theory seems particularly appropriate for the transplant population because the factors involved in transplantation education. In the initial meeting with a patient and family, transplant coordinators begin the **exposure** to the transplantation process. **Guided learning** becomes an important part of teaching patients and families about self-care because of the complexities associated with medications and long-term follow-up. Helping patients achieve **independence** in their care occurs in the discharge-teaching phase, and **mastery** is the goal of successful long-term self-care in transplant education.

6. Describe the education that should take place in the exposure phase of learning.

Exposure occurs during the first interaction between any member of the transplant team and the patient and/or family. During this phase the learning begins for the process of transplantation from the referral through follow-up care. The quality of this first interaction is important in setting the tone for the relationship between the patient-family unit and the transplant team. In most transplant programs, the transplant coordinator initiates education about transplantation. Explaining the evaluation process for becoming a candidate for transplantation begins the education that will lead to the patient and family's understanding of the complexities of care following transplantation.

The actual content presented to patients being evaluated for transplantation may vary considerably from center to center and is dependent on the type of transplant involved. Topics providing an overview of transplantation are typically discussed during the evaluation. The nature of this material is diverse and the content relatively vast—an easy combination for overwhelming the patient. Providing information and addressing misperceptions helps patients to formulate questions for the physicians and consultants who will be conducting the evaluation.

Outline of Topics to Discuss with Patients Being Evaluated for Transplantation

I. Overview of specific organ transplantation	V. Surgery
II. Evaluation process for transplantation	VI. Length of stay in the hospital
Tests	VII. Medications to prevent rejection
Consultations	VIII. Post transplant complications
Blood work	Infections
III. Waiting for a new organ	Rejection
Staying healthy while waiting	Malignancy
Diet and exercise	IX. Quality of life after transplantation
When to call the transplant center	X. Follow-up visits to the transplant center
IV. The allocation system	

7. What education should be presented to patients awaiting transplantation?

The content of patient education during the waiting period depends on the organ(s) to be transplanted, patient acuity, and the specific policies of the transplant program. Most renal transplant candidates return to their home dialysis center. Although blood work for panel reactive antibodies or cross matching and quarterly reports on the patient's health are sent to the transplant center on a regular basis, most renal patients have little or no contact with the transplant center until they are called for the surgery. Renal coordinators should work closely with dialysis centers to determine the educational needs of these patients.

Outpatients awaiting liver, intestine, heart, or lung transplantation may be seen on a regular schedule for monitoring of their disease status at the transplant center until they are transplanted. In addition to routine pretransplant care, many programs provide ongoing patient education programs. Lung transplant candidates, for example, are usually required to participate in exercise programs several times a week while they wait. Heart, lung, liver, and intestine transplant candidates who are not hospitalized may be required to participate in support groups that incorporate educational activities. Selected educational topics relevant to the waiting period are listed in the following table.

Topics for Candidate Education Programs During the Waiting Period

1. The allocation system	8. Preventing infections after transplantation
2. Medications after transplantation Immunosuppression Over-the-counter Prescriptions Herbal medications	9. Traveling with a transplant 10. Staying healthy while waiting Diet and exercise
3. Insurance/financial issues	11. The surgery
4. Complications after transplantation	12. When to call the coordinator after transplantation
5. Panel of recipients to talk with candidates about "life after transplantation"	13. Quality of life after transplantation 14. Returning to work after transplantation
6. Panel of spouses of recipients to talk about "life with someone on steroids"	15. Dental care after transplantation 16. Sex after transplantation
7. Panel of children of recipients to talk with children of candidates	17. Marriage and the family: emotional roller coasters 18. Communication with donor families

8. How can one provide education for transplant candidates who are hospitalized?

Hospitalized candidates who are well enough may also participate in some educational activities. This activity is valuable because it allows patients to meet other patients experiencing the need for transplantation. Heart transplant candidates are often ambulatory on intravenous medications or mechanical assist devices. Support groups or regularly scheduled education programs help this unique group cope with long hospitalizations. Find a conference room, establish a time, and have a list of topics suggested by patients and families. Various team members from surgeons to pharmacists and dieticians can present educational programs for inpatients and their families. Inclusion of operating room nurses to describe their roles and the process the patient will experience is often well received.

9. What educational topics are used for returning patients to independence and self-care?

Education at this stage is more in-depth as patients begin to participate in their care with guidance from the nurse. Before discharge from the hospital after transplant surgery, patients should demonstrate a certain level of independence in their care. They should be able to meet the goals of self-medication, answering important questions about their medications (e.g., what, how, when, and side effects), and they must be able to describe the signs and symptoms of rejection and infection.

Audiovisual aids such as slides that review medications, diet prescriptions, signs and symptoms of rejection and infection, and when to call the transplant center are used to summarize information that the patient has already received. Providing the patient with printed copies of these slides allows for note taking and serves as a handy reference after discharge. Suggested topics for education prior to discharging a transplant recipient from the hospital are listed in the following table.

Topics for Discharge Education

1. Wound care	8. Self-care and self-monitoring at home
2. Medications	9. Travel
3. Signs and symptoms of rejection	10. Working outside
4. Signs and symptoms of infection	11. Exercise
5. Follow-up blood tests and trough levels	12. Sexual relations
6. Follow-up clinic visits	13. Returning to work
7. Dental visits	14. Writing to the donor family

Encouraging self-care and self-monitoring while the patient is hospitalized communicates the expectation of independence. If the patient will require the services of a home health nurse, inviting him or her to the hospital to participate in discharge teaching is an ideal way to reinforce education that must continue when the patient is at home.

10. How is completed patient education communicated among team members?

In the immediate postoperative period and until discharge, the new transplant recipient may have many nurses and many disciplines providing care and education. Educational maps serve as a guide for nurses and other team members to communicate the progress in patient education. Bedside nurses often provide the bulk of patient and family education. Before discharge, however, a transplant coordinator usually meets with the patient and family to review the information, evaluate patient readiness for discharge, and discuss plans for follow-up care. Documentation of all education serves as a communication tool among team members. Documentation can be recorded in the multidisciplinary progress notes or on the patient education map.

11. How is mastery defined in terms of transplant patient education?

Mastery is a process that begins once patients are discharged from the hospital and return to the transplant clinic for follow-up care. Mastery is characterized by appropriate self-care activities becoming automatic. Immediately after discharge, patients and families often call the transplant center or the on-call coordinator for assurances about medications and symptoms. Each clinic visit is filled with education that reinforces discharge teaching. Once patients become more confident about their care, mastery levels of understanding enable them to live life more fully with greater self-care and self-confidence.

12. How does one assess the patient's ability to understand transplantation?

Assessments of patient and/or family characteristics that could affect their ability to learn should be done before beginning educational activities and should cover the following:

- Cognitive status   • Patient goals
- Learning style   • Learning environment
- Readiness to learn   • Background knowledge of transplantation
- Physical health   • Cultural, spiritual, and religious beliefs and practices
- Emotional health

13. How does one teach patients with a poor cognitive status?

Various conditions may prevent patients from participating in educational activities. Patients may be cognitively impaired for a number of reasons depending on their underlying disease. Severe congestive heart failure causes a decrease in cardiac output and ultimately a poorer oxygenation of blood supply to the brain. Patients find concentration very difficult and are often consumed by fatigue. The decrease in cardiac output also contributes to renal dysfunction, resulting in poor filtering of nitrates from the kidneys. As the blood urea nitrogen (BUN) increases, the mental status further deteriorates.

Patients with liver failure also have problems concentrating and may develop a hepatic coma. End-stage organ disease often leaves a patient fatigued and unable to concentrate. Providing brief periods of teaching may be beneficial; however, most patients with cognitive disorders related to end-stage organ disease may not be able to concentrate or comprehend. Education may need to be deferred until after transplantation.

14. Are there any special teaching strategies for illiterate patients?

The illiterate patient requires special teaching strategies to ensure compliance with the complex medical regimens after transplantation. Some illiterate patients have such well-developed compensatory mechanisms that their illiteracy may not be discovered until after transplantation. Slides and pictures are excellent resources for teaching illiterate patients. Adhesive-backed pictures of commonly used transplant medications are available from several pharmaceutical companies. Such pictures can be attached to medication bottles and to the medication list to aid the patient in taking the correct doses of medications at the right times. Keeping an updated copy of the medication list in the patient's chart can help the transplant coordinator readily respond to questions from the patient or family about medications.

15. Are there any special teaching strategies for visually impaired patients?

Taped recordings of the discharge teaching information can be used with visually impaired patients. Patients can take the tapes home and replay them as needed to reinforce learning. In addition, if the patient knows Braille, the pharmacist can use a Braille label-maker to label medication bottles. The labels can also be attached to medication lists. Family members are very important in the education of patients with cognitive or special needs. They should be included in education sessions with the patient and should be educated about the strategies being used to enable them to assist the patient.

16. How does one determine a patient's learning style?

The teacher must evaluate how an individual learns best. Asking a patient the preferred method for learning usually helps to identify the best strategies for teaching. Some individuals learn best by reading whereas others rely on visual descriptions of concepts. Asking family members may help to determine the best approach to teaching a particular patient the much-needed information on self-care in transplantation.

17. How does one assess a transplant patient's readiness to learn?

Readiness to learn depends on several factors. For most patients who are newly diagnosed with end-stage organ disease, acceptance of the diagnosis must come first. It may not be possible to teach about transplantation if a patient believes his or her health will improve without the transplant. Nurses can provide additional education about the disease process and can provide the patient with outcome data on the appropriate type of end-stage disease. A patient's general health status and well-being also must be considered when determining readiness to learn. Symptoms such as pain, fatigue, and nausea are not conducive for learning. Having symptoms alleviated before teaching promotes the patient's capacity for learning. Anxiety, depression, and anger interfere with information processing and must also be addressed before effective teaching/learning can take place.

18. How does the environment affect learning?

Where we learn can be almost as important as how we learn. Some people learn well in a classroom environment, whereas others do not do well in a traditional setting. And it is unlikely that anyone receiving intravenous medications with telemetry attached to his or her chest, with people constantly walking in and out of the room, and continual interruptions from overhead speakers or alarms beeping can effectively process any new information. Yet this may be the environment in which the patient is expected to learn. Teaching should be postponed for patients who are acutely and critically ill until their condition is stable and they are in an environment more conducive to learning.

19. How does one evaluate background knowledge and perception versus fact?

Patients and families often bring preconceived ideas with them from experiences or information they have received from the media or friends. Therefore, it is important to evaluate their baseline knowledge of and explore their perceptions (accurate and false) about transplantation. Mishel and Murdaugh found that families' expectations were based on beliefs that life would return to normal after heart transplantation. As the reality of unpredictable posttransplant events become more evident, spouses and partners began to redefine *normal* with adaptive management strategies such as modification of roles and expectations. Patients may believe that transplantation will restore them to their pre-illness state. Still others believe that they will assume characteristics of their donor. Reality-based teaching is therefore important to help patients understand the risks and benefits of transplantation and to debunk myths and misperceptions.

20. How do cultural and religious practices affect learning?

Family members may attempt to direct teaching to themselves rather than to the patient, based on a belief that the patient be spared stressful information or bad news. Or an overprotective family member may request that teaching be deferred until the patient is in better health, not fully understanding that this is not likely to occur until after transplantation. It may be helpful in these situations to provide patient and family education separately. It should be explained to the family that patients must make an informed decision about transplantation and that an understanding of the risks as well as the benefits is essential to an informed decision and commitment to posttransplant care responsibilities.

A patient's cultural practices may prevent teaching at certain times of the day or on certain days. Religious practices such as Judaism may prohibit teaching at during certain times (i.e., the Sabbath). However, emergency medical interventions may pave the way for exceptions. Consulting with a Rabbi or religious leader may help the patient and the nurse to establish appropriate times for education and care. The patient who is a Jehovah's Witness will undoubtedly be concerned about blood transfusions during and after surgery. Information on performing transplants without blood products is available in the literature.[6]

21. Are there any standard educational materials for transplant patients?

Most people need more than a booklet and a handful of brochures to provide them with the information they need on transplantation. There are no recognized national standards for patient education for transplantation; educational programs vary from organ to organ and are center-specific. Some programs provide formal education programs in which patients participate in group activities on a regular basis, whereas others provide individualized, patient-specific programs on the various phases of transplantation from evaluation through discharge after transplantation. The time from evaluation to actual transplantation, however, may extend from months to years. Consequently, patients may be required to participate in education programs throughout the waiting period.

22. Being notified of a transplant can be very emotional. How does one prepare patients for the call?

Patients who are not hospitalized while awaiting transplantation may carry a pager so that they can be easily and readily contacted when a donor organ becomes available. Patients and families may need instructions on how to use the pager, depending on the type. Paging devices vary; some simply beep whereas others also display a number to call. Instructions should include information about how and who to contact from the transplant center when the pager beeps and about reporting to the transplant center when an organ is available. This call can be very stressful for patients and families, but written instructions can decrease anxiety associated with being called for transplant. Patients also need to understand that their pager may beep in error, the so-called "false alarm," and may need additional support when this happens.

23. Should teaching continue in long-term follow-up care appointments?

Yes, frequent clinic appointments at the transplant center for the first few months after surgery serve as excellent opportunities to reinforce patient and family teaching. During this time, patients are caring for themselves at least to some extent, depending on their specific situations.

Providing feedback to patients reinforces their new knowledge and skills and clarifies misunderstandings. Self-care skills that patients should be able to demonstrate in order to achieve mastery are listed in the following table.

Reinforcing Transplant Education

1. When to call the coordinator	4. Calling for refills of medications at appropriate times
2. Maintaining contact with the transplant center	5. Exercise and diet maintenance
	6. Traveling with a transplant
3. Follow-up appointments	7. Balancing work and family life

Patient education may be one of the most important roles of transplant nurses and coordinators. Teaching strategies need to be adapted to individualized patient learning needs. Research in the area of patient education must be incorporated into practice. By utilizing the four stages of learning and applying them to phases of transplant education, outcome research can demonstrate the effectiveness of nursing education in contributing to the long-term success of transplantation.

BIBLIOGRAPHY

1. Applebaum PS, Roth LH, Lidz CW, et al: False hopes and best data: Consent to research and therapeutic misconceptions. Hastings Cent Rep 17:20–24, 1987.
2. Blanchard W: Teaching an illiterate transplant patient. Am Nephrol Nurses Assoc J 25:69,76, 1998.
3. DeGeest S, Dobbels F, Martin S, et al: Clinical risk associated with appointment noncompliance in heart transplant recipients. Prog Transplant. 2000; 10: 162-168
4. Giacoma T, Ingersoll GL, Williams M: Teaching video effects on renal transplant outcomes. Am Nephrol Nurses Assoc J 26:29–33,81, 1999.
5. Grady KL, Jalowiec A, White-Williams C: Patient compliance at one year and two years after heart transplantation. J Heart Lung Transplant 17:383–394, 1998.
6. Grogan TA: Bringing bloodless surgery into the mainstream. Nursing 29(11):58–61, 1999.
6. Gubby L: Assessment of quality of life and related stressors following liver transplantation. J Transplant Coord 8(2):113–118, 1998.
7. Hauser M, Williams J, Strong M, et al: Predicted and actual quality of life changes following renal transplantation. Am Nephrol Nurses Assoc J 18(3):295–304, 1991.
8. Mishel MH, Murdaugh CL: Family adjustment to heart transplantation: Redesigning the dream. Nurs Res 36:332–338, 1987.
9. Muirhead J, Meyerowitz BE, Leedham B, et al: Quality of life and coping in patients awaiting heart transplantation. J Heart Lung Transplant 11(2):265–272, 1992.
10. Partovi N, Chan W, Nimmo CR: Evaluation of a patient education program for solid organ transplant patients. Can J Hosp Pharmacol 48: 72–78, 1995.
11. Reif SF: How to reach and teach ADD/ADHD Children: Practical techniques, strategies and interventions for helping children with attention problems and hyperactivity. West Nyack, NY, The Center for Applied Research in Education, 1993, p 53.
12. Setley S: Taming the Dragons: Real Help for Real School Problems. St. Louis, Starfish Publishing, 1995.
13. Steinberg T, Diercks MJ, Millspaugh J: An evaluation of the effectiveness of a videotape for discharge teaching of organ transplant recipients. J Transplant Coord 6(2):59–63, 2001.

INDEX

Page numbers in **boldface type** indicate complete chapters.